Clinical Competencies in Occupational Therapy

Cindy A. Kief, COTA/L, AP

Instructor and Advisor

Occupational Therapy Assistant Program

Cincinnati State Technical and Community College

Cincinnati, Ohio

Carol R. Scheerer, MEd, OTR/L

Assistant Professor

Department of Occupational Therapy

Xavier University

Cincinnati, Ohio

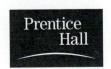

Prentice Hall

Upper Saddle River, New Jersey 07458

Library of Congress Cataloging-in-Publication Data
Kief, Cindy A.
   Clinical competencies in occupational therapy/Cindy A.
Kief, Carol R. Scheerer.
      p. ; cm.
   Includes bibliographical references and index.
   ISBN 0-8385-1248-8
   1. Occcupational therapy—Handbooks, manuals, etc. 2.
Occupational therapy—Problems, exercises, etc. I. Scheerer,
Carol R. II. Title.
[DNLM: 1. Occupational Therapy. 2. Clinical
Competence. WB 555 K47c 2000]
RM735.3.K54 2000
615.8'515—dc21   00-029819

Publisher: Julie Alexander
Acquisitions Editor: Mark Cohen
Editorial Assistant: Melissa Kerian
Director of Manufacturing
 and Production: Bruce Johnson
Managing Editor: Patrick Walsh
Production Editor: Tonia Grubb, York Production Services
Production Liaison: Cathy O'Connell
Manufacturing Manager: Ilene Sanford
Director of Marketing: Leslie Cavaliere
Marketing Manager: Kristin Walton
Marketing Coordinator: Cindy Frederick
Creative Director: Marianne Frasco
Cover Design: Joseph Sengotta
Composition and Interior Design: York Production
   Services
Printing and Binding: Banta, Harrisonburg

Prentice-Hall International (UK) Limited, *London*
Prentice-Hall of Australia Pty. Limited, *Sydney*
Prentice-Hall Canada Inc., *Toronto*
Prentice-Hall Hispanoamericana, S.A., *Mexico*
Prentice-Hall of India Private Limited, *New Delhi*
Prentice-Hall of Japan, Inc., *Tokyo*
Prentice-Hall Singapore Pte. Ltd.
Editora Prentice-Hall do Brasil, Ltda., *Rio de Janeiro*

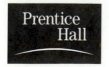

10 9 8 7 6 5 4 3 2 1
ISBN 0-8385-1248-8

This book is dedicated to:
Mary Jo Ellis
and
Virginia (Ginny) Scardina
Two occupational therapists, who by their dedicated example,
their thirst for knowledge, and their energetic spirits,
have inspired us, touched us,
and influenced the lives of so many.
We are forever grateful.

Contents

Foreword

Occupational therapy has long needed a comprehensive delineation and learner's guide for occupational therapy clinical competencies, in a form easy to use by educators and students alike, that can be adapted for use across professional- and technical-level education. This book is just such a comprehensive document. It will be of great value not only for the occupational therapy student, but also for the occupational therapist or occupational therapy assistant who has been out of the field and is returning to practice or who is changing practice areas. This manual takes key information for occupational therapy and distills it into the essential basic clinical competencies that will be needed by the occupational therapist and occupational therapy assistant.

Clinical competencies can be defined as the set of skills, knowledge, and attributes that, minimally, an occupational therapist and occupational therapy assistant needs to deliver effective services to clients and their families. The active learning activities and exercises presented in this manual are designed for the spirit of practice and are intended to lay the foundation for a practitioner's successful career. This manual presents information using a variety of teaching and learning techniques. Many of these techniques are cooperative and action oriented, and have originated from the first author's experiences as well as an understanding of cooperative learning from the field of education.

An element of play and playfulness has also been designed into the teaching and learning techniques presented in this manual. Remember that play is a fundamental part of occupational therapy. The authors have created a manual that conveys a sense that it is okay to have fun while learning. Indeed, much of learning in occupational therapy should really be fun!

A developmental frame of reference has been employed as the authors' philosophical base in this manual. Clinical competencies are developed when higher-level skills are built on the mastery of skills at a lower level. This approach evolved from many years of teaching experience on the part of the first author in an accredited occupational therapy assistant education program. The second author assisted the first author in the refinment and operationalization of the vision and content of the manual. The second author is currently teaching in an accredited occupational therapy educational program.

This manual, like most all of us, is a work in progress. It will provide the user with valuable information. If you are an instructor, take the information, use it, and adapt it as necessary so that each one of your students receives the best education possible. If you are a student, apply the information you learn to your specific situation. Analyze and synthesize the contents of the manual as you prepare to become an occupational therapist or occupational therapy assistant. If you are an occupational therapist or occupational therapy assistant who is just now returning to practice or who is changing practice areas, select the content that is most applicable to your needs. In all cases, however, this manual should serve as a stepping stone to continued learning and development in the field of occupational therapy throughout your career.

Charlotte Brasic Royeen, Ph.D, OTR, FAOTA
Associate Dean for Research and Professor in Occupational Therapy
School of Pharmacy and Allied Health Professions
Creighton University, Omaha, Nebraska

Preface

This manual is intended as an interactive manual for use by future occupational therapy (OT) practitioners. It is appropriate for use within an instructional setting, either as an alternative to lecturing or in a lab-type class, within an educational program that is accredited by the Accreditation Council for Occupational Therapy Education (ACOTE) of the American Occupational Therapy Association. Each student in a class should have a manual for his or her own use.

Fieldwork educators might also use this manual as they supervise students in a practice setting. Specific sections may be selected to supplement and augment the students' experiences. Additionally, this manual may serve as a learning tool for the OT practitioner who is returning to practice as well as the practitioner who is changing practice settings, as it reflects current content of the OT profession. In such a case it would be appropriate to use it as an independent study tool or in conjunction with the assistance of a mentor.

As OT practitioners we are charged with obtaining and maintaining competency. "Ensuring competency is key to both individual success and the continued success of the occupational therapy profession as a whole" (AOTA, 1998, p. 693). Currently there is no one suggested measure of competence but rather, as suggested by Salvatori (1996), a variety of methods are needed to do so. This manual presents such a variety of methods and represents the "can" level of Salvatori's (1996) "know-can-do" model. It teaches the basic knowledge, skills, and attributes that practitioners need to deliver effective services to clients. The professional behavior and judgments that an occupational therapy practitioner needs are many and varied. Herein is provided a solid foundation of the necessary beginning competencies needed by an OT practitioner.

Clinical reasoning and consideration of the context of practice are essential for occupational therapy, as you will see throughout this manual. You will be introduced to clinical reasoning attributes, especially the tacit knowledge to which Mattingly and Fleming (1994) refer. The information that is often taken for granted in the field of occupational therapy is enunciated clearly with the necessary components presented. However, advanced clinical reasoning is beyond the teaching scope of this book. Advanced clinical reasoning will become part of a practitioner's expertise with advanced practice and education.

A thorough review of the issues related to competency can be found in *Developing, Maintaining, and Updating Competency in Occupational Therapy: A Guide to Self-Appraisal* written by the Competency Task Force of the AOTA (1995). Additionally, the reader is directed to the *American Journal of Occupational Therapy*'s special issue on professional competency (October 1998), in which experts from across the field detail the critical importance of competency as it relates to the viability of the individual practitioner and the profession. The emphasis on achieving, maintaining, and updating competency is evident throughout this significant journal issue.

Content Development

The content of this manual was developed by the first author's experience as an educator. Course content from many years of experience teaching occupational therapy assistant classes in an ACOTE-accredited program has been included. Visiting local facilities during a recent teaching sabbatical to include current ideas, theories and techniques used, solidified the content. It was then modified accordingly and aligned with the "Standard for an Accredited Education Program for the Occupational Therapy Assistant" (ACOTE of AOTA, 1998a) and the "Standards for an Accredited Education Program for the Occupational Therapist" (ACOTE of AOTA, 1998b). As such, this manual represents current clinical practice in the field.

Throughout this manual the words *occupation* and *activity* are often used interchangeably. At times, the field of occupational therapy differentiates between these two words, and here it is assumed that activity is purposeful and meaningful, while occupation represents the essence and the most powerful tool of the profession. The words *assessment* and *evaluation* are used as defined in the Standards of Practice for Occupational Therapists (AOTA, 1998). *Assessment* refers to the specific tool used and evaluation is the entire process of collecting data. The words *intervention* and *treatment* are also used interchangeably; this is the authors' preference rather than a recommended or recognized delineation.

In the field of occupational therapy the occupational therapy assistant (OTA) and the occupational therapist (OT) work together. The OT considers the OTA an important and vital team member. The OTA depends on the supervision of an OT. The relationship between the two professionals needs to be collaborative, mutually respectful, and interactive (Neidstadt and Creapeau, 1998). This manual exemplifies that relationship.

Purpose

The purpose of this manual is to give the future occupational therapy practitioner, including both the OTA and the OT, a hands-on method of learning. The OTA's role in the field of occupational therapy is primarily that of intervention and "doing," so this manual meets the learning needs of the OTA. The content is commensurate with his or her main function. For the OT this manual puts the practical aspects of practice in the forefront. At times OT students are inundated with theory during their course of study. This manual provides a welcome breath of fresh air and an enjoyable way of integrating aspects of the curriculum content that are germane to occupational therapy. Therefore, this manual meets the needs of both the OTA and the OT as they learn how to use occupation in therapy.

It is the goal of this manual to provide the occupational therapy practitioner with the following:

- A comprehensible and enjoyable way of obtaining knowledge, skills, and attributes in preparation for the role of an OT practitioner.
- A user-friendly way for students to learn the occupational therapy curriculum content found in accredited OTA and OT programs.
- A format for the OT practitioner who is returning to practice or changing practice areas to learn the necessary basic and essential competencies of the profession.

Description

This manual has six chapters. The first two chapters deal with the fundamentals of OT. The remaining four are divided into main practice areas of OT: pediatrics, physical disabilities, mental health, and geriatrics. The content has been arranged in a developmental hierarchy, introducing basic OT concepts in the beginning and building on those concepts with differing degrees of difficulty throughout.

Each of the six chapters contain exercises that focus on the basic competencies of OT. There is a quote at the beginning of each exercise. These quotes have been collected from a variety of sources and are intended as food for thought. The quotes can be examined and dissected. Their meaning can be incorporated as part of the exercise.

Objectives of each exercise follow the quotes and are listed before the introduction of each exercise. A description and explanation of the exercise follow. Preparation for the activity of the exercise is to be accomplished by completing the readings listed and the study questions posed. The study questions take on a variety of formats, and most can be answered when the suggested readings are completed. The suggested readings are not intended to be all-inclusive but rather reflect an academic setting in which students may have access to some of the more recognized and commonly available textbooks. Specific pages where the answers to the study questions can be found have not been included. Rather, it is felt that if the student determines where in a source the content of the study questions is found, critical thinking skills are used and improved in doing so.

At least one and frequently several activities follow the study questions to put into practice the information contained in that exercise. The materials needed to complete each activity are listed, as well as instructions for doing so. A follow-up section directing the student to further evaluative and introspective activities is found at the end of each exercise.

Following the exercises, at the end of each chapter is an Application of Competencies section. Students are directed to turn to this section after doing each exercise to record the learning of at least one important application concept related to client intervention.

Following the Application of Competencies section is the Performance Skill section. The performance skills suggested in this section are specifically designed to provide further experience, reinforcement, and evaluation of the competencies the student has acquired. These activities pull together and synthesize the content just learned. These forms can be used to help provide feedback about one's professional behavior and skill performance. In determining final grades for all or parts of an instruction course, instructors may use the varied performance skills.

Students are directed to compile a portfolio, an ongoing display of their work. A portfolio can be used as an evaluative measure for grading purposes or as a way of documenting skills for a prospective employer. Content from the Application of Competencies and Performance Skills can be used for inclusion in such a portfolio.

At the very end of each chapter is a selection of case studies. The case studies have been taken from actual client charts. The case studies represent real-life scenarios, although the identity of the individuals has been changed. The diagnosis and abbreviations have purposefully been left in to further challenge the student's learning. The culture/religion and insurance information has been left unspecified so that variations can be added at will. As these situations change, it will then be clear how the occupational therapy process needs to change reflective of one's culture and reimbursement agency policies.

The case studies for the pediatric section follow a format that is typical in the educational system, in which a child's strengths and weaknesses are considered. The case studies for the other sections contain information that is typically available in hospital-based charts, including the client's social and medical history. All cases can be used as suggested and/or rearranged to be used with different exercises.

A list of references at the end of each chapter includes the full reference of items in the suggested reading list as well as those used in the exercises. This list should serve as a starting point for the resources that a future OT practitioner will need.

The perforated pages of this manual are intended to allow for selected removal of certain pages for review by an instructor in an academic program. The pages could also be removed for inclusion in a portfolio as suggested earlier.

A teacher's instructional guide accompanying this manual is available. Additional information available to supplement the suggested exercises can be found there along with the location of the answers to the study questions.

Summary

The content of this manual is designed to facilitate the learning of basic competencies needed in the field of occupational therapy by the OTA and OT. It exemplifies the collaborative teamwork inherently needed between the OTA and the OTR in clinical practice. On completion of the study questions and unique activities, a solid foundation for the occupational therapy practitioner will be laid. It is anticipated that this foundation will encourage and promote enjoyment of the lifelong learning process in one of the most exciting and rewarding career fields.

References

Accreditation Council for Occupational Therapy Education of the American Occupational Therapy Association. 1998a. *Standards for an Accredited Education Program for the Occupational Therapy Assistant.* Bethesda, MD: American Occupational Therapy Association.

Accreditation Council for Occupational Therapy Education of the American Occupational Therapy Association. 1998b. *Standards for an Accredited Education Program for the Occupational Therapist.* Bethesda, MD: American Occupational Therapy Association.

American Journal of Occupational Therapy. October 1998. Special Issue on Professional Competence. Bethesda, MD: American Occupational Therapy Association.

American Occupational Therapy Association. 1998. *Official Documents of the American Occupational Therapy Association.* 7th ed. Bethesda, MD: Author.

Competency Task Force. 1995. *Developing, Maintaining, and Updating Competency in Occupational Therapy: A Guide to Self-Appraisal.* Bethesda, MD: American Occupational Therapy Association.

Mattingly, C., and M. H. Fleming. 1994. *Clinical Reasoning: Forms of Inquiry in a Therapeutic Practice.* Philadelphia: F. A. Davis.

Neidstadt, M. E., and E. B. Crepeau. eds. 1998. *Willard and Spackman's Occupational Therapy.* 9th ed. Philadelphia: J. B. Lippincott.

Salvatori, P. 1996. "Clinical Competence: A Review of the Health Care Literature with a Focus on Occupational Therapy. *Canadian Journal of Occupational Therapy,* 63(4): 260–271.

Acknowledgments

We thank our colleagues at both Cincinnati State and Xavier University for all their help and support during the writing of this book. We especially acknowledge Anne Zobay, Academic Fieldwork Coordinator; Claudia Miller, Program Chair and Academic Staff; Jude Norton, Academic Staff and Physician's Assistant; Janelle Gohn, Program Chair of Clinical Laboratory; Marianne Kirsmer, Dean of Health Technology Division from Cincinnati State; Joann Estes, Department Chair and Assistant Professor; Georgianna Jorary Miller, Academic Fieldwork Coordinator and Academic Staff; Barb Sarbaugh, Academic Staff; Eileen Kempf, Lab Technician from Xavier University.

We are grateful for fellow practitioners and team members who are continually a source of ideas and support: Beatriz Merkelz, Michael Zaret, Carolyn Dehner, Patrick Brunner, Barb Homlar, Geri Vehr, Mary Anne Curtis, Jeanne Mack, and Joan Dostal. We also acknowledge Nick Puhlman and Tony Bartel, who have given of themselves as well as their time and expertise in creating optimal student learning experiences. Countless other occupational therapy practitioners have always been willing to share their expertise whether as a presenter or participant at many workshops throughout the years. Everyone who practices has a great idea to share. Friends and professionals from the following facilities shared significant information regarding clinical practice: Drake Memorial Hospital, Jewish Community Hospital, Breyer School, Cincinnati Occupational Therapy Institute, Children's Hospital and Medical Center, Ft. Hamilton Hughes Hospital, Bethesda Work Capacity Center, Clermont Mercy Hospital, University of Cincinnati Hospital, Redwood School and Rehabilitation, and St. James School. We are also grateful to the countless number of students who have contributed to the refinement of these exercises as they have evolved over the years. Additionally they need to be commended for not being deterred by photo opportunities that occurred on bad hair days.

Charlotte Brasic Royeen's initial interest and excitement in this project provided the impetus to forge ahead. We appreciate her for her reviewing and editing expertise. We also express gratitude to the following editors who have prodded and encouraged us along the way: Lin Marshall, Mark Cohen, and Anne Seitz. Tonia Grubb as project coordinator pulled this altogether. Thanks to Kim Davies for walking in the door and believing in this project.

Over the years many clients have contributed to our growth and development as professionals. We are indebted to all of them.

Finally, our families have been an ongoing source of support. Cindy's husband Bill has put up with household imperfections and continual schedule changes, but always maintained support. We give thanks to Cindy's children: Rob, who approaches life with a sensitive spirit and a thirst for knowledge and achievement: Krista, who loves life and spreads the joy wherever she goes: Corrie, who can always make others laugh and has an abundance of love to share; they have provided encouragement, support, and much pride in the anticipation of a published book. Carol's husband Dan has shown continued patience, support, and forbearance in her many endeavors. Our families' love has inspired and allowed us to bring this book to completion, and our parents have believed in us and encouraged us along the way in whatever we pursued. We couldn't have done this without them.

Thanks to Mary Anne Schlewinsky, who shared her creative talent for drawing and creating, and Tonya Brinson for her ability to make sense out of scribbles that launched this book on its way. Her computer expertise is greatly appreciated.

Our thanks to God for his many gifts and blessings received and to St. Anthony who has helped us find everything from a lost pencil to a lost chapter!

About the Authors

Cindy A. Kief, COTA/L, AP   Cindy has been working in the field of occupational therapy for 25 years in a variety of practice areas. Her experience includes work in acute care, rehabilitation, skilled nursing, home health, pediatric outpatient, school system, long-term psychosocial, and education. She has been teaching in an accredited Occupational Therapy Assistant program for 10 years and is currently full-time faculty at Cincinnati State Technical and Community College, Cincinnati, Ohio. Her duties include teaching courses in all areas of practice as well as serving as advisor to the American Student Occupational Therapy Association student club. Cindy is on the executive committee of the American Association of University Professors and serves on the advisory board for the occupational therapy assistant program and the geriatric activities coordinator program. She was one of the first COTAs to receive the Advanced Practice (AP) credentials from the American Occupational Therapy Association in the area of education. The Accreditation Council for Occupational Therapy Education has recently appointed her to the Roster of Accreditation Evaluators.

Carol R. Scheerer, MEd, OTR/L   Carol practiced as an occupational therapist in the school system for 18 years. She is certified in the Test Administration and Interpretation of the Sensory Integration and Praxis Tests and serves as a Sensory Integration Praxis Test Administration Observer for Sensory Integration International. Carol is currently an assistant professor at Xavier University, Cincinnati, Ohio, teaching full time in the Occupational Therapy Department. She also serves on the Advisory Board for Xavier University's Occupational Therapy Department. During the summer, Carol teaches in the Clinical Study Program of Sensory Integration at the Cincinnati Occupational Therapy Institute. Carol is the author of "Perspectives on an Oral Motor Activity: The Use of Rubber Tubing as a 'Chewy'," published in the *American Journal of Occupational Therapy* in 1992. She is also the author of a book entitled, *Sensorimotor Groups: Activities for School and Home,* published by Therapy Skill Builders. Carol earned a Bachelor of Science degree in occupational therapy at Indiana University in 1979 and a Master of Education degree at the University of Cincinnati in 1991. She is currently in the process of obtaining her doctoral degree from the University of Cincinnati in the Department of Education with a focus on curriculum and instruction.

Fundamentals I

CHAPTER ONE CONTENTS

EXERCISES

Exercise 1	Creating a Vision Statement
Exercise 2	Explaining What We Do
Exercise 3	Prevention and Wellness
Exercise 4	Cultural Awareness
Exercise 5	Learning Your Association's Official Documents
Exercise 6	Ethics in Practice
Exercise 7	Learning the Jargon
Exercise 8	AOTA: Your Professional Organization
Exercise 9	Essential Functions of Occupational Therapy Practitioners
Exercise 10	Frames of Reference
Exercise 11	Occupational Therapy Process
Exercise 12	Practice Guidelines
Exercise 13	Purposeful Occupation
Exercise 14	Occupation: Adaptation
Exercise 15	Occupation: Gradation
Exercise 16	Planning Intervention
Exercise 17	Role Delineation

APPLICATION OF COMPETENCIES

PERFORMANCE SKILLS

Performance Skill 1A	Craft Completion
Performance Skill 1B	Occupational Analysis
Performance Skill 1C	Adapting an Occupation
Performance Skill 1D	Developing Your File
Performance Skill 1E	Cultural Explanation

CASE STUDIES

Case Study 1
Case Study 2
Case Study 3
Case Study 4
Case Study 5
Case Study 6
Case Study 7

REFERENCES

Exercise 1

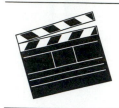

"Nothing is more terrible than activity without insight."

THOMAS CARLYLE

CREATING A VISION STATEMENT

OBJECTIVES

✔ Examine the American Occupational Therapy Association's (AOTA) mission statement
✔ Compose a class mission or vision statement
✔ Write a personal mission or vision statement

DESCRIPTION

This exercise will allow you and your classmates to write a mission or vision statement. A vision statement is born out of one's philosophy, beliefs, and values. A vision statement is the "doing" part—the putting into action and practice of one's core beliefs and values. It is appropriate for both individuals and institutions to create a mission statement, as this will guide their actions and beliefs. Different individuals, facilities, institutions, and organizations may use different descriptive terms for the same document. Designing a class vision statement will begin to create cohesiveness among your classmates. It will help to give your class a sense of purpose and direction.

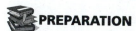PREPARATION

Suggested Readings

> AOTA Web site: *http://www.aota.org*
> Covey (1989)
> Mission or vision statement from your host facility, institution, and/or department

Study Questions

1. Write AOTA's mission statement here. Obtain this mission statement from AOTA's Web page.

2. Write your host institution's vision or mission statement here.

3. Write your program or department's vision or mission statement here.

4. Read the book entitled *Seven Habits of Highly Effective People* (Covey, 1989). Write your personal vision or mission statement here. Incorporate information that you learned from this reading.

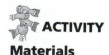ACTIVITY

Materials

Blackboard or overhead projector.

Instructions

1. Compose a class vision or mission statement with your instructors, program chair, and fellow students. Use a blackboard, flip chart, and/or overhead projector to record your classmates' ideas. Combine, arrange, reorder, synthesize, analyze, and integrate the views for which consensus is obtained. Record your class vision or mission statement here. Post it for all to refer to and adhere to for the duration of your education. Note that a mission statement is a work in progress, so you will need to be vigilant throughout your educational tenure and initiate changes and modifications as needed.

Mission Statement

FOLLOW-UP

✔   Complete the Application of Competencies at the end of this chapter.

EXPLAINING WHAT WE DO

Exercise 2

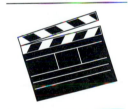

OBJECTIVES

✔   State the official definition of occupational therapy (OT)
✔   Define OT for the layperson
✔   Prepare and present a role-play promoting the understanding of the profession of OT

DESCRIPTION

This exercise will help you to understand the philosophical base of OT as well as give you a working definition of OT. It is important that you understand and are able to communicate the philosophy of occupational therapy. Many times over the course of your career you will be asked to explain the philosophy and definition of OT to your clients, other health professionals, friends, and the general public. It is your definition that will help your clients to understand your profession and the services you will provide. It is your definition that will differentiate you from the other health care professionals with whom they will interact.

"Knowledge speaks, but wisdom listens."

OLIVER WENDELL HOLMES

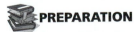PREPARATION

Suggested Readings

AOTA (latest edition)
AOTA Web site: *http://www.aota.org*
Moyers (1999)
Neidstadt and Crepeau (1998)
Read and Sanderson (1999)

Study Questions

1. Describe in your own words the official statement of philosophy of OT.

2. Summarize, in 25 words or less, the official AOTA definition of OT from the AOTA Web page.

3. Describe in your own words the profession's most current definition of occupation.

4. Describe in your own words the psychosocial aspects of OT.

5. Select a position paper from the *Reference Manual of the Official Documents of the AOTA* (latest edition) and briefly describe its contents.

6. Combining your descriptions in Study Questions 1–5, define OT in your own words.

7. Describe how you might define OT to the following people. Use terminology that each person will understand given his or her background, training, and education. Supplement your definition with examples to which each person can relate.
   a. Colleague

   b. Client

   c. Physician

   d. Insurance company

   e. Administrator

   f. Friend

8. Write a brief outline and summary of *The Guide to Occupational Therapy Practice* (Moyers, 1999).

9. List the principles of occupations as stated in *The Guide to Occupational Therapy Practice* (Moyers, 1999) and give one example that you can think of for each principle.

10. Briefly summarize how the practitioner may use *The Guide to Occupational Therapy Practice* (Moyers, 1999) in explaining what we do.

11. Explain the concept of occupational science as an academic discipline.

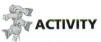 **ACTIVITY**

Materials

None.

Instructions

1a. Divide into small groups. As a group, decide how you would answer the questions in the following continuing scenario. With your group, role-play the responses to the scenarios for your classmates. After each role-play presentation, discuss Question 1c with your classmates.

Scenario

You have been assigned to work with a 22-year-old male named Charles who has been in an accident and sustained a spinal cord injury. He is paralyzed from the waist down. On entering the clinic, the patient appears very angry. He says to you, "What is occupational therapy and why do I have to come here?" You answer:

_____

_____

_____

_____

1b. Charles responds, "You can't help me. I will never want to do anything in this condition. I don't really care what happens to me now. Wouldn't it be better if I just had my parents do everything for me? You say:

_____

_____

_____

_____

1c. What philosophy and definition of OT were shared in terms to which this client could relate?

_____

_____

_____

_____

FOLLOW-UP

✔ Complete the Application of Competencies at the end of this chapter.

Exercise 3

"Would you tell me, please, which way I ought to go from here?' 'That depends a good deal on where you want to get to,' said the Cat."

LEWIS CARROL, *ALICE'S ADVENTURES IN WONDERLAND*

PREVENTION AND WELLNESS

OBJECTIVES

✔ Define prevention and wellness as it relates to occupational therapy (OT)
✔ Prepare a presentation on a topic in the area of prevention and wellness
✔ Assess your own state of wellness

DESCRIPTION

This exercise will give you a more thorough understanding of prevention and wellness as they relate to OT. It is important for you to stay healthy and well so that you can teach others to do so. You may find your educational experience taxing on your health. Many of you will be holding down a job and have various family responsibilities at the same time you are a student. Therefore, now is the best time to learn and practice wellness principles. You need to be able to practice these principles before you can effectively pass them on to your clients.

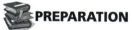**PREPARATION**

Suggested Readings

American Occupational Therapy Association (AOTA) (latest edition)
Christiansen and Baum (1997)
Health risk behavior prevention information from your local health clinic, such as a booklet or pamphlet on sexually transmitted disease, smoking, drug/substance abuse, or self-defense.

Study Questions

1. Define the following terms:
    a. Prevention

    b. Primary prevention

    c. Secondary prevention

    d. Tertiary prevention

    e. Health

    f. Health education

    g. Health promotion

    h. Health promotion and disease prevention

    i. Secondary conditions

2. List the objectives of "Healthy People 2000" from the U.S. Surgeon General's Report (as cited in Christiansen and Baum, 1997), which is aimed at people with disabilities.

3. Summarize AOTA's position on health promotion and prevention.

4. List basic competencies that all OT practitioners should have attained by the year 2005 according to the Pew report "Healthy America: Practitioners for 2005" (as cited in Christiansen and Baum, 1997).

5. Describe the general role the OT practitioner should take in the area of prevention and health promotion.

6. Describe specific means by which the OT practitioner may use health and promotion of wellness with the following individuals or in the following settings:

    a. Parent and child health

    b. Adolescence

    c. Independent living

    d. Cross-cultural community programming

    e. Worksite programs

    f. Self-help with chronic illness

    g. Older adults: fall prevention

    h. Older Adult Services and Information System (OASIS)

7. Prepare information to be presented in class on one of the assigned topic areas of primary prevention intervention including health risk behaviors (e.g., sexually transmitted disease, smoking, drug or substance abuse, self-defense). Work with a partner or a small group. Obtain your information from local health clinics and/or the health clinic of your host campus.

    a. Prevention intervention topics

    b. Information obtained to be shared with the class.

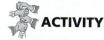 **ACTIVITY**

Materials

Items for presentations, such as photos, overhead projector.

Instructions

1. Share the information on your assigned primary prevention topic, using visual aids to emphasize important points. Take notes on the information presented by your classmates.

2. After the presentations, take a few minutes to assess the state of your wellness by answering the next six questions. Share this information with at least one other student.

    a. What do I currently do to stay well?

    b. What do I do that interferes with wellness?

    c. What do I choose to change? Write a goal for each change you seek—for example, "I will eat three vegetables a day adding one new one every week for two months."

    d. What resources are available on my campus or in my fieldwork setting that can be used for health and wellness (e.g., exercise facilities, counseling, seminars on health-related issues)?

    e. If you are a student with a disability, what services are available to help you succeed?

    f. What is my plan for changing?

FOLLOW-UP

✔ Complete the Application of Competencies at the end of this chapter.

CULTURAL AWARENESS

Exercise 4

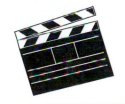

OBJECTIVES

✔ Identify cultural and religious differences in various groups
✔ Diagram the physical, mental, and spiritual aspects of your culture
✔ Examine the impact of various cultures and religious affiliations on health practices

DESCRIPTION

This exercise is designed to help you understand the impact of culture and religious affiliations on health. Before you work with clients of different cultures and religious affiliations, it is important to understand your own views on health. What are your personal beliefs and values toward maintaining and restoring health? As you articulate your own values and beliefs, you will also begin to see the importance and impact of cultures and religious affiliations that are different from your own. Your client's cultural and religious background will influence all interactions you have with them. Understanding your client's culture will enhance your effectiveness as an occupational therapy (OT) practitioner. This will be an ongoing process during your therapeutic interactions.

"Culture is a unified whole even unto psychosis and death."

JYLES HENTRY, *CULTURE AGAINST MAN*

PREPARATION

Suggested Reading

Davis (1998)
Neidstadt and Crepeau (1998)
Spector (1996)

Study Questions

1. Complete a Personal Cultural Chart (adapted from Spector, 1996) as it relates to you and your family. Use your parents, grandparents, and living relatives as sources of information. Refer to the sample personal culture chart completed below to assist you. Use the Personal Cultural Chart categories as your guidelines.

Fig. 1-1

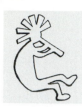

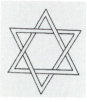

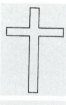

SAMPLE PERSONAL CULTURE CHART

CONTEXTUAL INFORMATION: <u>Married female, age 40</u>

CULTURE/RELIGION: <u>German American, Catholic, large family</u>

	PHYSICAL	MENTAL	SPIRITUAL
Maintain/protect health	Take daily vitamins Get 8 hours of sleep a day Dress warmly Stay dry outdoors Don't go to bed with wet hair Don't drink from the cup of a sick person Get all childhood shots See a doctor regularly	Eat dinner together as a family for support Do what the authorities say It's good to play sports Don't eat meat on Fridays in Lent	Go to church every Sunday Pray the rosary Don't sin, especially mortal sin Belief in one God Belief in saints to assist in disease prevention Must be baptized soon after birth
Restore health	Eat chicken noodle soup Drink honey, tea, and whiskey Apply vapor rub on chest and wrap the area with cloth Drink fluids, rest	Mother in charge of health care	Go to confession Get blessed with holy water Go to healing service at church Pray to saints to assist in various needs

PRACTICES CONCERNING DEATH AND MOURNING:
It is believed the person's soul leaves the body immediately after death. A body will be viewed by friends and family the night before burial. A full Mass will be performed at the funeral, which usually occurs in the morning. This process generally occurs two or three days after death.

PERSONAL CULTURAL CHART

CONTEXTUAL INFORMATION: _____

CULTURE/RELIGION: _____

	PHYSICAL	MENTAL	SPIRITUAL
Maintain/ protect health	(foods and food combinations, symbolic clothing, practices concerning bodily eliminations, childhood inoculations)	(avoid certain people who cause illness, family activities)	(religious customs, superstitions, wearing symbols to delay sources of harm)
Restore health	(homeopathic remedies, foods, massage, acupuncture, use of touch, medicine, services of a physician)	(relaxation, exorcism, traditional healers, family members in charge of health care)	(religious rituals, special prayers, meditation, traditional healings, exorcism)

PRACTICES CONCERNING DEATH AND MOURNING:

2. Briefly summarize what culture is and what it is not.

3. Define the following terms as they relate to culture:

    a. Myth

    b. Stereotype

    c. Xenophobia

    d. Generalizations

4. Describe what is meant by the term *cultural competence*. Explain why this is important for OT practitioners.

5. Describe what is meant by high-context and low-context cultures.

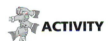 **ACTIVITY**

Materials

Chairs, flip charts, markers.

Instructions

1. Arrange chairs in the shape of two circles, one inside the other, with equal number of chairs in the center circle facing outward as in the outer circle facing inward. Take a seat in any chair. Share your personal cultural chart with the person you are facing and have that person do the same. Have the people in the inner circle move one chair to the right and repeat the sharing process. Answer the following questions in the allotted sharing time:

    a. What are some of the similarities between yourself and the people with whom you shared?

    b. What are some of the differences between yourself and the people with whom you shared?

c. Who did you share with that was most like you? Who was least like you?

d. Who did you not get to share with that you would have liked to? Why?

2. Identify yourself with a cultural group that exists in your class (e.g., groups based on religion, gender, sexual preference, race, occupation). Join the group with which you most closely identify. With your group, decide on answers to the following questions. Present your answers to the class. Use the flip chart provided to display your information.

   a. What distinguishes you as a cultural group?

   b. What do you most like about being associated with this cultural group?

   c. What do you least like about being associated with this cultural group?

   d. What do other people say about your group? Address both positive and negative stereotypes. What are three things you wish no one would ever say again about your cultural group?

   e. What did you learn from this exercise?

3. What do you need to work on to improve your cultural competence? Make a plan in the chart below.

IDENTIFIED NEEDS	GOAL	PLAN

FOLLOW-UP

✔ Complete the Application of Competencies at the end of this chapter.
✔ Complete Performance Skill 1E on Cultural Explanation.

LEARNING YOUR ASSOCIATION'S OFFICIAL DOCUMENTS

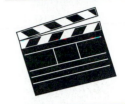

OBJECTIVES

✔ Become familiar with the *Reference Manual of the Official Documents of the American Occupational Therapy Association* (AOTA, latest edition)
✔ Identify specific topical content from the *Reference Manual of the Official Documents of the American Occupational Therapy Association* (AOTA, latest edition)
✔ Prepare a persuasive commercial to "sell" an official occupational therapy document

Exercise 5

"He who would climb the ladder must begin at the bottom."

ENGLISH PROVERB

DESCRIPTION

This exercise is designed to give you the opportunity to become competent in the use of the *Reference Manual of the Official Documents of the American Occupational Therapy Association* (AOTA, latest edition). The documents in this manual govern and guide the practice of occupational therapy. It is important that you familiarize yourself with them as quickly and thoroughly as possible. These documents are revised annually to reflect the changing and evolving profession. You will need to keep apprised of the changes as they occur.

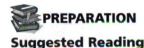

PREPARATION

Suggested Reading

AOTA (latest edition)

Study Questions

1. List the document or section in which each of the following topics is found.

TOPICS	DOCUMENT AND/OR SECTION
a. Standards for an accredited program for the occupational therapist	
b. Standards for an accredited program for the occupational therapy assistant	
c. Uniform terminology	
d. Philosophy of OT	
e. Case managing and OT	

2. Find the answers to the following questions and statements. Give the document title and the section in which it was found.

QUESTIONS/ STATEMENTS	ANSWER	DOCUMENT	SECTION
a. Name and number of the principle of patient confidentiality.			
b. Qualifications to work in neonatal intensive care unit			
c. What is service competency?			
d. Evaluation areas that must be performed by the OT			
e. Definition of close supervision			
f. Definition of occupational therapy practitioner			
g. Can an OT be a member of a hospice team?			
h. On what premise is service delivery based?			
i. Document that describes occupation as the common core of occupational therapy			
j. What is Principle IV in the Code of Ethics?			
k. What are the core values and attitudes of OT?			
l. Purpose of the Representative Assembly			
m. Definition of policy			
n. What is the definition of evaluation?			
o. What are the practitioner's roles regarding research?			
p. Definition of clinical reasoning			
q. Role of OT			
r. Role of OTA			

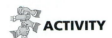 **ACTIVITY**

Materials

Poster board, markers, flip chart.

Instructions

Prepare to present to your classmates one or two assigned sections of the first eleven sections (denoted by Roman numerals) of the Reference Manual of the Official Documents of the AOTA (AOTA, latest edition). Do so in the format of a television commercial. Divide into small groups of two to five individuals per group. Assume that the class has to buy each section of the manual separately and your group wants to make sure other class members buy your section(s), as you are OT entrepreneurs who want to make as much money as possible. Be creative so that your presentation will be memorable. Prepare your commercial below. Use the presentation chart provided to record points earned and important information from other commercials presented in class. Score each group's presentation based on a total of 25 points possible, awarding up to 5 points for each of the following categories: creativity, communicativeness, clarity of information, persuasiveness, and use of humor.

Plan

Section _____

Information that needs to be presented:

Format of presentation:

Section _____

Information that needs to be presented:

Format of presentation:

	NOTES	A	B	C	D	E	TOTAL
PRESENTATION							
Section 1							
Section 2							
Section 3							
Section 4							
Section 5							
Section 6							

	NOTES	A	B	C	D	E	TOTAL
Section 7							
Section 8							
Section 9							
Section 10							
Section 11							

Key: A = creativity; B = communicativeness; C = clarity; D = persuastiveness; C = use of humor

FOLLOW-UP

✔   Complete the Application of Competencies at the end of this chapter.

Exercise 6

"The great and glorious masterpiece of humanity is to know how to live with a purpose."

MONTAGUE

ETHICS IN PRACTICE

OBJECTIVES

✔   Describe the ethical principles that guide the practice of occupational therapy
✔   Determine the standards of practice that relate to specific tasks of the occupational therapy practitioner
✔   Define the jurisdiction of the National Board for Certification of Occupational Therapy

DESCRIPTION

This exercise is designed to help you become more familiar with several of the documents and organizations that govern the practice of occupational therapy (OT). The Occupational Therapy Code of Ethics (American Occupational Therapy Association (AOTA), latest edition) binds OT practitioners to providing their clients with services in an appropriate and just manner. The Standards of Practice for Occupational Therapists (AOTA, latest edition) delineates the steps from the beginning to the end of the OT process when working with a client. The National Board for Certification of Occupational Therapy (NBCOT) is an independent certification board that grants certification to both registered occupational therapists (OTR) and certified occupational therapy assistants (COTA) on completion of the national certification examination.

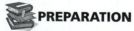**PREPARATION**

Suggested Reading

AOTA (latest edition)
NBCOT Web site: *http://www.nbcot.org*

Study Questions

1.   Locate the following documents and describe what each contains.

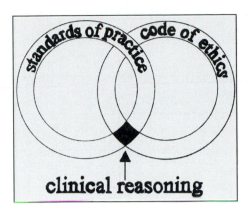

Fig. 1-2 The Standards of Practice and Code of Ethics both must be considered in making clinical decisions.

a. Occupational Therapy Code of Ethics

b. Standards of Practice for Occupational Therapy

2. Following are examples of adherence to and violations of the Occupational Therapy Code of Ethics. State the specific principle that is related.

PRINCIPLE

_____ A therapist orders equipment for his patients from a company that he owns.

_____ A therapist who continually overcharges her patient's time is reported by her supervisor.

_____ An OT practitioner must keep all patient information confidential.

_____ Patients and/or caregivers must be involved in setting goals.

_____ All practitioners must report a breach of the code.

_____ All safety measures must be taken to avoid harm.

_____ A supervisor must provide the appropriate amount of supervision.

_____ A patient has the right to refuse treatment.

_____ A therapist promises that the treatment will make the patient more independent.

_____ An OT practitioner refuses to treat patients who have AIDS.

_____ A practitioner must abide by all rules to keep his or her license.

_____ A therapist treats a patient for drug addiction when the issue arises during treatment for a head injury. The therapist must report this to the patient's physician.

_____ A student supervisor discusses the previous student's performance with his or her current student.

3. From the OT Standards of Practice (AOTA, latest edition) determine the role of the OTA in the OT process. It is understood that the OT is able to do all parts of the process. Identify the standard and number that answers each question.

4. What are the possible disciplinary actions that the AOTA may administer for a vi-

QUESTION	ANSWER	STANDARD
a. Can an OTA accept a referral?		
b. Must all practitioners be knowledgeable about research done in their area of practice?		
c. Must notes be written within a certain time frame?		
d. Can an OTA educate other professionals?		
e. Can an OTA document recommendations in the discharge plan?		
f. Can an OTA prepare a transition plan?		
g. Must the goals be written to reflect the philosophy of OT?		
h. Are there state laws that govern the amount of supervision an OTA must receive?		
i. Can an OTA participate in the process to determine whether a patient is in need of OT services?		
j. Can an OTA perform standardized tests?		

olation of the code of ethics?

5. List and describe the guidelines outlined in the document "Guidelines to the Occupational Therapy Code of Ethics" (AOTA, latest edition).

6. What are the responsibilities of the NBCOT?

7. What are the general requirements to be eligible to take the NBCOT exam?

8. What are NBCOT's specific requirements to obtain OTR and COTA status?

9. Describe the NBCOT's procedure for disciplinary action.

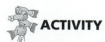 **ACTIVITY**

Materials

Copy of "Standards of Practice for OT" and "OT Code of Ethics," from which the game host (instructor) will read the examples. Study questions can also be used to develop similar questions.

🎲 GAME

Instructions

As a class, divide into two teams. Play a game based on the TV program *Name That Tune*. The object of the game is to identify the specific standard of practice or code of ethic along with the corresponding number and/or letter before the other team does. As on *Name That Tune,* the value of the correct response drops as more information is given. Have your instructor begin reading a sentence that describes one of the principles or standards. If a team can identify the correct standard of practice or code of ethic, the team receives three points. Each time your instructor reads another clue, the value drops one point. Keep a running tally of your team's points.

Team Points _____

FOLLOW-UP

✔ Complete the Application of Competencies at the end of this chapter.

LEARNING THE JARGON

OBJECTIVES

✔ Identify jargon related to occupational therapy
✔ Interpret a sign language message
✔ Decipher a jargon-contained sentence typically found in medical records

DESCRIPTION

This exercise will give you experience in deciphering the jargon related to the profession of occupational therapy (OT). Jargon includes the various medical words, symbols, and acronyms that are associated with the profession. In an OT setting, jargon will often be used to communicate with your colleagues quickly and efficiently. Jargon may also be used in documenting services provided. When communicating with clients and/or those unfamiliar with OT, you will need to avoid the use of jargon and make sure you explain in full any abbreviations and concepts that are not universally known.

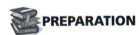PREPARATION

Suggested Readings

Costello (1994)
Jacobs (1999)
Neidstadt and Crepeau (1998)
Smith (1994)

Study Questions

1. Decipher the following text:

Dear OT student:

I hope you get to visit the *OT* _____ department tomorrow at the hospital. They have a large staff, with six *OTRs* _____

and five *COTAs* _____, who are all members of the *AOTA*

_____. They are also training three *OTAS* _____

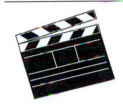

Exercise 7

"One loses many laughs by not laughing at oneself."

SARA JEANETTE DUNEAN

and two *OTS* _____. Some of the things you will observe

will be *ROM* _____ *tx* _____

done with the *pts* _____ who are seen *bid* _____

_____. They are seen in the mornings for *ADL* _____.

The pts. are also assisted with meals unless they are *NPO* _____

per doctor's orders.

If you are $\bar{c}$ _____ the COTA when he is doing ROM,

see whether you can tell whether the ®*UE* _____ has the

same ✔ _____ and /_____ as the

Ⓛ*UE* _____. It will be important for you to see *PT*

_____, *RN* _____,

MD _____, *SLP* _____, and *RT*

_____ *2°* _____ to the team ap-

proach used at most facilities. $\bar{S}$ _____ teamwork the pt.

will not receive the best care, no matter how many *x* _____

you see the patient.

Some of the pts. you will see while visiting include those pts. with *TBI*

_____, *CVA* _____,

THR _____, *Ca* _____,

COPD _____, *RA* _____,

AIDS _____, *SCI* _____,

IDDM _____, *MS* _____,

MD _____, *CP* _____,

MR _____, *TIA* _____,

and *ALS* _____. You will not be seeing a ♂ _____

pt. *Dx*_____ with *PMS*_____!

Remember that to be a really great practioner and ↑ _____,

your knowledge you must study ≈ _____*t.i.d.* <

_____ that will only ↓ _____

your chances and make it ? _____ if you will succeed. It

certainly doesn't matter if you are > _____ 25 *y/o*

_____, as long as your grades are *WNL* _____.

I hope you don't *c/o* _____ too much about homework

because there will be a great deal, and we want to *R/O* _____ whin-

ers. You will most certainly notice a △ _____ in your balance of

occupations, which may at times require you to have *SBA* _____.

When treatment involves a patient who has had a *CVA* _____,

you may need to use some *NDT* _____, *PNF* _____

_____, and screen them with the *ACL*. For *tx* _____

_____ you may use a *BTE* _____ work

simulator. Another test to try is the *MVPT* _____ and

check their *FIM* _____ score also. Make sure you read the

AJOT _____ for the latest information written by a prac-

tioner who is also a *FAOTA* _____ and a *ROH*_____.

The children you work with will normally have an *IEP* _____

_____ or an *IFSP* _____, especially if

they have *LD* _____, *AD/HD* _____,

ADD _____ or if they have a low *IQ* _____.

If a *SIPT* _____ was completed, it may not tell you

whether the child can *don* _____ or *doff* _____

_____ their shirt.

Agencies you will need to deal with in your profession from time to time are

HCFA _____, *HMO* _____,

NIMH _____, *WFOT* _____,

NARC _____, *JCAHO* _____,

CARF _____, and *NBCOT* _____.

You must document in the *POMR* _____ the results

of your *SI* _____ Tx, your *MMT* _____,

the use of the *CPMM* _____ , and any *PROM* _____

_____ you have to do to the *BLEs* _____.

Be careful in your documentation because they will grade you on the *FWE*

_____.

The HMO may develop a *DRG* _____ for your pa-

tients to determine their *LOS* _____. If you write so

much that your *MCP* _____, *PIP* _____

_____, and *DIPs* _____ get sore, you may

need a pencil grip.

If you are working in a psychiatric setting, you may work with an *AT* _____

_____. You may document progress in the *SOAP* _____

_____ format when discussing results of the *KELS* _____

_____ or the *BaFPE* _____. Your re-

search may take you to the *DSM-IV* _____ to see whether

your pt. has *PTSD* _____ and whether an *ECT* is standard

tx. If your pt. is an alcoholic, he/she may need to go to *AA* _____

_____, a group called *SAMI* _____, or

even *ALANON* _____.

Next, make sure you search through the *CINAHL* _____

_____ for the latest copies of *OTJR* _____, *OTMH*

_____, *OTHC* _____, *POTG*

_____, *POTP* _____, and the *CJOT*

_____. It will help in your research. *Hint*: For acronyms

that are not found in the suggested sources, try to guess what the answers might be

using the context cues given. As a last resort, ask your instructor to help you out.

2. Interpret the sign language message.

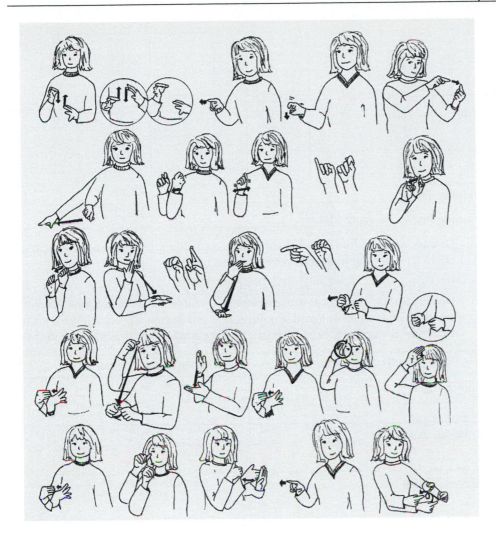

Fig. 1-3 Decipher this message.

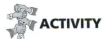 **ACTIVITY**

Materials

Poster board or paper.

GAME

Instructions

Divide into teams to play a Jargon Jeopardy game as prepared by your instructor. Fill in the abbreviations and answers as they are uncovered. After playing the game, discuss the questions presented.

1.

$400

$300

$200

☐ ☐ ☐ ☐

$100

☐ ☐ ☐ ☐

Winning Team: _____

Winning Prize: Bragging Rights _____

2. Discuss when and under what circumstances it is appropriate and not appropriate to use OT jargon. Record your thoughts below.

3. Divide into small groups. Decipher a sentence written on the chalkboard by your instructor that is typically found in a medical record document. The first group to decipher the sentence will be given points. Use the space below to complete your work.

MEDICAL RECORD SENTENCE	DECIPHERED SENTENCE
Sentence One	
Sentence Two	
Sentence Three	
Sentence Four	

Winning Team: _____

Winning Prize: Bragging Rights _____

FOLLOW-UP

✔   Complete the Application of Competency at the end of this chapter.

Exercise 8

"The task ahead of us is never as great as the power behind us."

RALPH WALDO EMERSON

AOTA: YOUR PROFESSIONAL ORGANIZATION

OBJECTIVES

✔   Become familiar with occupational therapy's national, state, and local organizations
✔   Become familiar with occupational therapy's professional publications
✔   Identify continuing education opportunities and responsibilities

DESCRIPTION

This exercise is designed to introduce you to some of your professional obligations. Part of professionalism is taking the initiative and responsibility to be a member of your state and national organizations as well as taking part in continuing education opportunities.

The American Occupational Therapy Association (AOTA) is the national organization of occupational therapy, and future practitioners have a duty and responsibility to join. Each state also has its own occupational therapy association with district subsections. It is imperative that you become and remain an active member. Among many other benefits, doing so will allow you to keep up to date and network with others. Continuing education opportunities are also a part of maintaining one's competency.

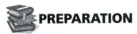 **PREPARATION**

Suggested Readings

American Journal of Occupational Therapy (any)
AOTA Web site: *http://www.aota.org*
Occupational Therapy Practice (any)
Advance for Occupational Therapy Practitioners (any)

Study Questions

1. Go to AOTA's Web site. Give a brief description of each of the following areas:
    a. AOTA's address, telephone, and fax numbers

    b. Accreditation

    c. Membership

    d. About AOTA

    e. Educational programs

    f. American Occupational Therapy Foundation (AOTF)

    g. Fieldwork

    h. The *Journal of Occupational Therapy Students*

2. The *American Journal of Occupational Therapy (AJOT)* is a scholarly journal that uses the process of peer review to determine the selection of works included. *Advance for Occupational Therapy Practioners* contains news and

employment opportunities. *OT Practice* contains information about specific practice areas with hands-on content. Review each publication and fill in the following information.

	TYPE OF ARTICLES	LIST OF CONTINUING EDUCATION OFFERS
AJOT		
Advance for Occupational Therapy Practitioners		
OT Practice		

3. Go to the AOTA web site.

   a. List and describe current news and events affecting OT.

   b. List the areas available to members and nonmembers.

4. Attend an occupational therapy district meeting in your area. Complete the following:

   a. What was the format of the meeting?

   b. List and describe the topics that were discussed or presented.

   c. How often are meetings held?

   d. What are the functions of the board?

   e. What is the relationship of the district OT association to the state association? To the national association?

   f. What is the purpose of the district association?

   g. How does one become a member?

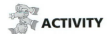 **ACTIVITY**

Materials

Large posterboard for each group, markers, construction paper, glue.

Instruction

1. Divide into small groups. Prepare a full-page color advertisement to entice students to join the AOTA. Use the space below to plan and prepare your group's advertisement.

    a. Information you want to include on poster.

    b. Examples of artwork that may be helpful to understanding and appealing to see.

    c. Sketch the outline of the poster below.

2. Hang each poster in the room and rate each one on the information contained therein and its appearance as indicated in the following scoring criteria. Use a score of 1–7, 7 being the highest rating, to rate each poster. Place that score in each box, then total the scores for that poster.

	PERTINENT INFORMATION INCLUDED	BENEFITS HIGHLIGHTED	PURPOSE OF AOTA	CLEAR, CONCISE WORDING	CREATIVE, ATTRACTIVE APPEARANCE	TOTAL POINTS
Poster 1						
Poster 2						
Poster 3						
Poster 4						
Poster 5						
Poster 6						
Poster 7						

FOLLOW-UP

✔ Complete the Application of Competencies at the end of this chapter.

Exercise 9

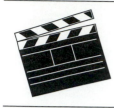

"The best career advice to give the young is find out what you like doing best and get someone to pay you for doing it."

KATHERINE WHILEHAEN

ESSENTIAL FUNCTIONS OF OCCUPATIONAL THERAPY PRACTITIONERS

OBJECTIVES

✔ Compare and contrast essential function requirements of educational and clinical settings

✔ Develop a plan to meet anticipated essential job functions in an educational and clinical setting

✔ Determine possible reasonable accommodations that may be needed for performance requirements in an educational and clinical setting

DESCRIPTION

The activities in this exercise give you an opportunity to explore and examine the essential function requirements of the educational and clinical settings. These are the physical, mental, sensory, emotional, and social performance skills necessary for competent performance in a particular setting. These essential functions are often included in the student handbook of an educational facility and/or job descriptions of a clinical facility. You need to be prepared to meet the demands of your educational program as well as the demands of your future career.

PREPARATION

Suggested Readings

Essential functions of host educational program
Job descriptions listing the essential job functions and performance requirements from local facilities
Sladyk (1997)
Americans With Disabilities Act of 1990 (P.L. 101–336)

Study Questions

1. List the essential function requirements of your host educational program.

2. List the essential functional requirements included in the job descriptions from local facilities.

3. Using the assigned job description from one clinical facility, summarize the essential job functions by listing the similarities and differences between the demands of the occupational therapist (OT) and the occupational therapy assistant (OTA).

SIMILARITIES	DIFFERENCES

4. Using documents from your host educational facility and the assigned clinical facility, list the essential functions outlined in both. Indicate your current performance and/or skill for each essential function. Place a checkmark next to your skills that are aligned with the requirements. Place an "E" next to those needed by your educational facility and a "C" by those required by your assigned clinical facility. See the sample below.

ESSENTIAL FUNCTIONS	CURRENT SKILL LEVEL	✔
Lift equipment weighing 40 lbs **E**	Able to lift 35 lbs. With difficulty	

5. Develop a plan to master these skills with a target date for completion. If you need assistance ask your instructor or counselor.

SKILLS TO DEVELOP	PLAN	MASTERY DATE

6. If there are skills that you cannot master because of a registered disability, what reasonable accommodations might assist you in being successful in your education or employment? Align these with the specifications of the Americans With Disabilities Act (ADA) of 1990.

SKILLS UNABLE TO DO	ADAPTATION OR ACCOMMODATION NEEDED

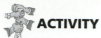 **ACTIVITY**

Materials

Essential job skills from the job descriptions of various occupational therapy settings, including pediatrics, physical dysfunction, mental illness, and geriatrics.

Instructions

1. Compare the job description documents from the various practice settings. As a class or in your small group, complete the following statements. Highlight the functions that are unique to the OT.

   a. List the essential job functions that are the same on all documents.

   b. Find the essential job functions that are unique between the documents. List those essential skills here and describe the facility that requires them.

   c. For each of the following practice areas, describe the physical requirements, including lifting.

PEDIATRICS	PHYSICAL REHABILITATION	PSYCHOSOCIAL	GERIATRICS

   d. For each of the following disciplines, describe the mental demands.

PEDIATRICS	PHYSICAL REHABILITATION	PSYCHOSOCIAL	GERIATRICS

   e. For each of the following practice areas, describe the sensory demands.

PEDIATRICS	PHYSICAL REHABILITATION	PSYCHOSOCIAL	GERIATRICS

f. For each of the following practice areas, describe the social and emotional demands.

PEDIATRICS	PHYSICAL REHABILITATION	PSYCHOSOCIAL	GERIATRICS

2. Using the information from all the occupational therapy practice settings, which other essential functions do you need to master to become a competent practitioner? What adaptations and accommodations might you need in accordance with the ADA?

FOLLOW-UP

✔ Complete the Application of Competencies at the end of this chapter.

FRAMES OF REFERENCE

Exercise 10

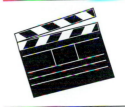

OBJECTIVES

✔ Describe the role and importance of a frame of reference in occupational therapy
✔ List the major frames of reference and the accompanying supporting theory
✔ Discuss the client population and environment for which a particular frame of reference might be used

DESCRIPTION

The purpose of this exercise is to familiarize you with the different frames of reference that may be used in occupational therapy. A frame of reference is a particular emphasis or focus. It is based in strong theoretical constructs. A frame of reference links theory to practice. Frames of reference are sometimes refered to as models, and they give us much information and guidance in treatment planning. They will continue to be critiqued for their usefulness in the years to come. Occupational therapists need to be competent in both using and interpreting frames of reference. Occupational therapy assistants need to be familiar with the frames of reference that are commonly used in occupational therapy treatment.

"Nothing contributes so much to tranquilize the mind as a steady purpose—a point on which the soul may fix its intellectual eye."

MARY WOLLSTONECRAFT
SHELLEY

PREPARATION

Suggested Readings

Cole (1998)
Neidstadt and Crepeau (1998)

Study Questions

1. Define a frame of reference.

2.   Define *theory*.

3.   Describe the function of a theory.

4.   Discuss the relationship between a theory and a frame of reference.

5.   List the steps in extrapolation that make a theory usable.

6.   Describe how to combine the compatible concepts of both a theory and a frame of reference to provide maximal therapeutic intervention for a client.

7.   List at least ten frames of reference or models that an OT practitioner may use in practice, as well as two postulates, beliefs, and/or assumptions of each frame of reference. Identify at least one related theorist and explain how the frame of reference can be used in clinical practice.

FRAME OF REFERENCE	POSTULATE/BELIEF/ ASSUMPTION	THEORIST(S)	USE IN PRACTICE

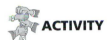 **ACTIVITY**

Materials

Posterboards, markers, book entitled *Psychosocial Components of Occupational Therapy* (Mosey, 1986).

Instructions

1a. Break into small groups of approximately four people. Gather as much information as you can about an assigned frame of reference. Describe your frame of reference with one-sentence statements, starting with broad concepts and narrowing the concepts with each respective turn that is taken. Word your statements so that the other teams have a difficult time figuring out which frame of reference you are describing. Make sure all statements are accurate and not misleading. Every time your team takes a turn and the frame of reference is not discovered, your team earns a point. Continue to take turns until all teams have taken one turn, then continue in a round-robin fashion until the frame of reference is discovered. Use the questions below to gather information about your assigned frame of reference and to plan the statements you will use for this game.

Frames of Reference: _____

- With what client population might this frame of reference be used?

- What would the population characteristics be (e.g., age, gender, diagnosis, cognitive status)?

- In what environment and/or context might you use your frame of reference?

- What activities might you use for intervention?

- Who are the leaders and proponents of this frame of reference?

- With what theoretical base(s) is your frame of reference most closely aligned?

- What researchable question might be generated from your frame of reference?

1b. Record highlights from the class presentation of your peers.
Frame of reference:

Frame of reference:

Frame of reference:

Frame of reference:

Frame of reference:

Frame of reference:

Frame of reference:

Frame of reference:

Frame of reference:

Frame of reference:

2. Gather further information about the four hierarchical components in your assigned frame of reference as described by Mosey (1986). Diagram this information on a poster, using descriptions and illustrations as needed. Display the posters for viewing by classmates and as a source to assist in learning.

   a. Theoretical base

   b. Function-dysfunction continuum

   c. Behaviors indicative of function-dysfunction

   d. Postulates regarding change and intervention

FOLLOW-UP

✔ Complete the Application for Competencies at the end of this chapter.

OCCUPATIONAL THERAPY PROCESS

Exercise 11

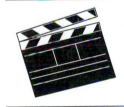

OBJECTIVES

✔ Identify the steps in the occupational therapy (OT) process
✔ Define and describe the evaluation component of the OT process
✔ Prepare and present a role-play depicting the OT process

DESCRIPTION

This exercise is designed to help you understand the occupational therapy (OT) process from beginning to end. The OT process can be defined as the steps set forth in the "Standards of Practice for Occupational Therapy" (AOTA, latest edition), which follow the client from entering the domain of OT services to exiting the services. The steps in that process include referral, screening, evaluation, intervention planning, intervention, transition, and discontinuation. Once a client gets to the evaluation component, a practitioner's skills are relied on to begin to determine the direction the intervention will take. The evaluation component lays the foundation on which the resulting OT services are built. Both occupational therapy assistants and occupational therapists need to be able to appropriately determine their client's progress through the entire OT process.

"In our art we touch, if only for a moment, the realness of each other."

ANNE CRONIN MOSEY

PREPARATION

Suggested Readings

AOTA (latest edition)
Asher (1996)
Christianen and Baum (1997)
Hinojosa and Kramer (1998)
Neistadt and Crepeau (1998)
Reed and Sanderson (1999)

Study Questions

1. Diagram the steps to the OT process, using the document "Standards of Practice for Occupational Therapy" (AOTA, latest edition) and identify two or three key concepts associated with each step.

2. Differentiate between evaluation and assessment.

3. Identify the purposes of the following three types of time-determined OT assessments:

   a. Initial

   b. Interim

   c. Discharge

4. Describe the following types of assessments:

   a. Medical records

   b. Skilled observation

   c. Interview

   d. Inventories and checklists

   e. Standardized tests

   f. Norm-referenced tests

   g. Criterion-referenced tests

5. Describe how objects in the client's environment might tell you about that client's interests and values. How might you use this information as part of your assessment and/or to help you establish rapport with the client.

6. Describe how narratives might be used as part of an evaluation to understand the clients' perspective.

7. Delineate the responsibilities of the different aspects of the evaluation/assessment process for the OT and the OTA.

8. Describe how the evaluation process is documented and communicated.

9. List the content in the following areas that needs to be documented in the evaluation report:
    a. Identification and background information

    b. Assessment results

    c. Intervention or treatment plan

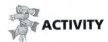 **ACTIVITY**

Materials

Props for role-playing, flip charts, markers, tape.

Instruction

1a. Divide into seven small groups. Represent your assigned step in the OT process in the form of a drawing. Be creative in trying to think of representations that will be informative and helpful in remembering what occurs in that step.

1b. Present your drawing to the class. Display the seven steps on the wall in order of occurrence. Note below the aspects of the drawing that will help you remember the entire OT process.

Referral

Screening

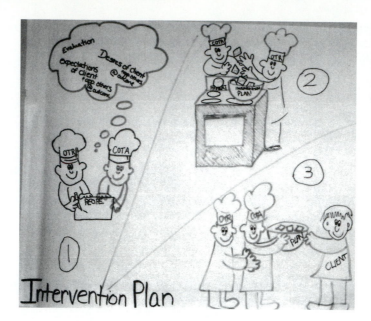

Fig. 1-4 Drawing of an intervention plan.

Drawing courtesy of Mary Klei, Tricia Carroll, Cathy Lampe, Tina Leap, and Jillian Joseph.

Evaluation

Intervention planning

Intervention

Transition

Discontinuation

2.   Your group is now the expert for the step to the OT process just presented. Write two test questions that cover the material in your step of the OT process. Give the questions to your instructor. As your instructor reads the questions aloud to the class, answer them, challenging yourself to see how much you know. Record below the areas of strength you have in remembering and understanding the OT process as well as areas of concern about your knowledge base.

STRENGTHS	AREAS OF CONCERN

3. Divide into small groups of three to five people. Designate a step in the OT process for each group to simulate. Pattern your role-play after a particular real-life scenario; for example, designate a client age, diagnosis, presenting problems, and context under which OT services are being sought. Members who are not participating in the role play will observe. After the presentation the observers will critique the participating group's performance, indicating the parts of the OT process that were well represented and those that were not well represented. Use the space below to record the information you gained from the role-playing scenario.

    a. Referral

    b. Screening

    c. Evaluation

    d. Intervention plan

    e. Intervention

    f. Transition

    g. Discontinuation

4. Divide into small groups. Create a logo to differentiate between the terms *evaluation* and *assessment*. Draw this logo on flip chart paper. Design it for ease in remembering these sometimes confusing terms. Share the logo with your class. Vote on the one that is the most likely to help you remember the difference between the two terms. Draw the winning logo below.

FOLLOW-UP

✔   Complete the Application of Competencies at the end of this chapter.

PRACTICE GUIDELINES

Exercise 12

OBJECTIVES

✔   Identify common terminology used within the profession
✔   Determine domains of concern in the performance areas, components, and contexts from a case study
✔   Communicate the scope of OT services to a client and external groups

"Stress is when your body doesn't agree with what your mouth just said."
ANONYMOUS

DESCRIPTION

This exercise will give you an opportunity to become familiar with common terminology and guidelines used within the profession. The scope of occupational therapy includes performance areas, performance components, and performance contexts. Understanding these terms and their subsets is important in communicating the scope and parameters of OT services with your client, other related disciplines, and external groups. Aligning OT terminology with International Classification of Functioning and Disability (ICIDH-2) terminology will assist in this process. This understanding will guide your practice.

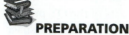

PREPARATION

Suggested Reading

AOTA, (latest edition)
Moyers (1999)
ICIDH-2 web site: http://www.who.int/icidh/

Study Questions

1a. Occupational therapy is defined as

b. Occupational therapy services include:

c. Occupational therapy intervention involves:

d. Achieving outcomes means:

2. Make a set of flash cards with a picture on each card symbolizing all the performance areas, components, and contexts terms as described in the latest edition of Uniform Terminology (AOTA). On each completed card include the term, definition of the term, performance title under which the term is located, and a symbolic picture. Obtain pictures from magazines or other printed sources, or draw your own.

3. Go to the ICIDH-2 web site. List and describe the areas of classification.

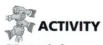

ACTIVITY

Materials

Index cards with uniform terminology terms on each, highlighter, Case Studies 2, 3, and 4 located at the end of this chapter.

Instructions

1. Divide into two groups. Take turns acting out a charade (an area, component, or context from the latest edition of Uniform Terminology (AOTA) or term used in ICIDH-2) assigned to you by your instructor. When it is your turn, your team members are to guess the meaning of the charade. If your team does not guess correctly, another team can guess and thereby steal a point. Keep a tally of the total points earned by each team. Record in the space provided the terms that you now understand and the terms that are still unclear to you. Include an example of how that term is used.

TERMS	✔ CLEAR	✔ UNCLEAR	EXAMPLE
Figure ground	✔		Finding a pen among a cluttered desk top

2a. Use the latest edition of Uniform Terminology (AOTA, latest edition) for the assigned case studies. After reading the case, highlight the concerns in the performance areas, performance components, and performance contexts. Use this information to determine appropriate treatment intervention as you think your client might prioritize. Fill out the following chart. An example from Case Study 1 (located at the end of this chapter) has been started for you.

CASE NO.	CONCERNS IN PERFORMANCE AREAS	CONCERNS IN PERFORMANCE COMPONENTS	CONCERNS IN PERFORMANCE CONTEXTS	SUGGESTED TREATMENT ACTIVITIES
1	Play/leisure performance	Interpersonal skills	Progression of Parkinson's disease is causing withdrawal	1:1 in OT with partner to play cards; make simple wood project in parallel group
	Feeding and eating	Fine motor coordination/ dexterity	Socially embarrassed to eat with people	Assess for adaptive equipment needs

CASE NO.	CONCERNS IN PERFORMANCE AREAS	CONCERNS IN PERFORMANCE COMPONENTS	CONCERNS IN PERFORMANCE CONTEXTS	SUGGESTED TREATMENT ACTIVITIES
2				
3				
4				

2b. Role-play with a partner how you would use *The Guide to OT Practice: Quick Reference* (Moyers, 1999) to describe the OT process your client may experience. Use this document to increase your client's understanding of the scope of OT services. As your classmates role-play use of this document, give them feedback to improve their effectiveness in communicating. Record how you plan to use this document and the feedback you received from your classmates.

PLAN:
FEEDBACK FROM CLASSMATES:

2c. Discuss how you might use this quick reference with an administrator, legislator, program developer, and/or third-party payer in relationship to the needs of your client.

FOLLOW-UP

✔ Complete the Application of Competencies at the end of this chapter.

PURPOSEFUL OCCUPATION

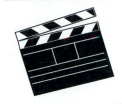

OBJECTIVES

✔ Describe the importance of using occupation
✔ Analyze an occupation and its inherent characteristics according to the occupational therapy performance areas, components, and contexts
✔ Select therapeutic occupations for a case study

DESCRIPTION

When you select therapeutic occupations with your client, they need to be appropriate, meaningful, and purposeful. A thorough occupational analysis can help determine the appropriateness of an activity by looking at the components and steps of the activity, the materials that will be needed, the implications for intervention, the evaluation potential, the frame of reference compatibility, as well as any possible contraindications to the activity. Additionally, the client's strengths, interests, and needs will determine activities that are meaningful and purposeful. The person and the meaningful activity will then be aligned with the environmental context to achieve maximal therapeutic benefits.

"While one person hesitates because he feels inferior, the other is busy making mistakes and becoming superior."

HENRY C. LINK

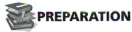**PREPARATION**

Suggested Readings

AOTA (latest edition)
Breines (1995)
Drake (1992)
Watson (1997)

Study Questions

1. Describe what is meant by activity, purposeful activity, and occupation.

2. Draw a diagrammatic and pictorial representation of the performance areas, performance components and contexts from the latest edition of Uniform Terminology (AOTA). In your drawings, represent the major categories in the document. A drawing of the performance contexts has been done for you. Add color to all three of the drawings to help you learn and remember this essential document.

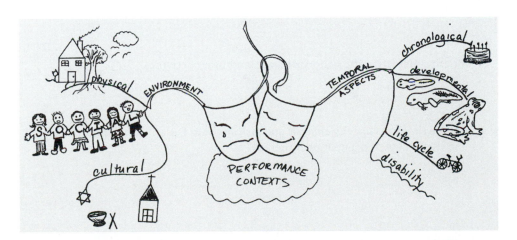

Fig. 1-5 Sample pictorial representation of performance context.

3. Summarize AOTA's position on the use of task, activities, and occupations.

4. Describe the use of purposeful activity or occupation in each of the following life stages:
    a. Childhood

    b. Adolescence

    c. Adult

    d. Senior

5. Why is it important for clients to be involved in the choice of occupations used for treatment?

6. Define the following terms as they relate to occupational performance:
    a. Role

    b. Task

    c. Activity

7. Describe what factors need to be considered in analyzing contexts.

8. Briefly summarize the history of crafts and other activities.

9. Define the terms *activity analysis* and *task analysis*. Describe the importance of using these tools in occupational therapy.

10. Describe how the process of activity analysis can be mastered.

11. How can task analysis be used during the screening and evaluation process?

12. Describe the use of crafts in each of the following frames of reference:
    a. Neurophysiologic

    b. Cognitive disabilities

    c. Developmental

    d. Role acquisition

    e. Biomechanical

    f. Life-style performance

    g. Rehabilitation

    h. Human occupation

13. Complete the following Occupational Performance Questionnaire on yourself, determining your strengths and areas of concern regarding each performance area, context, or area as listed in the latest edition of Uniform Terminology (AOTA). Add your level of interest or need in regard to the same area. Do likewise with the performance components and performance context, completing the chart in all applicable areas. Afterward, complete the Occupational Performance Questionnaire on one other person who is in a different stage of life than you. Find someone who is considerably younger or older than you and of a different culture. A sample has been provided for you to begin each section.

OCCUPATIONAL PERFORMANCE QUESTIONNAIRE (SELF)			
PERFORMANCE AREAS	STRENGTHS	AREAS OF CONCERN	INTERESTS OR NEEDS
Sensory	Keen sense of smell; love to taste different foods	Very poor vision; hate to spin	Love to read; need to get new glasses

PERFORMANCE AREAS	STRENGTHS	AREAS OF CONCERN	INTERESTS OR NEEDS
ADL	All independent	Increasing weight gain as aging	Adapting lifestyle to meet changing metabolism

PERFORMANCE CONTEXTS	STRENGTHS	AREAS OF CONCERN	INTERESTS OR NEEDS
Chronological	42 years old— enjoy this age	Joints starting to hurt	Need to keep physically fit

OCCUPATIONAL PERFORMANCE QUESTIONNAIRE (OTHER)			
PERFORMANCE COMPONENTS	STRENGTHS	AREAS OF CONCERN	INTERESTS OR NEEDS

PERFORMANCE AREAS	STRENGTHS	AREAS OF CONCERN	INTERESTS OR NEEDS

PERFORMANCE CONTEXTS	STRENGTHS	AREAS OF CONCERN	INTERESTS OR NEEDS

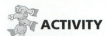

ACTIVITY

Materials

See and Say™, Playdoh™, finger paint and paper, Chutes and Ladders™, cards with topics for charades, Pictionary™, Boggle™, Scruples™, Scattergories™, The Ungame™, a deck of cards, material for a craft activity such as basket weaving or making a tile trivet or a cooking activity such as making a cake, latest edition of Uniform Terminology (AOTA), Case Studies 2, 3, 4, and 5 located at the end of this chapter.

Instructions

1a. Divide into small groups. Summarize and discuss the strengths, areas of concern, and interests or needs of yourself and the person on whom you filled out the questionnaire. Compile a written summary based on the information obtained from yourself and other members in your small group. Fill in the following chart accordingly. When all the information from your small groups has been compiled, compare and contrast similarities and differences among and between the age groups as well as the genders.

SUMMARY CHART FOR CHILDREN		
	MALE	FEMALE
Areas Strengths Areas of concern Interests/needs		
Components Strengths Areas of concern Interests/needs		
Contexts Strengths Areas of concern Interests/needs		

SUMMARY CHART FOR ADOLESCENTS		
	MALE	FEMALE
Areas Strengths Areas of concern Interests/needs		
Components Strengths Areas of concern Interests/needs		
Contexts Strengths Areas of concern Interests/needs		

SUMMARY CHART FOR ADULTS		
	MALE	FEMALE

Areas
  Strengths
  Areas of concern
  Interests/needs		

Components
  Strengths
  Areas of concern
  Interests/needs		

Contexts
  Strengths
  Areas of concern
  Interests/needs		

SUMMARY CHART FOR SENIORS		
	MALE	FEMALE

Areas
  Strengths
  Areas of concern
  Interests/needs		

Components
  Strengths
  Areas of concern
  Interests/needs		

Contexts
  Strengths
  Areas of concern
  Interests/needs		

1b. Discuss and record below your impressions of the influences of the cultures represented on the individual's functional performance.

1c. Join the entire class and share your findings. Record how you plan to use this information for intervention.

2a. Each person in your small group will be assigned different categories from the latest edition of uniform terminology (AOTA) for which you are to become the expert. List the performance components or contexts below for which you will be responsible.

2b. Meet with other "experts" in the same area(s) you have been assigned. Discuss your areas and become familiar with the terms. List below the subcomponents of the area for which you are responsible and add a brief description of each.

Fig. 1-6 Playing
"Chutes and Ladders"©.

Photo courtesy of Michelle Perkins, Kim Guffey, Anita Terry, Gary Gibbons, Kim Kendall, and Sara Karcher.

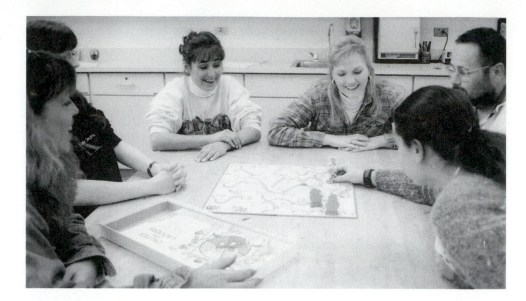

2c. Rejoin your original group and participate in the activities available (e.g., a craft, game, or cooking activity as listed in the Materials section). Focus on analyzing the component(s) and or context(s) you were assigned. Once the activity has been completed or the time allotted has expired, briefly discuss the components and context of each activity as a group. Contribute your "expert" input. Fill in the Abbreviated Occupational Analysis Form (found in Appendix A) for each activity, indicating the degree to which the component or context is involved. Briefly describe that involvement to complete the total analysis of each activity.

3a. Participate in an instructor-led task that involves new learning. Analyze that task to determine its therapeutic value by using the Occupational Analysis form (found in the Appendix A).

3b. Once you have completed the analysis, join with a partner or small group. Fill in areas on the analysis you may have missed. After a group discussion, list the strengths and areas of concern regarding your competence in completing an occupational analysis.

STRENGTHS	AREAS OF CONCERN

4. Participate in a second instructor-led task and analyze the task to determine its therapeutic value by using the Occupational Analysis form (found in Appendix A), this time completing the form not as a class but by yourself.

5a. Given an assigned case study, with a partner and using the latest edition of Uniform Terminology (AOTA) determine concerns in the performance areas, performance components, and performance contexts displayed by the individual in your case study.

5b. Brainstorm with your partner a list of occupations that may be used with this client for intervention. To do this, go back to the information collected in Study Question 13 and add the summary information from a client of the same age and gender specified as part of the profile of your case study.

5c. Select two appropriate and therapeutic occupations from the list and record the rationale for their selection.

CLIENT	OCCUPATION 1	RATIONALE	OCCUPATION 2	RATIONALE
Case 1				
Case 2				
Case 3				
Case 4				
Case 5				
Case 6				
Case 7				

5d. Repeat parts a–c for all four case studies.

5e. Join the class and share your ideas. Record below any ideas you wish to remember for future use in activity selection.

FOLLOW-UP

✔ Complete the Application of Competencies at the end of this chapter.
✔ For each completed activity, fill out an Analysis of Self found in Appendix B.
✔ Complete Performance Skill 1B on Occupational Analysis.

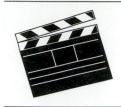

Exercise 14

"Do what you can where you are with what you've got."

THEODORE ROOSEVELT

OCCUPATION: ADAPTATION

OBJECTIVES

✔ Invent methods to use common household items as adaptive devices
✔ Describe the relationship between the person-occupation-environment-fit and adaptation
✔ Suggest adaptations for specific purposeful activities and/or occupations

DESCRIPTION

Occupations that are purposeful and meaningful will motivate a client to participate in them. For an occupation to be purposeful and meaningful, it often needs to be adapted or made easier for the client. As an occupational therapy practitioner you will need to be able to adapt common household items. Additionally, occupations that have multiple components or steps may need to be further arranged and broken down into even smaller steps so that the client can complete the occupation successfully. Often a simple adaptation to an occupation can make the difference between that occupation not being appropriate for the client and the same occupation, once adapted, providing maximal therapeutic benefits to the client. The ability to adapt the occupation, person, or environment is an essential competency for all OT practitioners.

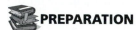**PREPARATION**

Suggested Readings

Neidstadt and Crepeau (1998)
Ryan (1995a)
Watson (1997)

Study Questions

1. Describe how an activity or occupation can be adapted.

2. Describe how activities or occupations can be adapted according to the following:
   a. Task demands

   b. Environmental parameters

   c. Individual's approach

3. Describe what is meant by the following terms:
   a. Performance discrepancy

   b. Skill deficit

c. Habit deficit

d. Adapt

e. Prevent

f. Create

g. Establish or restore

4. Give one example of intervention to increase function in an individual with a skill or habit deficit.

SKILL DEFICIT	HABIT DEFICIT
a. Adapt	f. Adapt
b. Alter	g. Alter
c. Prevent	h. Prevent
d. Create	i. Create
e. Establish/restore	j. Establish/restore

5. Define the term *adaptive equipment*.

6. Describe the following terms as they relate to the construction of adaptive equipment:
   a. Criteria

   b. Precautions

   c. Design

   d. Size

e. Cost

f. Appearance

g. Safety

h. Comfort

i. Maintenance

7. Describe the steps and equipment needed to design adaptive equipment.

8. Gather odds and ends from home to bring to lab. Suggested items: bolts, screws, sponges, hooks, blocks of wood, and the like.

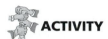 **ACTIVITY**

Materials

Hardware supplies, odds and ends from homes, supplies for one or two craft projects, card game Go Fish™, Pictionary™, checkers, Connect Four™, baseball bat, ball, baseball glove, toothbrush, toothpaste, cup.

Instructions

1. Bring various items from home or the local hardware store to class. As a class, discuss how these and other similar materials commonly found in your home or a hardware store may be used to adapt activities. List the items, as well as suggestions for using the items in an adaptive manner, in the following chart. An example is provided for you.

ITEM	SUGGESTED USE/S
Washcloth	Wrap it around a hammer to facilitate grip; wrap it around a utensil to increase ability to grip; wet it and place it under a bowl to keep the bowl from sliding on the counter or table

2. Pass around an activity given to you by your instructor (e.g., checkers or Connect Four™). When you receive the item, describe one way in which it can be adapted for a client who is unable to use it in the usual manner. Continue passing the activity from student to student, with each student adding his or her ideas for adaptation. If a student cannot think of an idea that hasn't already been said, he or she is out. The winner will be the student who is left when all other students have exhausted their ideas. List the ideas you would like to remember.

3. With a partner or small group, plan adaptations for the following activities. Assume that the deficits listed below exist in a particular client. Make adaptations to the task, the environment, or the individual's approach.

ACTIVITIES	ONE HAND	LOW VISION	POOR FINE MOTOR	POOR COGNITIVE FUNCTION	SOCIAL/ EMOTIONAL DIFFICULTY
a. Go Fish™					
b. Pictionary™					
c. Baseball					
d. Brushing teeth					
e. Other					

4. Participate in an instructor-led craft or activity, such as basket weaving or fabric painting. After completion of the activity, fill out an Occupational Analysis form (found in Appendix A). List several possible adaptations for each component involved.

FOLLOW-UP

✔ Complete the Application of Competencies at the end of this chapter.
✔ For each completed craft activity fill out an Analysis of Self found in Appendix B.
✔ Complete Performance Skill 1C on Adapting an Occupation.

Exercise 15

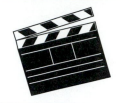

"Four steps to achievement—plan purposefully, prepare prayerfully, proceed positively, pursue persistently."

WILLIAM WARD

OCCUPATION: GRADATION

OBJECTIVES

✔ Describe the relationship between the person-occupation-environment-fit and gradation
✔ Analyze a craft activity, including components of gradation
✔ Suggest gradations for specific purposeful and/or occupations

DESCRIPTION

Gradation of an occupation is as important as adaptation in making the occupation therapeutically beneficial to your clients. Gradation involves challenging the client so that improvements in function are realized. This can be done either by increasing the complexity of a sequence of different tasks in which the client engages or by increasing the complexity of a single task. In either way, goal acquisition is facilitated by making the intervention continually more of a challenge. In doing so, it will be critical to keep your clients motivated in reaching their goals. There is often a fine line between challenging a client and frustrating a client. You will use your observation skills, clinical reasoning skills, and experience to introduce the right challenge at the right time in the right way to your clients.

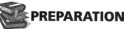PREPARATION

Suggested Readings

Neidstadt and Crepeau (1998)
Watson(1997)

Study Questions

1. Describe what is meant by grading an activity or occupation.

2. Describe how an activity or occupation can be graded.

3. Describe how activities or occupations can be graded according to the following:
    a. Task demand

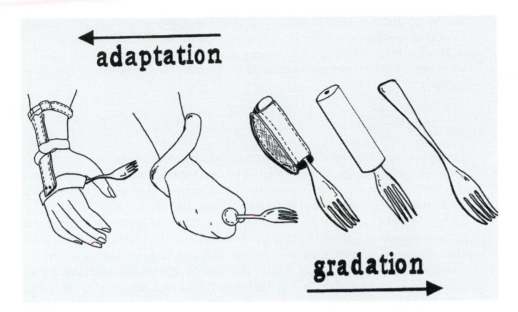

Fig. 1-7 The arrows indicate how a utensil might be adapted for independence and graded as the client gains skill.

b. Environmental parameters

c. Individual's approach

4. What can happen to a client if you grade an activity or occupation too quickly? What should be done to prevent this?

5. How does the number of treatment sessions affect the speed with which you grade your activities or occupations?

6. Using your own ideas, list the progressive steps of meal preparation for a person who is totally dependent in this area.

7. Describe how context may be used in the graded treatment program.

 ACTIVITY

Materials

Checkers, Connect Four™, flip charts, craft materials for selected project.

Instructions

1. Pass around the activity given to you by your instructor, such as checkers or Connect Four™. When it is your turn to hold the activity, state one way in which it

can be graded and used in therapy to promote improvements in your clients. Continue passing the activity from student to student. If a student cannot think of an idea, he or she is out. The winner will be the student who is left when all other students have exhausted their ideas. List the ideas you would like to remember.

2. Divide into small groups. Each small group will be assigned one of the following activities: golf, taking a shower, playing bridge, making tacos, bowling. Assume that accomplishment of this activity is the ultimate goal of your client, who is weak, has low endurance, and is cognitively impaired to the point of having forgotten the steps in performing this activity. Introduce and gradually teach the basic components of this activity to your client as he or she is able to learn and tolerate treatment. Describe an activity you will use to begin intervention. List activities as well as methods of grading this activity. The environment and the approach may also be graded. Record your ideas below, then put them on a flip chart and share them with your class.

3. Participate in an instructor-led craft activity. Following completion of the craft activity, fill out an Occupational Analysis Form (found in Appendix A). List several possible gradations for each component involved.

FOLLOW-UP

✔ Complete the Application of Competencies at the end of this chapter.
✔ For each completed craft activity fill out an Analysis of Self found in Appendix B.
✔ Complete Performance Skill 1B on Occupational Analysis.
✔ Complete Performance Skill 1D on Craft Completion.

Exercise 16

"In the power to change yourself is the power to change the world around you."

ANWAR SADAT

PLANNING INTERVENTION

OBJECTIVES

✔ Formulate one long-term goal and two short-term goals for a selected target area
✔ Plan intervention to meet targeted goals
✔ Document progress toward accomplishing the goals

DESCRIPTION

This exercise is designed to help you develop an intervention or treatment plan for your clients. Before a plan can be developed, assessment data must be gathered. Once the information is gathered, it is then appropriate to (a) determine areas of need, (b) write goals for the areas of need, (c) select activities to meet the goals, and (d) document progress toward the goals. Goal writing occurs at the end of the evaluation process and before treatment begins. Goals direct therapeutic intervention and provide a "road map" of how to get to the end point of functional change. Once goals are written, occupations are selected and the intervention begins. Throughout this process, documentation is an important component.

PREPARATION

Suggested Readings

AOTA (latest edition)
Neistadt and Crepeau (1998)
Reed and Sanderson (1999)

Study Questions

1. Summarize the occupational therapy process model.

2. List the contents of an intervention or treatment plan.

3. Describe the components necessary to include in long-term functional goals.

4. Describe the components necessary to include in short-term functional goals.

5. Describe what is meant by each of the following hallmarks of a behavioral objective goal:
    a. Behavior

    b. Condition

    c. Criteria

    d. Time frame

6. List and describe the meaning of the letters in the acronym RUMBA as they relate to goal writing.

R	
U	
M	
B	
A	

7. What guidelines are available to assist a practitioner in selecting problem areas to address during intervention?

8. List and describe teaching methods, therapeutic approaches, and adapted techniques that are used in occupational therapy.

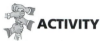 **ACTIVITY**

Materials

Dynamometers, Minnesota Rate of Manipulation Test (University of Minnesota Employment Stabilization Research Institute, 1933), Purdue Pegboard (Purdue Research Foundation, 1948), stopwatches, textbook, tape measure.

Instructions

1a. Invite a student in the class a year ahead of you to gather data from you about the information contained in the following Personal Data Sheet. Record your data on the chart below.

PERSONAL DATA SHEET

Name _____

To practice evaluation and recording of results, please complete the following form. It is important that you evaluate and record accurately because information will be averaged for comparison purposes.

		Right	**Left**
1.	**Grip Strength** (average of three trials, standard position)	_____ lb.	_____ lb.
2.	**Coordination**		
	Minnesota Rate of Manipulation Test (time to place $\frac{1}{2}$ board)	_____ seconds	_____ seconds
	Purdue Pegboard (number of pegs placed in 30 seconds)	_____ pegs	_____ pegs
3.	**Upper-Extremity Strength**		
	Number of push-ups (from the knees)	_____	
4.	**Abdominal Strength**		
	Number of stomach crunches (arms crossed over chest, knees bent, lift shoulders off floor)	_____	
5.	**Endurance**		
	Time that dominant upper extremity can hold a textbook parallel to the floor (shoulder abducted, elbow extended, hand pronated)	_____ seconds	
6.	**Range of Motion**		
	Maximum trunk flexion with knee extension (distance measured in inches from nose to knee)	_____ inches	

Taken from: Everly, J. S. 1996. A goal-setting experiential for the classroom. Education Special Internet Section Newsletter, 6(4), 2, 4. Used with permission.

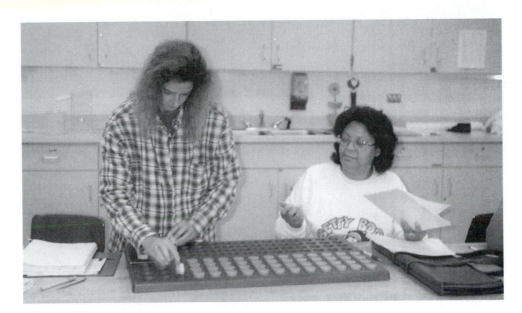

Fig. 1-8
Administering the Minnesota Rate of Manipulation.
Photo courtesy of Michelle Moore and Renee Davis.

1b. Select an area from your Personal Data Sheet that you would like to improve. Fill out the following intervention plan, structuring your long-term goal within the time frame assigned by your instructor. Determine the time frame for achieving the two short-term goals accordingly. Write an evaluation summary. Continue to track and document your progress toward your goals as outlined.

INTERVENTION PLAN

FINDINGS FROM PERSONAL DATA SHEET:

Target Area _____

Present Functioning Level _____

LONG TERM GOAL:

Behavior (_____)   Measurement (_____)

Condition (_____)   Date (_____)

SHORT-TERM GOALS:

1. Behavior (_____)   Measurement (_____)

   Condition (_____)   Date (_____)

2. Behavior (_____)   Measurement(_____)

   Condition (_____)   Date (_____)

ACTIVITIES TO BE USED:

METHOD AND FREQUENCY:

1c. Track your progress over the next several months, using the following progress chart.

PROGRESS CHART					
DATE	ACTIVITY	MET	PARTIALLY MET	NO PROGRESS	COMMENTS

1d. Write a discharge summary on the progress made toward reaching your goals. Include in your summary the activities you used to meet your goals, the degree to which your goals have been achieved, and any functional outcomes you observed.

1e. After writing your discharge summary, record your feelings about this assignment. Analyze your compliance with your initial plan to reach the goals. Add any other comments as appropriate.

2a. Begin to develop functional goals. Think of unique skills you have that you would be able to teach others, such as playing a musical instrument, tai-chi, public speaking, writing poetry, sewing, cooking, or throwing a football pass. List your name with the accompanying skills on the chalkboard. Review the talents of your classmates, determining several skills you would like to learn. Record below accordingly.

SKILLS YOU CAN TEACH	SKILLS YOU WANT TO LEARN

2b. Pair with a partner from whom you would like to learn a skill he or she can teach and who is interested in learning the skill you can teach. Determine the task components of the skill you will teach. Record those components below. An example of the tasks involved in playing a guitar are provided for you as an example.

Skill (example) Playing a song on a guitar	**Skill**
Tasks String guitar Tune guitar Read music Play cords Strum guitar	**Tasks**

2c. Interview your partner to determine his or her current skill level. Write below the component tasks already mastered and those yet needed to be competent in the skill.

SKILLS MASTERED	SKILLS YET TO LEARN

Long-term goal

2d. Write one long-term goal for the skill you are teaching. For playing a song on a guitar, a goal might read as follows: Jason will play the song "Twinkle, Twinkle, Little Star" reading sheet music by October 15.

1.

Short-term goals

2e. Write three short-term goals that will lead up to your long-term goal. For the guitar-playing example, three goals might read as follows:

1. Jason will apply 2 strings to the guitar with assistance of minimal verbal cueing by Oct. 2.
2. Jason will tune the guitar completing 5/5 strings correctly with assistance of minimal verbal cueing by Oct. 5.
3. Jason will demonstrate correct finger placement 4/5 times for cords C, G, Em, and D using written instructions by Oct. 10.

1.

2.

3.

2f. Write an initial evaluation summary and a discharge summary. Record your feelings and analyze your compliance.

2g. Repeat 2b through 2e, switching roles.

2h. Meet with your partner outside class to teach the identified skill. Record your progress below, summarizing your results.

FOLLOW-UP

✔ Complete the Application of Competencies at the end of this chapter.
✔ Complete a Therapeutic Use of Self Analysis (found in Appendix B) on your intervention planning performance.
✔ Complete Performance Skill 1 D on Developing Your File.

ROLE DELINEATION

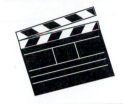

✔ Discuss the supervisory relationship between the occupational therapist (OT) and the occupational therapy assistant (OTA)

✔ Identify similarities and differences between OT and OTA accredited programs of study

✔ Interview an OT/OTA team to obtain insight on the teamwork involved in this relationship

"Kind words can be short and easy to speak, but their echoes are truly endless."

MOTHER TERESA

DESCRIPTION

This exercise will help you to understand the role delineation between the OTA and the OT. The OTA and the OT work together as a team, with the OT supervising the OTA at some level. The relationship between the two practitioners needs to be ongoing, mutually respectful, and collaborative. Open communication and joint problem solving are also critical to enabling the OTA/OT team to work together effectively. Understanding the skills each practitioner will bring to the relationship begins with understanding their respective program requirements. Drawing on each other's strengths will enable the team to provide the best possible service to your clients.

PREPARATION

Suggested Reading

American Occupational Therapy Association (AOTA) (latest edition)
Moyers (1999)
Ryan (1995b)

Study Questions

1. What are the educational and certification requirements to become an OTA? To become an OT?

2. List the tasks in the occupational therapy process that the OT cannot delegate to the OTA.

3. List the occupational therapy roles and a major function of each.

4. Assuming that the OT is able to assume all roles listed below, circle which of the following roles an OTA is unable to perform:

   Practitioner   Fieldwork coordinator
   Educator   Program director
   Fieldwork educator   Researcher/scholar
   Supervisor   Administrator
   Consultant   Entrepreneur
                           Faculty

5. Find the role you will fill on graduation from an accredited OT or OTA school. Describe the major functions and scope of this role.

6. Describe the OT/OTA relationship.

7. Describe the effect communication has on the OT/OTA relationship.

8. Describe the role and responsibilities of the experienced OTA.

9. Detail your state requirements (e.g., licensure, registration, certification) regarding OT/OTA supervision. Cite the specific section and article.

10. Define the responsibilities of the supervisor and supervisee in relationship to the following:

   a. Medicare/Medicaid

   b. Joint Commission on Accreditation of Healthcare Organization (JCAHO)

   c. Commission for the Accreditation of Rehabilitation Facilities (CARF)

   d. AOTA

 ACTIVITY

Materials

Program curriculum from an accredited occupational therapy school and an occupational therapy assistant school, textbooks from said programs, current standards for an accredited OT and OTA school and information collected from study questions of this exercise.

Instructions

1. Meet and interview a student from another program. If you are a student in an OT program, interview a student in an OTA program and vice versa. Conduct your interview in person or by phone, e-mail, or postal mail. Obtain the following information. Compare the information you obtained about your interviewee's program of study to your own program.

My Program: _____	Other Program: _____
	Student: _____
A. LENGTH OF PROGRAM	

B. FIELDWORK LENGTH AND REQUIREMENTS	

C. OT COURSES REQUIRED	

D. OTHER COURSES REQUIRED	

E. NUMBER OF STUDENTS IN PROGRAM	

F. NUMBER OF FACULTY	

G. DESCRIPTION OF TYPES OF REQUIRED ASSIGNMENTS	

H. REQUIRED TEXTBOOKS	

I. CURRENT KNOWLEDGE ABOUT THE ROLE OF OTA/OT	

J. REASON STUDENT ENTERED THE PROFESSION	

K. FUTURE JOB INTERESTS (POPULATION, SETTING, PRACTICE AREA)	

L. AOTA'S ESSENTIALS AND GUIDELINES FOR ACCREDITED EDUCATIONAL PROGRAMS	

2. With your partner, summarize and record the similarities and differences in your programs.

SIMILARITIES	DIFFERENCES

3a. With this same partner, discuss methods that may assist in improving relationships between the students and the programs of the two schools. Plan a proposal addressing one or both of these issues.

Goal(s) you would like to accomplish:

Ideas for activities:

3b. Present your ideas to your classmates. Summarize all of the ideas presented. Select one or two of the best ideas and a student representative to present these ideas to your department. Check with your instructor to determine to whom these ideas would best be presented. Record the best ideas below.

4. Invite at least one OTA/OT team to your class as guest speakers. Using the chart provided, compile a list of the roles and specific functions of both OT practitioners. Describe their relationship. Include how they maintain service competency. Critique the methods they use. Go to the Professional Practice Records found in Appendix C and further discuss how the Supervision Log for OTA and OT Collaboration and Service Competency forms might be used in future practice.

	ROLES	FUNCTION	RELATIONSHIP	SERVICE COMPETENCY
OTA				
OT				
OTA				
OT				

Application of Competencies

After completing each exercise, write one thing you learned and how that learning will influence your treatment of clients.

Exercise 1   Creating a Vision Statement
Application:

Exercise 2   Explaining What We Do
Application:

Exercise 3   Prevention and Wellness
Application:

Exercise 4   Cultural Awareness
Application:

Exercise 5   Learning Your Association's Official Documents
Application:

Exercise 6   Ethics in Practice
Application:

Exercise 7   Learning the Jargon
Application:

Exercise 8   AOTA: Your Professional Organization
Application

Exercise 9   Essential Functions of Occupational Therapy Practitioners
Application:

Exercise 10   Frames of Reference
Application:

Exercise 11   Occupational Therapy Process
Application:

Exercise 12   Practice Guidelines
Application:

Exercise 13   Purposeful Occupation
Application:

Exercise 14   Occupation: Adaptation
Application:

Exercise 15   Occupation: Gradation
Application:

Exercise 16   Planning Intervention
Application:

Exercise 17   Role Delineation
Application:

Performance Skill 1A

CRAFT COMPLETION

Make a list of the crafts to which you have been introduced in this section. Use the chart to indicate the practice area(s) in which each craft can be used. Write a term paper describing how those crafts can be used in the four traditional practice areas.

CRAFTS	PEDIATRICS	PHYSICAL REHABILITATION	PSYCHOSOCIAL	GERIATRICS

OCCUPATIONAL ANALYSIS

Performance Skill 1B

Complete the following occupational analysis on a craft or occupation as assigned by your instructor. Detail the materials needed, characteristics of the activity, treatment implication, steps to completion, and the identified components inherent in the craft or occupation. Fill out the outline and forms below as you go.

Descriptors:

Name: _____

Activity: _____

Cost: _____

General Characteristics: _____

Time (Are different sessions needed? If so, break up the time needed for each session.):

_____

Materials needed (including tools and equipment):

Characteristics of equipment, tools, materials (resistance, control, cleanliness):

Contraindications of occupation (precautions, danger):

Intervention implications (How could this activity best be used in each practice area?):

    Pediatrics

    Physical rehabilitation

    Mental health

    Geriatrics

Evaluation possibilities (How might this craft/occupation be used as part of the evaluation process?):

Frame of reference compatibility (With which frame(s) of reference does the activity best align?):

STEPS TO COMPLETION

Fill in the following columns indicating the major steps and the necessary instructions to complete the task along with applications.

MAJOR STEPS (usually only 3 or 4 steps)	INSTRUCTIONS (details of step by step instructions)	APPLICATION (include hints, nonessential, yet helpful information)

Using the chart below as a model, create a computer generated Performance Component and Context Chart using the definitions in the latest edition of uniform terminology (AOTA). Make as many component and context boxes as needed. Determine how much the component or context is involved in the activity. Circle the amount of involvement as appropriate: minimal (min), moderate (mod), maximal (max), not applicable (N/a). In the Describe Involvement column state how that component or context is involved. In the Adapted and Graded columns, state how the activity can be adapted and graded. Fill out the different columns as assigned by your instructor. See the following example for making a birdhouse. One component has been completed for you.

PERFORMANCE COMPONENT AND CONTEXT CHART

Component Title:

DESCRIBE INVOLVEMENT		ADAPTED	GRADED
Tactile			
Min Mod Max N/a	To determine that sanding is complete, it is necessary to feel the smoothness of the wood.	Pre-sand the wood for the client.	Make a more complicated birdhouse with intricate designs.

Component Title:

DESCRIBE INVOLVEMENT	ADAPTED	GRADED
Tactile		
Min Mod Max N/a		
Min Mod Max N/a		
Min Mod Max N/a		
Min Mod Max N/a		

Component Title:

DESCRIBE INVOLVEMENT	ADAPTED	GRADED
Min Mod Max N/a		
Min Mod Max N/a		
Min Mod Max N/a		

Performance Skill 1C

ADAPTING AN OCCUPATION

Select an occupation for which you will create adaptations so that it could be used by someone who is unable to participate in the activity. Make at least three physical changes to the occupation. State the performance component addressed in the activity, a description of the adaptation, the materials used, and the cost of the materials. Total the cost of the three adaptations and include that number at the top of the graph. Use this page as your worksheet. Bring your completed project to class and present it to your peers along with a handout describing how to make the adaptation. An example is presented below for making one physical change in adapting a puzzle, an occupation enjoyed by many children.

Activity _____   Total Cost of Adaptations _____

COMPONENT	DESCRIPTION OF ADAPTATION	MATERIALS USED	COST OF MATERIALS
Fine motor	Attached short dowel rod handles to each piece	Drill, screws, dowel rods, sand paper	$5.00

DEVELOPING YOUR FILE

Performance Skill 1D

Search and select occupations or purposeful activities that would be appropriate to use in a variety of settings. Type a paper on each occupation, compiling the needed information listed in the following chart. Assemble these pages and proceed with a table of contents. Add to this file throughout your educational tenure. As you finish gathering the information on a particular occupation, check each box to indicate that you have included that component in your write-up. Use at least three different references and a variety of media, including but not limited to groups, games, crafts, and activities of daily living. Include at least three occupations that would be appropriate for clients of cultures other than your own.

(✔) Check as you complete each section							
OCCUPATION	RATIONALE	PERFORMANCE CONTEXT	SUPPLIES/ MATERIALS	STEPS TO PERFORM	ADAPTATIONS	PRECAUTIONS	REFERENCES

Performance Skill 1E

CULTURAL EXPLANATION

With a small group, select a cultural group or religious affiliation from the lists below and complete a study on that group's beliefs about physical, mental, and spiritual health. Obtain information through library sources and Internet searches. Once you have a basic understanding of the culture, find people to interview who belong to that culture to further your study on a more in-depth level. Attend services and/or celebrations that are significant to the culture.

Prepare a presentation for your class. Use the chart below, taken from Spector (1996), to begin planning, by assigning each student in your group a section of information, as indicated in the chart, for which to be responsible. Use the second cultural chart to make notes about the information you are going to obtain. Prepare the information in a handout format to be given out during your presentation. Additionally, during the presentation, use a variety of media to facilitate your classmates' learning, including costumes and props when appropriate. After the class presentation, rate each group, using the rating form supplied.

Cultures

American Indian, African American, Hispanic American, European American, Asian/Pacific Islander American.

Religions and philosophies

Jehovah's Witness, Judaism, Mennonite, Seventh-Day Adventist, Unitarian/Universalist, Christian Science, Church of Jesus Christ of Latter Day Saints, Roman Catholic, Hindu, Islam, Bahaii, Buddhist, atheist, Baho'i, Shinto, Tao Voodoo, Church of Scientology, Christianity, existentialism.

CULTURAL CHART STUDENT ASSIGNMENTS			
Culture:			
	PHYSICAL	MENTAL	SPIRITUAL
Maintain/ protect health			
Restore health			
Practices concerning death and mourning			

CULTURAL CHART			
Culture:			
	PHYSICAL	MENTAL	SPIRITUAL
Maintain/ protect health			
Restore health			
Practices concerning death and mourning			

Rate each group's presentation according to the following criteria: A total of 100 points is possible.

PERFORMANCE CRITERIA

1. Well-prepared   (20 points)
2. Handout neat and organized   (20 points)
3. Props and visual aids used effectively (20 points)
4. Presented in a professional manner   (20 points)
5. Presentation complete for all categories (20 points)

PRESENTER(S) NAME(S)	CRITERIA					TOTAL POINTS
	1	2	3	4	5	

CASE STUDY 1

GERIATRIC

Type:
Geriatric, Retirement Setting

Age:
80 years old

Sex:
Male

Culture/Religion:

Insurance Information:

Diagnosis:
Parkinson's disease

Social History:
William lives in a retirement community in an independent living situation. He is responsible for obtaining breakfast and lunch in his apartment. Dinner is provided in a dining room down the hall from his room. Housecleaning services are provided, but William is responsible for his personal laundry.

William has been withdrawing from activities and social interactions lately. He has even been asking for dinner in his room, as he is embarrassed to eat in the dining room.

William used to go to resident council meetings, participate in the wood shop, and play cards occasionally.

Medical History:
William has been noted to be stumbling when he walks. His gait is shuffling, and he attempts to use a cane.

His face appears to be expressionless and has a slight waxy appearance. His tremors appear to be getting worse, interfering with his ability to cook, eat, and participate in activities.

CASE STUDY 2

PEDIATRIC

Type:
Pediatric, School-Based

Age:
6 years old

Sex:
Male

Culture/Religion:

Insurance Information:

Diagnosis:
Down's syndrome

Family Situation:
Derrick has two parents who have five other children, all older by at least fourteen years. His parents were in their mid-forties when Derrick was born. Derrick has normal active ROM in all extremities. He is able to feed himself independently and likes to eat. He has good family support and follow-through with any suggestions at home.

Problems:
Derrick has generalized low muscle tone and poor pelvic tilt, slumps forward, and tends to seek support to get up from the floor. He postures with his knees bowed to compensate for poor tone. He has decreased balance responses with delayed to no protective responses.

He is not toilet trained and requires much assistance to get dressed. Derrick uses both hands but tends to avoid crossing the midline. He has decreased pre-writing skills, much difficulty holding scissors, and poor grasp patterns.

Derrick does not play well by himself and parallel plays with children. He frequently loses his temper when unable to relate to other children and throws toys across the room or at staff.

CASE STUDY 3

ADOLESCENT PSYCHOSOCIAL

Type:
Inpatient

Age:
14 years old

Sex:
Male

Culture/Religion:

Insurance Information:

Diagnosis:
Dysthymic disorder, major depression, dysfunctional family, A-DHD

Social History:
Ryan lives with his father, who is recently divorced. Ryan's mother and sister live together. Ryan and his father moved to a condominium. Ryan says he hates his new house, there is nothing to do, and he is bored all the time.

Ryan is a student in the eighth grade, which he is repeating.

Medical History:
Ryan was admitted because of a suicide attempt. He states that school is a major problem; he says life isn't worth living. Ryan has been identified with the following problems: suicidal ideation, poor impulse control, intellectual impairment, poor attention span, hyperactivity, problems with authority figures, disturbance in conduct, eating disturbance, depression, low self-esteem, ineffective coping skills, and inadequate leisure skills. Since admission, Ryan has been uncooperative and is verbally abusive.

CASE STUDY 4

ADULT PHYSICAL REHABILITATION

Type:
Outpatient

Age:
30 years old

Sex:
Female

Culture/Religion:

Insurance Information:

Diagnosis:
TBI due to MVA

Social History:
Sarah lives with her parents at this time. She is married but is living with her parents because of their ability and time to care for her. The bathroom and bedroom are downstairs, and her parents are always at home.

Sarah previously worked as an attorney for a large firm. Her leisure interests are cards and tennis. She enjoys music and television.

Medical History:

Sarah suffered trauma from a motor vehicle accident three months ago and has received therapy on an impatient and outpatient basis. Physically, she has all return with some fine and gross motor impairment. All her sensation is intact. She tends not to use her right upper extremity many times. Her sitting balance is good, and her standing balance is fair. She requires SBA for transfers to tub and commode; all other transfers are independent. She has a narrow adult Quickie Wheelchair and is receiving physical therapy to help with walking.

Cognitively, Sarah is unable to recall yesterday's events and is able to describe her present living arrangement with 90% accuracy. She scored a 4.0 on the ACL. During the evaluation performing a cooking activity, she demonstrated deficits in task organization, attention to multiple tasks, safety awareness, and problem solving. Sarah is cooperative and pleasant.

CASE STUDY 5

ADULT PHYSICAL REHABILITATION

Type:
Acute Care

Age:
50 years old

Sex:
Female

Culture/Religion:

Insurance Information:

Diagnosis:
Lung cancer

Social History:

Joann lives alone in a two-story home. She is divorced and has two children who are living on their own. She has one cat, of which she is very fond. She has enjoyed crafts, flower arranging, and gardening in the past.

Joann has been on disability for six months. She worked as a manager of an insurance company.

Medical History:

Joann was admitted with extreme shortness of breath and inability to care for herself. She tires quickly and is unable to ambulate and transfer to all surfaces in her home. She was found to be partially dehydrated and has not been eating well. She complains of nausea almost constantly.

New mediation and O_2 will be attempted to see whether symptoms can be alleviated. Joann wishes to return to her home for as long as possible. She wants to die there.

OT has been ordered to see whether any recommendations can be made.

CASE STUDY 6

PEDIATRIC

Type:
Pediatric, School Based

Age:
2 years, 8 months

Sex:
Male

Culture/Religion:

Insurance Information:

Diagnosis:
Cerebral palsy (spastic quadriplegia) and bilateral hearing impairment

Family Situation:
Ishmel has recently moved to this area with his parents. He is an only child. He has reportedly been receiving therapy since six months of age.

Strengths:
Ishmel appears to be very motivated and attempts to actively explore his environment. He gets around in prone by using quick, froglike movements of his LEs; the weight is then shifted forward to his face. He does roll from prone to supine with the initiation of head and neck hyperextension. When Ishmel is positioned in his wheelchair with a lap tray, he is able to weight bear on his forearms and swipe. He occasionally grasps items within his reach. Ishmel eats all food presented to him and takes fluids easily from the bottle.

Problems:
Ishmel has increased muscle tone throughout extremities which fluctuate at rest and also with effort. He has learned to compensate for his lack of postural control by elevating the shoulders to positionally stabilize his head, by rounding the lower back with a posterior tilt, and by hunching the upper trunk forward.

Ishmel has upper trunk expansion, and the UEs are limited in external rotation, abduction, and shoulder flexion. He also has tightness of the hamstrings and limited pelvic mobility. Primitive postural reflexes continue to be present and interfere with midline orientation and postural control.

He is not able to maintain floor sitting. His reach does not appear to be visually monitored, and he seems to rely on asymmetrical tone for UE reach. He has difficulty reaching bilaterally or unilaterally in midrange.

CASE STUDY 7

ADULT PSYCHOSOCIAL

Type:
Chronic, State Institution

Age:
31 years old

Sex:
Male

Culture/Religion:

Insurance Information:

Diagnosis:
Chronic paranoid schizophrenic, alcohol dependent

Social History:
When not hospitalized, John lives with his father. He is separated from his wife and four children. He has been accused of domestic abuse. He has seven siblings including a brother who committed suicide within the past four years. John does not work, and he collects disability. He previously attended one year of college, then took a job as a truck driver, which he did for several years.

Medical History:
John was first hospitalized five years ago. He has been jailed ten times for offenses relating to DUI, disorderly conduct, burglary, and assault. John presents as being very depressed

and frequently speaks of others who are out to get him, especially by poisoning him.

John does not shower, shave, or wash his clothes; his room is a mess. John does not respond to reminders but requires maximum assistance to participate in any self-care.

REFERENCES

American Occupational Therapy Association. *American Journal of Occupational Therapy*. Bethesda, MD: Author.

American Occupational Therapy Association Web site: *http://www.aota.org*.

American Occupational Therapy Association. *OT Practice*. Bethesda, MD: Author.

American Occupational Therapy Association. latest edition. *Reference Manual of the Official Documents of the American Occupational Therapy Association, Inc.* Bethesda, MD: Author.

Americans with Disabilities Act of 1990. U.S. PL. 101–336. 42 U.S.C. 12101. *Federal Register,* 56:144, 35543–35691.

Asher, I. E. 1996. *Occupational Therapy Assessment Tools: An Annotated Index*. 2d ed. Bethesda, MD: American Occupational Therapy Association.

Breines, E. 1995. *Occupational Therapy Activities: From Clay to Computers*. Philadelphia: F. A. Davis.

Christiansen, C., and C. Baum. 1997. *Occupational Therapy: Enabling Function and Well-Being*. 2d ed. Thorofare, NJ: Slack.

Cole, M. B. 1998. *Group Dynamics in Occupational Therapy: The Theoretical Basis and Practice Application of Group Treatment*. 2d ed. Thorofare, NJ: Slack.

Costello, E. 1994. *Random House American Sign Language Dictionary*. New York: Random House.

Covey, S. 1989. *Seven Habits of Highly Effective People*. New York: Simon and Schuster.

Davis, C. M. 1998. *Patient Practitioner Interaction: An Experiential Manual for Developing the Art of Health Care*. Thorofare, NJ: Slack.

Drake, M. 1992. *Crafts in Therapy and Rehabilitation*. Thorofare, NJ: Slack.

Everly, J. S. 1996. A goal-setting experiential for the classroom. *Education Special Interest Section Newsletter,* 6(4): 1–2.

Hinojosa, J., and P. Kramer. 1998. *Evaluation: Obtaining and Interpreting Data*. Sterling, VA: World Composition Services.

International Classification of Functioning and Disability (ICIDH-2) web site: *www.who.int/icidh/*.

Jacobs, K. 1999. *Quick Reference Dictionary for Occupational Therapy*. 2d ed. Thorofare, NJ: Slack.

Merion Publications. *Advance for Occupational Therapy Practitioners*. King of Prussia, PA: Author.

Mosey, A. D. 1986. *Psychosocial Components of Occupational Therapy*. New York: Raven Press.

Moyers, P. A. 1999. *The Guide to Occupational Therapy Practice*. Bethesda, MD: American Occupational Therapy Association.

National Board for Certification of Occupational Therapy Web site: *http://www.nbcot.org*.

Neistadt, M. E., and E. B. Crepeau. 1998. *Willard and Spackman's Occupational Therapy*. 9th ed. Philadelphia: J. B. Lippincott.

Purdue Research Foundation. 1948. *Purdue Pegboard Test*. Bolingbrook, IL: Samons Preston.

Reed, K. L., and S. N. Sanderson. 1999. *Concepts of Occupational Therapy*. 4th ed. Philadelphia: J. B. Lippincott.

Ryan, S. E. ed. 1995a. *The Certified Occupational Therapy Assistant: Principle, Concepts, and Techniques*. 2d ed. Thorofare, NJ: Slack.

Ryan, S. E. ed. 1995b. *Practice Issues in Occupational Therapy: Intraprofessional Team Building*. Thorofare, NJ: Slack.

Slaydk, K. 1997. *OT Student Primer: A guide to College Success*. Thorofare, NJ: Slack.

Smith, V. 1994. *Occupational Therapy: Transition from Classroom to Clinic-Physical Disabilities Fieldwork Applications*. Bethesda, MD: American Occupational Therapy Association.

Spector, R. E. 1996. *Cultural Diversity in Health and Fitness*. Stanford, CT: Appleton and Lange.

University of Minnesota Employment Stabilization Research Institute. 1933. *Minnesota Rate of Manipulation Test*. Bolingbrook, IL: Samons Preston.

Watson, D. 1997. *Task analysis: An Occupational Performance Approach*. Bethesda, MD: American Occupational Therapy Association.

Fundamentals II

CHAPTER TWO CONTENTS

EXERCISES

APPLICATION OF COMPETENCIES

PERFORMANCE SKILLS

CASE STUDIES

REFERENCES

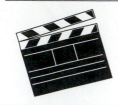

Exercise 18

"Imagination is more important than knowledge."

ALBERT EINSTEIN

THE TEACHING/LEARNING PROCESS

OBJECTIVES

✔ Discuss the role of the occupational therapy practitioner in the teaching/learning process
✔ Critique performance in giving and receiving directions
✔ Formulate a lesson plan to teach a new and unfamiliar activity to a potential client

DESCRIPTION

Ryan (1995a) discusses the teaching/learning process. This process is a significant component in occupational therapy. As an occupational therapy (OT) practitioner, you will teach clients, caregivers, and students as well as other health care professionals. Your teaching will relate to many different aspects of OT, ranging from conveying a simple concept to explaining a complicated procedure. A lesson plan is a tool that can assist you in your teaching. A lesson plan helps you to organize the activity and the environment so that the information can be presented in an easily understood manner. A well-thought-out lesson plan will guide you each step of the way, ensuring that all components of the learning process are addressed.

PREPARATION

Suggested Readings

Ryan (1995a)
Purtilo and Haddad (1996)

Study Questions

1. Describe the role of occupational therapy in teaching.

2. Describe each of the following terms as it relates to learning:
   a. Conditioning

   b. Reinforcement

   c. Shaping

   d. Behavior modification

   e. Assimilation

   f. Accommodation

   g. Reflective method

3. Describe several conditions that affect learning.

4. What is the one primary reason a client does not follow a health professional's instructions as communicated?

5. List four factors that determine the success of verbal communication.

6. Briefly describe how each of the following variables should be considered and/or used in communicating verbally with a client:
   a. Mental status

   b. Vocabulary

   c. Clarity

   d. Organization of ideas

   e. Attitudes

   f. Useful humor

   g. Destructive humor

   h. Tone

i. Volume

j. Effective listening

7. Describe the characteristics of the learning task.

8. List and describe the components in the teaching process:

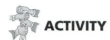 **ACTIVITY**

Materials

Plain paper, markers, tape to hang pictures around the room, materials for a small craft or activity.

Instructions

1a. Pick a partner and sit back to back. Participate in a drawing activity. Assume the role of teacher. Have your partner draw a picture that you are drawing at the same time. Do not tell your partner to draw a particular object or item, but rather describe the lines necessary to depict that object or item. For example, if you want your partner to draw a circle, tell him or her where to start on the paper as well as the direction in which you want the line

Fig. 2–1 Students participating in back-to-back drawings.

Photo courtesy of Jenny Mueller and Kelli Prather.

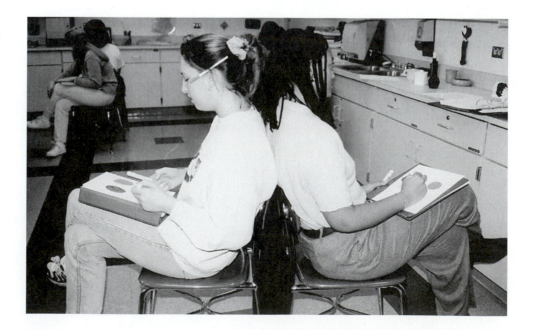

curved and distance. Include information about size. Do not allow your partner to ask questions to clarify what was said or meant. When the pictures are completed, compare your partner's drawing with yours. Display them on the wall.

1b. Switch roles with your partner. Repeat Activity 1a, using a different object or item to draw.

1c. Repeat Activity 1a. This time, allow your partner to ask questions to clarify your directions.

1d. Switch roles with your partner. Repeat 1c, using a different object or item to draw.

1e. Answer the questions on the following form for both of the activities you completed.

	NOT ASKING CLARIFYING QUESTIONS	ASKING CLARIFYING QUESTIONS
How did it feel to follow instructions?		
How did it feel to give the instructions?		
Which method (not asking clarifying questions or asking clarifying questions) was easier? Describe.		
How clear were your partner's instructions?		
What could have been communicated more clearly?		
How often did you jump to conclusions?		
What did you learn about yourself by doing this exercise?		
How can you apply what you learned about yourself to clinical practice?		

1f. What did you learn about communication? About communication being a two-way process?

2a. As a class, participate in an instructor-led small craft or activity. Afterward, critique your instructor's performance in each of the ten steps that are part of the teaching process (Ryan, 1995a). Did your instructor cover each area? If not, how could it have been included?

TEACHING PROCESS PLAN			
	YES	NO	COMMENTS
Learning objectives			
Content			
Modifications			
Steps of activity			
Materials assembly			
Workspace arrangement			
Client or group preparation			
Instruction presentation			
Trial run of task			
Performance assessment			

2b. Write a teaching process plan for performing an unusual or uncommon activity, such as making a paper airplane, using the following components as your guide:

TEACHING PROCESS PLAN

a. Learning objectives

b. Content

c. Modifications

d. Steps of activity

e. Materials assembly

f. Workspace arrangement

g. Patient or group preparation

h. Instruction presentation

i. Trial run of task

j. Performance assessment

2c. Select a partner and hand him/her your teaching process plan. Have your partner make a paper airplane following your written directions. Observe how your written directions are interpreted. Take notes while you are observing and record them in the space provided.

OBSERVATION NOTES:

Fig. 2–2 Following a lesson plan to make a paper airplane.

Photo courtesy of Jennifer Snell and Anna Sharpsheir.

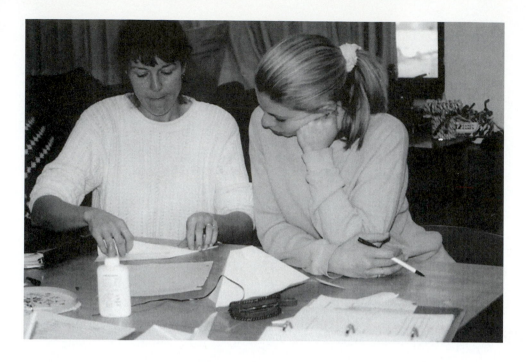

2d. Revise your teaching process plan on the basis of your observations. This time, add the use of demonstrations, illustrations, and visual cues as needed.

REVISED TEACHING PROCESS PLAN

  a. Learning objectives

  b. Content

  c. Modifications

  d. Steps of activity

  e. Materials assembly

  f. Workspace arrangement

  g. Client or group preparation

h. Instruction presentation

i. Trial run of task

j. Performance assessment

2e. Form groups of three people and use your revised teaching process plan. Teach one group member (a different classmate) how to make your paper airplane while using the revised lesson plan. Have the third group member observe and give you feedback about your performance. Continue to switch roles until all group members have had the opportunity to be a teacher. After each teaching session, give feedback to the teacher. Use the space below to record the feedback you received from your partners about your strengths and areas of concern when you were the teacher.

STRENGTHS	AREAS OF CONCERN

FOLLOW-UP

✔ Complete the Application of Competencies at the end of this chapter.
✔ Complete a Therapeutic Use of Self Analysis (found in Appendix B) on your ability to give and follow verbal and written directions.
✔ Complete Performance Skill 2A on Teaching an Occupation.

GROUP OBSERVATION

Exercise 19

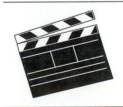

OBJECTIVES

✔ Observe and record the behavior of peers participating in a group activity
✔ Compare and contrast observation notes with the class
✔ Critique your behavior in the groups as participant and observer

DESCRIPTION

This exercise is designed to build your observation skills as a group leader when leading occupational therapy (OT) groups. As an OT practitioner, you will find yourself leading many different types of groups, in many settings, with clients of many varied diagnoses. As an OT practitioner group leader, you will need to have very good observation skills so that you can synthesize and analyze both the content and the process that occur in a group situation. This will need to be an ongoing endeavor so that you can guide your group toward therapeutic goals.

"Go confidently in the direction of your dreams."

HENRY DAVID THOREAU

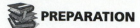 **PREPARATION**

Suggested Readings

Cole (1998)
Howe and Schwartzberg (1995)

Study Questions

1. What is the definition of a group?

2. List several benefits of using groups as a therapeutic modality.

3. Describe what is meant by the term *group process*.

4. Describe what is meant by the term *group dynamics*.

5. List the stages of group development and identify the theorist(s) who have described those stages.

6. Define group norms and differentiate between an explicit norm and an implicit norm. Give three examples of each.

7. Describe the following methods of observation according to Howe and Schwartzberg (1995):

   a. Sociogram

   b. Interaction process analysis

   c. Member role observation

   d. Content and process analysis

   e. Analysis of group behavior

8. Identify the stage of group formation that most closely fits your class at the present time. Provide support for your conclusion.

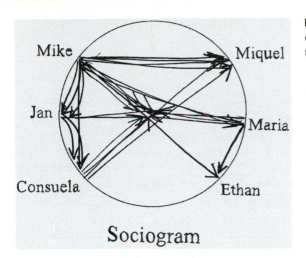

Sociogram

Fig. 2–3 This is the beginning of a sociogram. Each comment is recorded from sender to receiver.

 ACTIVITY

Materials

Posterboard, name tags, markers, paints, scissors, construction paper, glue, broken squares (provided by instructor).

Instructions

1a. As a class, divide into two groups. If you are in group 1, as a group activity, select a name for your group and draw a representation of the name on a posterboard. This representation should encompass the personalities of all members of the group. If you are in group 2, participate in a directed observation of group 1. If you are in group 2, draw a sociogram as suggested by Howe and Schwartzberg (1995) to show the lines of communication you observe in group 1. On the outside of the following circle, write the names of the members of the group. Draw an arrow leading from each person who speaks toward the person at whom the communication was directed. When communication is directed toward the entire group, indicate this by drawing the arrow from that person to the dot in the center of the circle.

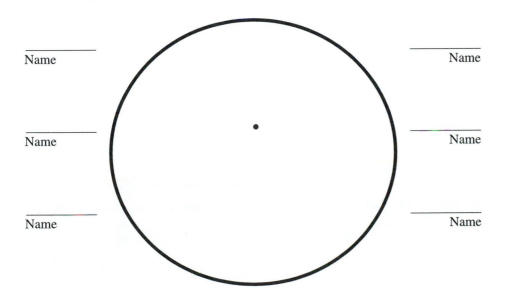

1b. Share and compare observations. What kind of information can be obtained from using a sociogram?

2. Switch roles. If you are in group 2, select a group name and illustrate this on a posterboard. If you are in group 1, observe group 2 as they participate in the group project. Write down your observations about each member's verbal and nonverbal communications that pertain to the content or the process of the group. Place comments that are made and behaviors observed that relate to the activity in the Content column. Place all other comments that are made and behaviors observed that do not relate to the activity in the Process column. Look at the following example.

NAME	CONTENT	PROCESS
Melinda	Melinda asked the group whether they wanted to use markers or finger paint.	
Marcus		Marcus rolled his eyes when Melinda brought up finger paint and said, "What do you think we are, a bunch of babies?"

NAME	CONTENT	PROCESS

2b. What kind of information can be obtained using content/process observations?

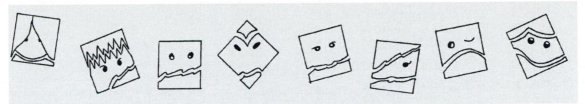

Fig. 2–4

3a. Participate in a group activity entitled Broken Squares (Rider and Rider, 1999). Five students volunteer to participate in the Broken Squares activity while the remainder of the class observes. If you are one of the five members participating, use your puzzle pieces to construct a square. Each member will construct one of five different squares. Follow the rules listed below. If you are an observer, answer the questions listed below the rules.

✔ Talking, pointing, or any other kind of communication is not allowed.

✔ Participants may *give* pieces directly to other participants but may not *take* pieces from other members.

✔ Participants *may not* place their pieces in the center for others to take.

✔ It is permissible for a member to give away all the pieces of the puzzle, even if she or he has already formed a square.

QUESTIONS FOR OBSERVERS TO ANSWER:

a. Who is willing to give away pieces of the puzzle?

b. Does anyone finish his or her own puzzle and then withdraw from the group problem solving?

c. Is there anyone who continually struggles with his or her pieces yet is unwilling to give any or all of them away?

d. How many people are actively engaged in putting the pieces together?

e. What is the level of frustration and anxiety?

f. Is there a turning point at which the group begins to cooperate?

g. Does anyone try to violate the rules by talking or pointing as a means of helping fellow members to solve the problems?

3b. If you were an observer, share your observations with your class, giving feedback to group members regarding their behavior.

3c. If you were one of the five participants, share with your class how it felt to be watched.

3d. How might you use an activity like this in the clinic? How might clients feel?

3e. How might you use this activity as part of your occupational therapy intervention? How might clients respond?

3f. How might you use this activity as an assessment? What information could you obtain?

FOLLOW-UP

✔ Complete the Application of Competencies at the end of this chapter.
✔ Complete a Therapeutic Use of Self Analysis (found in Appendix B) on your group observation and participation performance.

Exercise 20

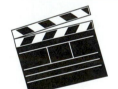

"We must live together as brothers or perish together as fools."

MARTIN LUTHER KING, JR.

GROUP LEADERSHIP

OBJECTIVES

✔ Identify task building/maintenance and anti-group/individual roles
✔ Differentiate styles of group leadership
✔ Facilitate a therapeutic group process

DESCRIPTION

This exercise will help you to understand the various roles your group members may assume and how you as a group leader might effectively handle those roles. When leading client groups, you will encounter members who exhibit group maintenance roles that are healthy and helpful for the group and members who exhibit anti-group roles that are detrimental to the group process. Your effectiveness as a group leader in dealing with these roles will influence your client's behavior and performance in a group setting. You will need to be very skillful in redirecting and limiting inappropriate behavior. At the same time you will need to be just as skillful in encouraging and facilitating appropriate behavior. To do so, you will need to become proficient at using a variety of leadership styles.

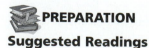 **PREPARATION**

Suggested Readings

Cole (1998)
Howe and Schwartzberg (1995)

Study Questions

1. Define task building/maintenance roles.

2. Define anti-group/individual roles.

3. Describe the following task building/maintenance roles, as described by Cole (1998). Circle the roles you see yourself in most often when participating in group situations.

TASK ROLES	DESCRIPTION
Initiator–contributor	
Information seeker	
Opinion seeker	
Information giver	
Opinion giver	
Elaborator	
Coordinator	
Orienter	
Evaluator-critic	
Energizer	
Procedural technician	
Recorder	
Encourager	
Harmonizer	
Compromiser	
Gatekeeper	
Standard setter	
Group observer	
Follower	

4. Fill in the following chart on anti-group/individual roles, as described by Cole (1998). Describe the behaviors an individual may display when taking on those roles. Describe the intervention you may use as a group leader to facilitate the group's goals and discourage the continuation of behavior that is detrimental to the group process. Circle any of the roles you see yourself in most often when participating in group situations.

ROLE TYPE	BEHAVIOR	INTERVENTION
Silent member		
Playboy		
Special interest pleader		
Blocker		
Dominator		
Aggressor		
Help seeker		
Recognition seeker		
Self-confessor		

5. Describe the following group leadership styles.

    a. Directive

b. Facilitative

c. Advisory

d. Co-leadership

6. List several effective techniques that set limits and can be used to redirect inappropriate behavior and facilitate appropriate behavior in a group.

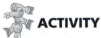 **ACTIVITY**

Materials

Books entitled *S.E.A.L.S. +Plus* (Korb-Khalsa, Azok, and Leutenberg, 1995b) and any of the Life Management Skills series by Korb-Khalsa, Azok, and Leutenberg, (1989, 1993, 1995a).

Instructions

1a. Participate in an instructor-led group activity. As a class, discuss and record several therapeutic factors that you experienced while participating in this group discussion.

1.

2.

3.

4.

5.

6.

7.

8.

1b. Discuss and record leadership qualities and techniques you observed that contributed to the effectiveness of this group. Discuss and record leadership qualities and techniques you observed that hindered the effectiveness of this group.

2a. Participate in a group activity while portraying various group roles as assigned to you by your instructor. Use the following chart to discuss the roles you believe students were playing, the behaviors they displayed to make you decide, what the leader did to redirect the behavior, and what the leader could have done differently. Divide into smaller groups and repeat this process, taking turns being the leader and having your group members role-play anti-group behaviors. Use limit-setting techniques as appropriate. Discuss and continue to complete the chart after each group activity in which you participate.

	NAME	ROLE PORTRAYED	BEHAVIOR OBSERVED	LEADER INTERVENTION	WHAT LEADER COULD DO DIFFERENTLY
GROUP ONE					
GROUP TWO					
GROUP THREE					
GROUP FOUR					

2b. Discuss different leadership styles and when they are appropriate to use. Discuss behavior management strategies and how they are appropriate to use. How did you see these used in the groups you observed?

FOLLOW-UP

✔ Complete the Application of Competencies at the end of this chapter.
✔ Complete a Therapeutic Use of Self Analysis (found in Appendix B) on your leadership skills.

GROUP TREATMENT

OBJECTIVES

✔   Prepare and actively participate in group discussions
✔   Develop a group treatment plan
✔   Analyze your leadership skills using feedback from instructor and peers

DESCRIPTION

This exercise is designed to give you practice in becoming a group leader. As a group leader, you will be responsible for both the process and the content of your groups. You will enable your clients to reach their therapeutic goals. The discussion and activities that occur during a group will facilitate your clients toward this end. Much planning and attention to detail are needed to lead a well-run group. In planning a group, using an established protocol will help to ensure your thoroughness. A well-planned group leads to effective group treatment. Use Cole (1998) as a reference.

"The true leader inspires in others self trust—guiding their eyes to the spirit, the goal."

BRONSON ALCOTT

PREPARATION

Suggested Readings

Cole (1998)
Mosey (1986)
Neidstadt and Crepeau (1998)

Study Questions

1.   Describe Mosey's (1996) six major types of activity groups.

2.   Briefly describe what happens in each of the seven steps in group leadership, as outlined by Cole (1998).

   a. Introduction
      (1)
      (2)
      (3)
      (4)
      (5)

   b. When selecting activity, determine the following:
      (1)
      (2)
      (3)
      (4)
      (5)

   c. Sharing

   d. Processing

   e. Generalization

f. Application

g. Summary

3. What can group leaders do to help people understand the purpose of their group?

4. Why is it important for you to experience group activities before you begin to lead them?

5. Describe the process you would use to make a theory usable in practice.

6. Describe leadership strategies that can be used to facilitate the following therapeutic factors:

a. Group cohesiveness

b. Interpersonal learning

c. Instillation of hope

7. How might you measure change in your group? What pre-assessment and post-assessment criteria might you use?

8. Using the brief group outline below, prepare a ten-minute group problem-solving discussion group that you will lead in lab. Select a problem topic that relates to everyone in the group. Use a problem topic that is pertinent to your college community, such as parking problems, food in the cafeteria, or theft. Generate questions that will facilitate discussion. When leading your group in class, have your members formulate a plan of action to solve the identified problem.

GROUP OUTLINE
Problem topic:
Format:
Questions to facilitate discussion:
Plan of action:

What type of leadership style will you use? Why?
What frame of reference will you use? Why?

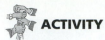 **ACTIVITY**

Materials

Books entitled *S.E.A.L.S. +Plus* (Korb-Khalsa, Azok, and Leutenberg. 1995b), *Life Management Skills III* (Korb-Khalsa, Azok, and Leutenberg, 1995a), and *Group Dynamics in Occupational Therapy* (Cole, 1998).

Instructions

1. With your class, discuss the role of a group leader. Write the highlights of the discussion below.

2. Lead a small group discussion about the problem identified in Study Question 8 using the Seven-Step Format (Cole, 1998). Assign group members task building/maintenance and anti-group/individual roles to assume. Solicit feedback from your peers and instructor on your leadership style, skills, and use of the seven steps. Record the feedback you received in the following chart.

WHAT DID YOU DO WELL?	WHAT COULD YOU HAVE DONE BETTER?
Leadership style: Leadership skills: Use of seven steps:	

3. Lead a small group activity using Cole's (1998) Seven-Step Process. Obtain ideas from the sources suggested in the materials section. As your classmates lead their groups, critique the leader, using the worksheets Cole (1998) provides on leadership evaluation. Record the feedback you receive as a group leader in the space provided.

WHAT DID YOU DO WELL?	WHAT COULD YOU HAVE DONE BETTER?

FOLLOW-UP

✔ Complete the Application of Competencies at the end of this chapter.
✔ Complete an Analysis of Self (found in Appendix B)on your leadership abilities.
✔ Complete a Therapeutic Use of Self Analysis found in Appendix B on your leadership skills.
✔ Complete Performance Skill 2B on Leading a Group.

MANAGED CARE

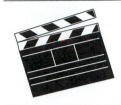

OBJECTIVES

✔   Define commonly used terms related to managed care
✔   Choose functional activities that may be used during intervention
✔   Reconfigure traditional exercises into purposeful activities or occupations

DESCRIPTION

This exercise will introduce you to managed care. In certain settings managed care has forced delivery of occupational therapy (OT) services to be provided in a shorter amount of time while still demanding the same outcomes. With shorter stays, each treatment session must try to address as much functional treatment as possible. This is critical to our service provision. In such an arena it is a challenge to meet the needs of our clients and to provide high-quality services within the constraints of managed care. Continual outcome studies are needed to validate the efficiency of our functional treatment choices.

"In all human affairs there are efforts, and there are results, and the strength of the effort is the measure of the result."

JAMES ALLEN

 PREPARATION

Suggested Readings

AOTA (1996)
Neidstadt and Crepeau (1998)

Study Questions

1. Fill out the Managed Care Crossword Puzzle, which contains commonly used definitions and terms associated with managed care. (See p. 106)
2. Describe how recent managed care guidelines have changed the delivery of occupational therapy services.

3. Contact a local clinician who is in managed care. Obtain information about current managed care regulations and guidelines. Identify at least six current terms, regulations, or guidelines with which you are not yet familiar.

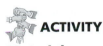 **ACTIVITY**

Materials

As many of the following as are available: cones, dowel rod, skateboard, washers, small dowel rods, shoulder ladder, pulley, Theraband®, pegboard.

Instructions

1. Divide into small groups. Participate in the following exercises that are used as treatment activities for clients. Determine a more functional, meaningful, and purposeful activity or occupation that could be used in treatment to meet the same goal in the identified practice setting. An example for each practice setting is provided for you.

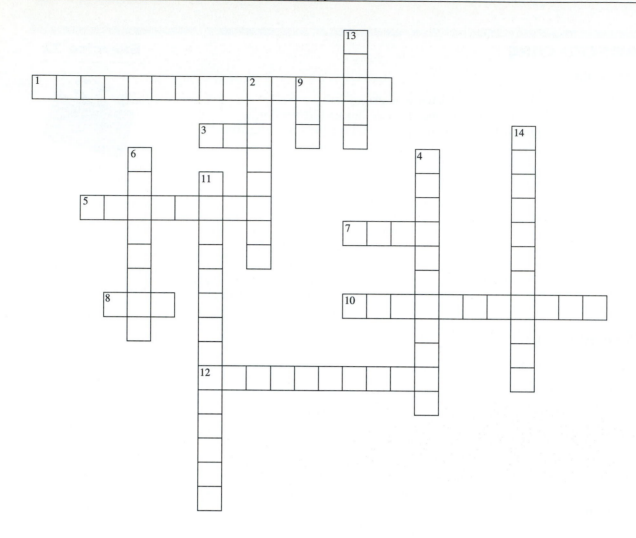

ACROSS

1. Defining essential events in care that provide the most care at the most economical price
3. Abbreviation for the network of providers that discount their charges for a high-volume of patients
5. Program for low-income people
7. Abbreviation for the department that administers Medicare and Medicaid
8. Abbreviation for the classification of illnesses that help to determine payment
10. Fixed price for one day including all supplies and services
12. A primary care physician who coordinates all services

DOWN

2. Who provides the care
4. Health cost containment approach
6. Program for persons over 65 or disabled
9. Abbreviation for the program that sets fees for a year and members receive all required care
11. Arrangement in which a person coordinates care process
13. Request to insurer for payment of insurance benefits
14. A deductible is part of this

a. Adult physical rehabilitation

GOAL OF ACTIVITY	PRESENT TREATMENT	SUGGESTED FUNCTIONAL TREATMENT
Increased range of motion (ROM)	Client is stacking cones sitting in a wheelchair while at the table.	Client is reaching to high shelves to obtain needed cooking ingredients and utensils.
Increased bilateral use	Client is lifting a dowel rod above head while seated on the mat.	
Increased assistive ROM	Client is moving a skateboard on the table with the weak extremity.	
Increased ROM; improved pincer grasp	Client is putting washers on the dowels for ROM.	
Increased ROM	Client is walking fingers up the shoulder ladder on the wall.	
Improved balance	Client is reaching to pick up cones from the floor.	
Increased hand strength	Client is squeezing and pulling putty.	
Increased upper extremity (UE) strength	Client is pulling and stretching a piece of Theraband®.	
Increased fine motor skill	Client is putting in/taking out pegs in a pegboard.	
Improved endurance	Calisthenics	
Other		
Other		
Other		

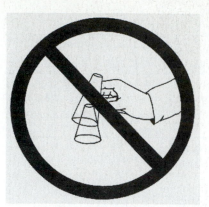

Fig. 2–5 Find something more purposeful!

b. Pediatric rehabilitation

GOAL OF ACTIVITY	PRESENT TREATMENT	SUGGESTED FUNCTIONAL TREATMENT
Increased ROM	Client is stacking cones while sitting in a wheelchair at the table.	
Increased bilateral use	Client is lifting a dowel rod above head while seated on the mat.	
Increased assistive ROM	Client is moving a skateboard on the table with the weak extremity.	Client is playing air hockey.
Increased ROM; improved pincer grasp	Client is putting washers on the dowels for ROM.	
Increased ROM	Client is walking fingers up the shoulder ladder on the wall.	
Improved balance	Client is reaching to pick up cones from the floor.	
Increased hand strength	Client is squeezing and pulling putty.	
Increased UE strength	Client is pulling and stretching a piece of Theraband®.	
Increased fine motor skill	Client is putting in/taking out pegs in a pegboard.	
Improved endurance	Calisthenics	
Other		
Other		
Other		

c. Geriatric rehabilitation

GOAL OF ACTIVITY	PRESENT TREATMENT	SUGGESTED FUNCTIONAL TREATMENT
Increased ROM	Client is stacking cones while sitting in a wheelchair at the table.	
Increased bilateral use	Client is lifting a dowel rod above head while seated on the mat.	
Increased assistive ROM	Client is moving a skateboard on the table with the weak extremity.	
Increased ROM; improved pincer grasp	Client is putting washers on the dowels for ROM.	
Increased ROM	Client is walking fingers up the shoulder ladder on the wall.	
Improved balance	Client is reaching to pick up cones from the floor.	Client is making a bed.
Increased hand strength	Client is squeezing and pulling putty.	
Increased UE strength	Client is pulling and stretching a piece of Theraband®.	
Increased fine motor skill	Client is putting in/taking out pegs in a pegboard.	
Improved endurance	Calisthenics	
Other		
Other		
Other		

d. Psychosocial

GOAL OF ACTIVITY	PRESENT TREATMENT	SUGGESTED FUNCTIONAL TREATMENT
Decreased stress	Client is participating in a discussion group.	
Improved time management	Client is reading handouts on time management techniques.	Client is making a personal schedule for the upcoming week

Increased self-esteem	Clients are taking turns complimenting each other.	
Increased reality orientation	Clients are referred to a calendar in each room.	
Improved anger management	Clients are discussing alternatives to deal with aggression.	
Increased assertiveness	Clients are listening to an assertiveness lecture.	
Improved self-care	Clients are told to take better care of themselves.	
Increased leisure interests	Client lists current engagement of leisure activities.	
Improved work habits	Clients discuss characteristics of good work habits.	
Improved endurance	Calisthenics	
Other		
Other		

e. Share your ideas with your classmates. Make note of any treatment suggestions you would like to remember.

GOAL OF ACTIVITY	PRESENT TREATMENT	SUGGESTED FUNCTIONAL TREATMENT
Increased ROM	Client is stacking cones while sitting in a wheelchair at the table.	
Increased bilateral use	Client is lifting a dowel rod above head while seated on the mat.	
Increased assistive ROM	Client is moving a skateboard on the table with the weak extremity.	
Increased ROM; improved pincer grasp	Client is putting washers on the dowels for ROM.	
Increased ROM	Client is walking fingers up the shoulder ladder on the wall.	
Improved balance	Client is reaching to pick up cones from the floor.	

Increased hand strength	Client is squeezing and pulling putty.	
Increased UE strength	Client is pulling and stretching a Theraband®.	
Increased fine motor skill	Client is putting in/taking out pegs in a pegboard.	
Improved endurance	Client is playing forward pass.	
Other		
Other		

2. For the psychosocial goals, list your classmates' functional treatment ideas on the blackboard. Vote on the best ones.
3. Decipher the acronyms contained in the following sentences: "You have a client admitted to your SNF, and you are working under PPS. You will be given the client's RUGS level, and the team members will help to fill out the MDS. Be certain to use the correct CPT and ICD-9 codes when documenting to get the best reimbursement." Discuss these and other managed care–related acronyms and their implications to clinical practice.

FOLLOW-UP

✔ Complete the Application of Competencies at the end of this chapter.

INTERNET

Exercise 23

OBJECTIVES

✔ Define terminology related to Internet use
✔ Assess Internet sites to obtain information that is relevant for occupational therapy
✔ Build directory of occupational therapy resources on the Internet

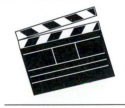

"Always put off until tomorrow what shouldn't be done at all."

AUTHOR UNKNOWN

DESCRIPTION

This exercise is designed to provide you with experience searching the Internet for valuable health care information. The Internet holds a wealth of information on many topics related to health care. In the pursuit of your education, as well as later, when you begin practicing occupational therapy, there will be many occasions when you will need to obtain and review related information. To obtain some of this information, you will need to be adept at using the Internet as a resource. When you obtain information from the Internet, be sure that the source is valid and the information contained therein is properly documented. Also, note that, unlike a library, the content of the Internet is not regulated or given any oversight. The selection of the information you decide to use is up to your own judgment.

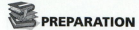

PREPARATION

Suggested Reading

Gibbs, Sullivan-Fowler, and Rowe (1996)
Neidstadt and Crepeau (1998)
Pomeroy (1997)
Reed and Sanderson (1999)

Study Questions

1. Define the following terms related to use of the Internet.

   a. Internet

   b. Web site

   c. Address

   d. World Wide Web

   e. Access provider

2. Describe the steps in surfing the Web.

3. What criteria can be used to determine the quality and reliability of a Web site?

4. Assume that you will be working with a client who has a diagnosis that is unfamiliar to you (your instructor will assign you the diagnosis). Working with a classmate, go to the Internet and print out the information you find on this diagnosis. Keep a record of all sites visited and the information found. Highlight the most useful sites to share with your class.

ACTIVITY

Materials

Printouts from students' Internet searches completed in Study Question 4, chart paper, Internet access via computer.

Instructions

1. Share the information found on the Internet about your assigned diagnosis. Record the uniform resource locations (URLs) of the sites and information available at the sites your peers visited.

2. Discuss as a class and list below other situations in which you may need to obtain information from the Internet.

3. In the computer lab, divide into teams of two or small groups. Find OT-related Web sites on the Internet. List on chart paper the sites found, providing the URL and a summary of the information found at each site. Designate a class member to be responsible for distributing the information to the class. Discuss how this information might be useful to you as an OT practitioner.

FOLLOW-UP

✔ Complete the Application of Competencies at the end of this chapter.

CLINICAL REASONING

OBJECTIVES

✔ Identify different types or facets of clinical reasoning
✔ Describe specific situations in which clinical reasoning will be used
✔ List the clinical reasoning steps to identify problems and select interventions

DESCRIPTION

This exercise will help you to understand and see the importance of clinical reasoning. Clinical reasoning is the essence of one's knowledge, thought processes, problem-solving and decision-making skills. Clinical reasoning skills will be needed and used continually to make decisions during the entire occupational therapy (OT) process. Your judgment and ability to put it all together will be challenged often. Your clinical reasoning skills will improve with experience. Even the most skilled therapist started out as a beginner.

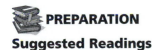 **PREPARATION**

Suggested Readings

Christianson and Baum (1997)
Mattingly and Fleming (1994)
Neistadt and Crepeau (1998)

Study Questions

1. Define the term *clinical reasoning.*

2. Define the term *tacit knowledge.*

3. Define the term *metacognition.*

Exercise 24

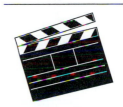

"Our plans miscarry because they have no aim. When a man does not know what harbor he is making for, no wind is the right wind."

Seneca

4. Detail the different types or facets of clinical reasoning:
    a. Procedural

    b. Interactive

    c. Conditional

    d. Scientific

    e. Narrative

    f. Pragmatic

    g. Ethical

5. Describe how clinical reasoning relates to the OT process.

6. Describe the therapist with the "three-track mind" (Mattingly and Fleming, 1994).

7. List the steps and characteristics of clinical reasoning in OT practice.

8. Outline the reflective framework for problem sensing and intervention (Bridge, Twible and Beltran, as cited in Christanson and Baum, 1997) that can be used to facilitate conscious reflection.

9. Describe the effects the following experiences have on clinical reasoning.
    a. Clinical experience

    b. Personal experience

c. Reflection on experiences

d. Education

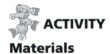 **ACTIVITY**

Materials

Flip chart or large paper.

Instructions

1. Divide into groups. Draw a picture on a piece of paper from the flip chart that illustrates the therapist with a "three-track mind" (Mattingly and Fleming, 1994). Be creative. Share your drawing with your classmates. Discuss the reasoning that contributed to your portrayal of such a therapist.

2a. Divide into small groups. Share the most difficult decision you have had to make at your fieldwork setting to date. Share the most difficult decision you have observed your supervising therapist have to make. Use the reflective framework for problem solving as detailed by Bridge, Twible, and Beltran as cited in Christianson and Baum 1997) and outline the steps to the decision-making process you encountered. Consider both the process you actually did go through and what you might have gone through. Repeat this procedure, using the scenario with your supervisor. Write out the steps for both scenarios. Share the scenarios and the reflective framework steps with the classmates in your small group.

YOUR DECISION IN YOUR FIELDWORK SETTING

REFLECTIVE FRAMEWORK STEPS:

a.

b.

c.

d.

e.

f.

g.

h.

i.

YOUR SUPERVISOR'S DECISION IN THE FIELDWORK SETTING

REFLECTIVE FRAMEWORK STEPS:

a.

b.

c.

d.

e.

f.

g.

h.

i.

2b. Decide as a small group which one of the shared scenarios best depicts the clinical reasoning process. Prepare a role-play for your small group to perform before the rest of the class using this scenario. Present the scenario either as it happened or as you think it should have happened. Be sure to tell your classmates which way you are presenting the scenario. Discuss the role-play as each group finishes.

FOLLOW-UP

✔   Complete the Application of Competencies at the end of this chapter.

TEAM MEMBERS

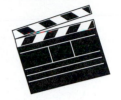

OBJECTIVES

✔   Differentiate models of team interaction
✔   Describe a team member's role in a team meeting
✔   Role-play a team member in a simulated team meeting

DESCRIPTION

This exercise is designed to acquaint you with the roles and responsibilities of the various team members with whom you will be working. As an occupational therapy (OT) practitioner you will be one member of a team providing services to your clients. It is important that you understand the roles and responsibilities of your team members so that you can work together more effectively. A smoothly running team is characterized by mutual support, respect, and cooperation, no matter what model of delivery is used. A smoothly running team delivers client care services to all concerned in a more satisfactory manner.

"We are not here merely to make a living. We are here to enrich the world, and we impoverish ourselves if we forget this errand."

WOODROW WILSON

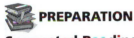PREPARATION

Suggested Readings

Neistadt and Crepeau (1998)

Study Questions

1.   Define a team approach.

2.   Discuss the difference between a multidisciplinary team, an interdisciplinary team, and a transdisciplinary team.

3.   List the team members with whom you may be working. Briefly describe the roles they play and the practice setting(s) in which you think they may be working.

TEAM MEMBER	ROLE	SETTING

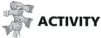 **ACTIVITY**

Materials

Role-playing props, Case Studies 8 and/or 9 located at the end of this chapter.

Instructions

1. Assuming the team member role assigned to you, participate in a mock team meeting to plan a course of intervention for the individual in Case Study 8 or 9. In your team meeting discuss the intervention area for which each team member will be responsible. Talk about the interventions you may use. Decide as a group how often the team will need to meet. Discuss who will provide intervention to your client in the overlapping areas and consider co-treatment options. Prepare for your meeting using part a below. Complete part b as you role-play your team meeting.

   a. Your team member role:

AREAS YOU WILL TREAT	INTERVENTIONS YOU WILL USE

b. Record other team roles here:

TEAM MEMBER	AREA TO TREAT	INTERVENTION USED

c. Reflect on your team meeting by answering the following questions:

   a. What were the overlapping areas of intervention?

   b. What determined who would provide intervention for these areas?

c. Was it determined that this client might benefit from any co-treatments?

d. If not, why not? If so, with which team members and why?

e. What type of relationship among team members will provide for the most effective client treatment?

2. As a class discuss, the emerging practice areas. What team members might be involved in these settings?

FOLLOW-UP

✔   Complete the Application of Competencies at the end of this chapter.

Exercise 26

"Nothing is more terrible than activity without insight."

THOMAS CARLYLE

DOCUMENTATION

OBJECTIVES

✔   Define the content of standard occupational therapy documents
✔   Compose documentation according to guidelines from the American Occupational Therapy Association (AOTA)
✔   Critique documentation for required elements per AOTA's guidelines

DESCRIPTION

This exercise is designed to familiarize you with the documentation process. As an occupational therapy practitioner, you will complete documentation relative to all aspects of client care. Although writing styles may vary, there are certain standard elements set forth by AOTA that should be included in writing all documents. In addition to these guidelines, the facilities, governmental agencies, and accreditation organizations of a particular setting may also have established guidelines for content inclusion. During the documentation process, the occupational therapist (OT) and the occupational therapy assistant (OTA) need to work together in a collaborative manner.

PREPARATION

Suggested Readings

>   Acquaviva (1998)
>   AOTA (2000)
>   AOTA (latest edition)

Study Questions

1. Identify four purposes of documentation.
   a.

   b.

c.

d.

2. Fill in the missing information in the following chart. The first one is done for you.

TYPE OF DOCUMENTATION	CONTENT	CLARIFICATION
Evaluation Report	Precautions and contraindications	May be identified by referral sources or occupational therapy practitioners.
		Prognosis and anticipated level of performance
	Activities, techniques, and modalities used	
		Functional limitations that must change
	Short-term goals	
		Include copy of home program
	Consumer/caregiver instruction	
		Results analyzed and compared with previous
	Follow-up plans	
	Referral source	
	Consumer's response to therapy	
		State new goals and rationale for change

3. What governing agencies require documentation to be countersigned?

4. Describe the relationship between the OT and the OTA in countersigning documentation.

5. List fundamental elements of documentation.

    a.

    b.

    c.

    d.

    e.

    f.

    g.

    h.

    i.

    j.

6. Describe the S.O.A.P. format of documentation and identify the individual letters in the acronym.

    a. S:

    b. O:

c. A:

d. P:

7. Describe the most frequent causes of denial for payment by Medicare.

8. Describe some tips for using diagnostic and procedural codes in documentation.

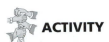 **ACTIVITY**

Materials

Transparencies and overhead projector, index cards, Case Study 10 located at the end of this chapter.

Instructions

1. With an assigned case study, work in a small group to write the following documentation papers.
   a. *Initial Note:* Develop an initial note from the case study assigned. Determine assessments that would be appropriate to give, predict results on the basis of those assessments, and compose treatment goals accordingly. Use the space below to plan and complete your work.

Case study name: _____ Gender:_____Age:___ Diagnosis: _____

ASSESSMENT GIVEN	RESULTS
Goals:	

Fig. 2–6 Document as if each note may one day be used in a court of law.

Write an initial note including the results of the assessment. Include treatment goals at the end of the narrative.

b. *Progress Note:* Use the information from the initial note and assume that the client has been involved in treatment for one week. Predict the results and compose a progress note.

c. *Discharge Summary:* Develop a discharge summary assuming that the client has been involved in OT treatment for three weeks. The amount of progress a patient has made depends on you.

2. Check your notes to determine whether or not the components listed below are included in them. These components are taken from the guidelines set forth in the document "Elements of Clinical Documentation (Revision)" (AOTA, 1998).

PROTOCOL	INITIAL NOTE			PROGRESS NOTE			DISCHARGE SUMMARY		
Organized									
Legible									
Concise									
Clear									
Accurate									
Complete									
Current									
Objective									
Correct grammar									
Correct spelling									
Fundamental elements									
Patient's full name									
Complete date									
Type of document									
Signature and credentials									
Signature directly at end									
Countersignature									
Confidentiality maintained									
Acceptable terminology									
Facility approved abbreviation									
Errors corrected with line and initials									

3. Have your notes reviewed by at least one other student using the protocol criteria outlined above. Record here your strengths and areas of concern regarding your documentation skills. Develop a plan for needed improvements in this area.

STRENGTHS	AREAS OF CONCERNS	PLAN

4. Write a goal on the index card provided by your instructor. Divide into three groups. Have two of the groups be defense and prosecution groups. Appoint one student in each group to be the attorney; the other students serve as witnesses. Have the third group serve as the jury. After your instructor writes one of the goals from the index cards on the chalkboard, take ten to twenty minutes to prepare your opening remarks, witnesses, and closing remarks (defense group or prosecuting group). If you are on the jury, use this time to make a list of the information you will look for to determine whether the goal is written correctly—for example, is the goal relevant, understandable, measurable, behavioral, and achievable (RUMBA)? Has the defense group defended the goal as correctly written? Has the prosecution shown proof or evidence that it is not correctly written? Proceed with the trial, with your instructor as judge. Change groups, players, and goals as time permits.

FOLLOW-UP

✔ Complete the Application of Competencies at the end of this chapter.

SERVICE COMPETENCY

Exercise 27

OBJECTIVES

✔ Define principles of service competency
✔ Develop service competency in a peer-taught task
✔ Compare and contrast service competency methods

DESCRIPTION

This exercise is designed to assist you in obtaining service competency. Throughout your professional career as an occupational therapy practitioner you will need to establish service competency in your clinical skills. Service competency will need to occur between the registered occupational therapist (OT) and the certified occupational therapy

"It's never too late to be what we might have been."

Geᴏʀɢᴇ Eʟɪᴏᴛ

assistant (OTA) as well as between the entry-level OT and the supervising OT. To achieve that competency, it is essential to develop plans that will lead to mastery of a particular task. A variety of methods can be used to do so, and it is important to track one's progress throughout the process. The use of magic tricks can be useful during treatment. Therefore, this exercise will use magic tricks to help you develop service competency.

PREPARATION

Suggested Readings

AOTA (latest edition)
magic trick book (any)
Ryan (1995b)
Thomson, Lieberman, Murphy, Wendt, Poole, and Hertfelder (1995)

Study Questions

1. Define the term *service competency*.

2. Describe guiding principles and patterns of supervision that are related to service competency.

3. List methods of achieving competency.

4. List common measures that are used to document competency.

5. Who has the ultimate responsibility to ensure that service competency is achieved and maintained between an OT and an OTA? Between the entry-level OT and the supervising OT?

6. Develop service competency in performing a magic trick with which you are not familiar. You will be performing this magic trick for your classmates and determining service competency by those who master your trick. In the following chart, record the methods used to achieve your competence in performing this trick. Methods to use in preparation of your competency may include, but are not limited to, reading related literature, attending a magic workshop, observing the trick being performed by someone else, and practicing with an individual who has mastered the trick. Preparing for this event may take several weeks. Document below your steps in preparation of competency. Include the date completed and the progress you are making.

COMPETENCY PLAN		
Magic Trick: _____		
METHOD	DATE COMPLETED	PROGRESS

ACTIVITY

Materials

Materials for magic tricks brought by students.

Instructions

1a. Divide into small groups. Perform your magic trick for your group. Teach the steps to master this trick to your group. Share the methods you used for learning the trick and achieving competency. Fill out the following chart, indicating the progress each member has made toward achieving service competency. Solicit and record feedback from your group members about your performance.

NAMES OF GROUP MEMBERS	PROGRESS REGARDING COMPETENCY

FEEDBACK

1b. Participate in the tricks your classmates demonstrate. Use the following chart to record each performer's tricks and the method used to achieve competency. Have the performer initial the appropriate box indicating that you have achieved service competency in the demonstrated trick. Record feedback on each performance and communicate your feedback to that individual verbally.

STUDENT PERFORMER	MAGIC TRICK	METHODS USED TO ACHIEVE COMPETENCY	INITIALED	FEEDBACK GIVEN TO PERFORMER

1c. As a class, discuss and record information on how this exercise relates to obtaining service competency in occupational therapy. Go to Appendix C and further discuss how the Service Competency forms might be used in future practice.

FOLLOW-UP

✔ Complete the Application of Competencies at the end of this chapter.

Exercise 28

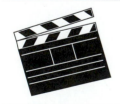

"Things which matter most must never be at the mercy of things which matter least."

GOETHE

SERVICE MANAGEMENT

OBJECTIVES

✔ Define terms related to service management
✔ Describe the policies and procedures within a department of occupational therapy (OT)
✔ Determine the relative placement of an OT practitioner in an organization flow chart

DESCRIPTION

This exercise is designed to help you understand the management of occupational therapy (OT) services. As a practitioner of OT you will be a part of your department and part of a larger facility. It is important to understand how you will fit into the order of the department and how the department fits into the order of the facility. It is also important to understand the policies and procedures for which you will be responsible once you are employed. Understanding your department and the entire organization will facilitate your effectiveness as an OT practitioner. Effective service management ensures efficient operation of an OT department.

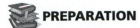 **PREPARATION**

Suggested Readings

Neistadt and Crepeau (1998)
Ryan (1995b)

Study Questions

1. Define the following terms as they relate to service management:

   a. Organizational patterns

   b. Tables of organization

   c. Job description

   d. Policies

   e. Procedures

   f. Productivity

2. List and describe the steps in the strategic planning process that are used in management of OT services.

3. Describe quality assurance and the process this involves.

4. List and briefly describe the components involved in service management operations.

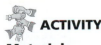 **ACTIVITY**

Materials

Guest speaker, a policy and procedure manual from the guest speaker's facility, transparency or handout of an organizational chart from the guest speaker's facility, overhead projector and screen.

Instructions

1a. Listen to a guest speaker who is the manager of an OT department of a general hospital. Briefly describe his or her facility and organizational setup. Through a question and answer time, solicit the following information about this facility.

1b. What are the duties of the occupational therapy manager?

1c. What are the policies or procedures for the following occupational therapy services?
   a. Response to referral

   b. Timeline for evaluation

   c. Personnel to perform evaluation

   d. Writing the evaluation

   e. Treatment

   f. Discharge

   g. Documentation

   h. Follow-up

   i. Referrals

   j. Accident/incident reports

   k. Billing

Organizational Charts
Lines of Authority and Communication

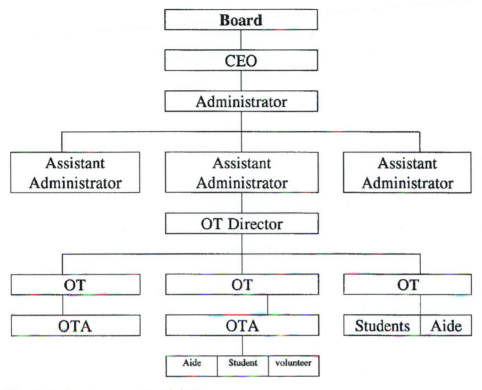

Fig. 2–7 Sample organizational chart.

l. Supplies/inventory management

m. Budget

n. Sick/vacation time

o. Quality monitoring

p. Continuing education

q. Research

r. Team planning

1d. As a new graduate, describe where you would fit into the organizational chart presented by the guest speaker.

2. Predict differences that will be on the organizational flowcharts from various other facilities, such as skilled nursing facilities, private practice, and schools. Discuss these predictions as a class.

FOLLOW-UP

✔ Complete the Application of Competencies at the end of this chapter.

Exercise 29

"The gift of a great teacher is creating an awareness of greatness in others."

JOHN HEIDER

SUPERVISION

OBJECTIVES

✔ Examine the functions of a fieldwork supervisor
✔ Critique your strengths and areas of concern as a supervisor
✔ Provide proactive suggestions for difficult supervisor/supervisee situations

DESCRIPTION

The purpose of this exercise is to familiarize you with supervision. Supervision affects every practitioner in occupational therapy. Generally, practitioners supervise and are supervised by others in one form or another. As students you will experience different levels of supervision on your various clinicals. On entering practice, you will most likely be supervised as an entry-level practitioner, and you may supervise occupational therapy aides and volunteers. With increasing experience, you will then assume supervisory duties with occupational therapy and occupational therapy assistant (OTA) students. If you are an OTA, you will receive at least routine supervision. If you are an OT, you may be supervised by someone within or outside the profession.

PREPARATION

Suggested Readings

AOTA (1991)
AOTA (latest edition)

Study Questions

1. Write a brief summary describing each of the four functions of a fieldwork supervisor:

   a. Administrative function:

b. Teaching function:

c. Consultative function:

d. Evaluative function:

2. To be an effective supervisor, it will be important to remember the experience of being supervised. Write notes to yourself that you want to remember when you are in a fieldwork or clinical supervisory capacity. Include notes on techniques that you have experienced to be helpful and those you have found to be not so helpful. Draw from the experiences you have had in an occupational therapy setting or in a related discipline setting.

MOST HELPFUL TECHNIQUES:	WHY?
LEAST HELPFUL TECHNIQUES:	WHY?

3. Describe how a good supervisory relationship affects the components identified in the balloon in the accompanying drawing and how a poor supervisory relationship influences those same components.

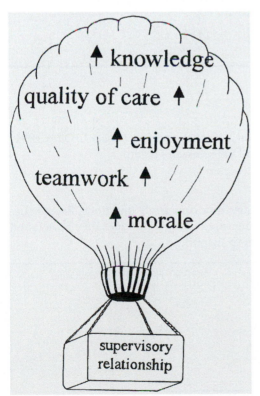

Fig. 2–8 The arrows indicate the positive impact a good supervisory relationship will have.

COMPONENT	GOOD RELATIONSHIPS	POOR RELATIONSHIPS
Knowledge		
Quality of care		
Enjoyment		
Teamwork		
Morale		

4. The AOTA has developed a program to assist in the education of fieldwork supervisors called *S.P.I.C.E.S.* (Self-Paced Instruction for Clinical Education and Supervision) (AOTA, 1991). Complete information on one of the worksheets on self-assessment in Unit One of that document. Include a summary of your supervisory strengths and areas of concern. Develop a corresponding action plan to continue to develop your strengths and improve your areas of concern.

STRENGTHS:	PLAN TO ACCENTUATE THESE FURTHER:
AREAS OF CONCERN:	PLAN TO IMPROVE:

ACTIVITY

Materials

S.P.I.C.E.S.: Self-Paced Introduction for Clinical Education and Supervision (AOTA, 1991) video and workbook, television monitor, and videocassette recorder.

Instructions

1. With your class, discuss the information from your study questions. Record suggestions from your classmates regarding supervisory techniques they have found helpful and those they have found not so helpful.

HELPFUL TECHNIQUES	NOT SO HELPFUL TECHNIQUES

2a. As a class, view selected scenes from the *S.P.I.C.E.S.: Self-Paced Introduction for Clinical Education and Supervision* (AOTA, 1991) video, using the space below to record the various skills you need to remember as they are portrayed in each scene.

SCENE	TEACHING FUNCTIONS	CONSULTANT FUNCTIONS	EVALUATIVE FUNCTIONS
One			
Two			
Three			

2b. Discuss and record here other information available in the S.P.I.C.E.S. (AOTA, 1991) program that you could use at a later date.

3. Role-play the following scenarios. Have your group or class observe the behavior of both student and supervisor giving proactive suggestions for the problem areas.

   a. Role-Play 1: The student is experiencing extreme anxiety and is feeling totally overwhelmed by the requirements of Level II fieldwork.

PROACTIVE SUGGESTIONS	
STUDENT	SUPERVISOR

   b. Role-Play 2: The student is always late to fieldwork even after the supervisor has reminded the student many times how important it is to be on time.

PROACTIVE SUGGESTIONS	
STUDENT	SUPERVISOR

c. Role-Play 3: The supervisor repeatedly talks negatively about the student to other members of the team.

PROACTIVE SUGGESTIONS	
STUDENT	SUPERVISOR

d. Role-Play 4: The student does what is required and nothing more. If a task is not given to the student, he or she sits and waits for the supervisor to direct the next step.

PROACTIVE SUGGESTIONS	
STUDENT	SUPERVISOR

FOLLOW-UP

✔ Complete the Application of Competencies at the end of this chapter.
✔ Complete a Therapeutic Use of Self Analysis found in Appendix B on your supervision skills.

Exercise 30

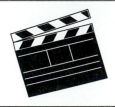

"Relationship is the mirror in which the self is revealed."

KRISHNAMURTI

PROFESSIONALISM

OBJECTIVES

✔ Analyze elements of professionalism in the field of occupational therapy (OT)
✔ Illustrate professional roles within the field of OT
✔ Identify professional behavior and characteristics

DESCRIPTION

This exercise is intended to assist you in understanding the professional behaviors and responsibilities of an occupational therapy practitioner. Within the profession of occupational therapy there are many roles that can be assumed. Each role contains a set of professional behaviors and responsibilities that are specific to that role. These behaviors and responsibilities need to be assumed as practitioners function in these roles. As your career unfolds over time, your roles may change. Additionally, it will probably not be uncommon for you to assume more than one role at a time. Throughout the assumption of these roles, exhibiting professionalism is imperative.

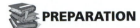 **PREPARATION**

Suggested Readings

AOTA (latest edition)
Purtilo and Haddad (1996)
Ryan (1995b)

Study Questions

1. In the following chart, list and describe the steps in the socialization process of the occupational therapy assistant (OTA).

STAGE	DESCRIPTION

2. Summarize the entry-level skills expected of the OTA and OT when they enter the field of occupational therapy.

3. Describe the integration of professional and personal qualities for effective practice.

4. Briefly describe the following terms regarding professional boundaries:
   a. Physical boundaries

   b. Unconsented touching

   c. Sexual touching

   d. Sexual contact

    e. Emotional-psychological boundaries

    f. Pity

    g. Overidentification

    h. Affection

5. List and describe how the virtues used to create professional closeness may be used in occupational therapy as they relate to patient treatment.

6. Briefly describe the professional responsibilities in each of the occupational therapy roles.
   a. Practitioner–OT

   b. Practitioner–OTA

   c. Educator

   d. Fieldwork Educator

   e. Supervisor

   f. Administrator

   g. Consultant

   h. Fieldwork Coordinator

   i. Faculty

   j. Program Director

   k. Researcher/Scholar

   l. Entrepreneur

7. List and describe the core values and attitudes of occupational therapy practice as taken from the document of the same name (AOTA, 1998).

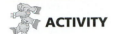 **ACTIVITY**

Materials

Flip charts or large posterboards, colored markers.

Instructions

1. Divide into small groups. Illustrate your assigned OT role (AOTA, 1998) on a large flip chart page. Consider using other professionals in your drawings as well as any objects that might help to depict the duties and responsibilities of the role. When your drawing is completed, identify the roles portrayed by the other groups in your class. Once the role has been identified, label the drawing and place it on the wall for display. Record information from your classroom drawings that may not have been included in your study questions.

2. As a class, discuss the following professional characteristics that will need to be displayed as a student in a clinical setting. Record information in the space provided.

   a. Dress

   b. Punctuality

   c. Organization

   d. Dependability

   e. Interpersonal skills

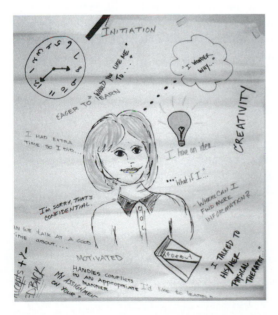

Fig. 2–9 One representation of an advanced clinician.

Courtesy of participants at a Clinical Educators Meeting.

f. Respect for staff

g. Confidentiality

h. Verbal communication

i. Nonverbal communication

FOLLOW-UP

✔   Complete the Application of Competencies at the end of this chapter.

Exercise 31

"Knowing is not enough; we must apply. Willing is not enough; we must do."

JOHANN WOLFGANG VON GOETHE

PUBLIC RELATIONS/SERVICE LEARNING

OBJECTIVES

✔   Identify community agencies that could benefit from receiving community service
✔   Participate in community service at an agency of your choice
✔   Promote occupational therapy through community service

DESCRIPTION

This exercise is intended to help you understand the importance of learning through participation in community service. A responsible member of any community should seek out and assist in filling the identified needs of that community. Community service can also be a time to help promote the profession of occupational therapy (OT). Occupational therapy is not a household term. Many people are still unfamiliar with the unique aspects of OT. Spreading the word about OT while performing community service is an effective way to teach others about the profession and at the same time build public relations. This service project will be a learning experience for you, too. Providing a needed community service provides much goodwill and facilitates cooperation and understanding among community members.

PREPARATION

Suggested Readings

Any American Occupational Therapy Association (AOTA) resources, such as the Web site *www.aota.org,* publications, or catalogues
Local community resource guide, such as a United Way pamphlet
Local newspaper for agencies seeking volunteers or stories that pertain to a needy organization
Local phone book

Study Questions

1. List agencies you identified from reviewing the documents on community resources that have a stated need.

AGENCY	NEEDS

2. Determine the relationship of the above agencies and needs to OT in anticipation of completing a service learning project. For example, a group of students identified a local health clinic as an agency in need. They determined that the children coming to the clinic were very much in need of an area to play with safe and age-appropriate toys, as there was nothing for the children to do while waiting for services. This often caused very uncomfortable conditions for children, adults, and staff. The students set out to seek donated materials and supplies to equip a play center. This project helped to educate the agency about OT, and at the same time the service very much related to the philosophy of OT. It emphasized the importance of play for children, a fundamental principle in OT.

   Select several agencies from your list and describe if and how their needs relate to OT.

AGENCY	RELATIONSHIP TO OT

3. Which month is designated as OT month? (Hint: The national AOTA conference is held in the same month.)

4. Consult AOTA resources for ideas to promote occupational therapy during OT month. List these ideas below.

 ACTIVITY

Materials

None.

Instructions

1. Share the findings of community needs from your study questions with your class. Participate in a brainstorming session to determine the needs in the community and the relationship of these needs to OT. List the agencies here that might be appropriate recipients of a service learning project.

AGENCY	NEEDS	RELATIONSHIP TO OT

2. Participate in a brainstorming session to determine the needs of the community in understanding the role of OT as it relates to legislative or reimbursement or agencies or individuals. For example, there may be a need to provide information about OT to a senator who is going to vote on new health care financing.

LEGISLATIVE OR REIMBURSEMENT ORGANIZATIONS	NEEDS	RELATIONSHIP TO OT

3. Divide into groups of four or five students and select an agency at which you will complete a public relations or service learning project. Coordinate your efforts of selecting the agency with the faculty of your host institution. List here the members of your group and the selected agency.

Agency: _____

Members of group: _____

Plan of action:_____

4. As a class, plan and prepare activities for OT month to be held at your host facility or institution. Designate the individuals who are responsible for completing the activities and the timeline for completion.

ACTIVITIES	PERSON	TIMELINE

FOLLOW-UP

✔   Complete the Application of Competencies at the end of this chapter.
✔   Complete Performance Skill 2C on Public Relations/Service Learning.

ADVOCACY

OBJECTIVES

✔   Define terms related to marketing occupational therapy (OT) services
✔   Present the benefits of OT to a service organization
✔   Compose a presentation for marketing occupational therapy services

DESCRIPTION

In this exercise you will look at the importance of marketing and advocating for occupational therapy (OT) services. The profession of occupational therapy has continued to expand, in part, because of the many practitioners who have been able and willing to market our services to various organizations. Such action is necessary, as there are still many people and organizations that are not familiar with the services an OT practitioner can provide. Throughout your career your will undoubtedly come across individuals or groups who could benefit from OT services. It will be your responsibility to advocate for the members of those groups so that OT services may be provided. As we educate the general public and advocate for our services, our profession will continue to expand and meet the needs of the community.

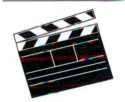

Exercise 32

"To be successful, the first thing to do is fall in love with your work."

SISTER MARY LAURETTA

PREPARATION

Suggested Readings

Neistadt and Crepeau (1998)
AOTA Web site: *www.aota.org*

Study Questions

1.   Define *marketing*.

2.   Define several *internal marketing* strategies.

3.   Define several *external marketing* strategies.

4. Describe how marketing is involved in every contact you make in which you are a representative of occupational therapy.

5. Why do you think marketing is so important to the profession of occupational therapy?

6. Describe what the American Occupational Therapy Association is doing in the area of advocacy and public awareness.

7. As a student, how do you think you can be involved in marketing?

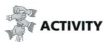 **ACTIVITY**

Materials

None.

Instructions

1. Divide into four groups. Using the following scenarios, present the need for occupational therapy services to your classmates.
   a. *Group 1:* Present to consumers of mental health services who meet in the community as a support group.
   b. *Group 2:* Present to a managed care representative (payer).
   c. *Group 3:* Present to a group of parents of preschoolers with disabilities.
   d. *Group 4:* Present to a group of medical residents on rotation at your hospital.
2. Use the space below to prepare your presentation and to record notes from your classmates' presentations.

   Group No.: _____

   Target audience: _____

   Presentation notes:

   Group No.: _____

   Target audience: _____

   Presentation notes:

   Group No.: _____

   Target audience: _____

   Presentation notes:

   Group No.: _____

   Target audience: _____

   Presentation notes:

3. Discuss the effectiveness of the presentations. Identify what seemed to be strengths and what appeared to be areas of concern for your group's presentation as well as your classmates' presentation. Be specific in your critique and give constructive suggestions for improvement.

STRENGTHS	AREAS OF CONCERN	SUGGESTIONS

FOLLOW-UP

✔   Complete the Application of Competencies at the end of this chapter.

RESEARCH

Exercise 33

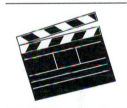

OBJECTIVES

✔   List the steps to the research process
✔   Formulate questions that may be appropriate to turn into a research project
✔   Access computer databases to obtain literature that provides pertinent information to a researchable question

DESCRIPTION

This exercise is designed to help you understand the research process. Part of the research process is doing a thorough literature review. As an occupational therapy practitioner, you will generate many questions about your practice when you are in the field. Some of these questions will be answerable only through research. Engaging in research at both the primary (actual systematic investigation) and secondary (reviewing the literature) level is part of our charge and challenge as occupational therapy practitioners. As we continue to actively engage in the research process to answer our research questions, our profession will survive and thrive.

PREPARATION

Suggested Readings

AOTA (latest edition)
American Occupational Therapy Foundation's Web site: *http://www.aotf.org*
Bailey (1997)
Neidstadt and Crepeau (1998)

Study Questions

1. Define and describe quantitative research.

"The man who does not read good books has no advantage over the man who can't read them"

MARK TWAIN

2. List and describe at least three quantitative research designs.

3. Define and describe qualitative research.

4. List and describe at least three qualitative research designs.

5. List and describe five different data collection techniques.

6. Differentiate the roles in the key performance areas for the different skill levels of occupational therapy practitioners who are functioning in the role of researcher/scholar.
   a. Entry-level

   b. Intermediate

   c. High-proficiency

7. List the steps in the research process.

8. Detail the purpose of a literature review and explain why it is important when doing a research project.

9. Explain the relevance of research for the academic discipline of occupational science and the profession of occupational therapy.

10. Go to the AOTF's Web site (*www.aotf.org*). Make a list of the content areas. For each content area, summarize the information contained therein and explain how that information might be used in conducting a literature review or engaging in the research process.

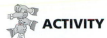 **ACTIVITY**

Materials

Flip chart, computer with online access to database resources of OT BibSys, Cumulative Index to Nursing and Allied Health Literature (CINAHL), MEDLINE, Educational Resources Information Center (ERIC), and PsychLit.

Activity

1. As a class, develop a top ten list of reasons to do research. Write down your top ten reasons; then combine, collaborate, and come to a consensus with your classmates about the best ten. Write the list on a flip chart. Title your list "Why Do Research, Why Study Research, Why Research Is Important," or use some other similarly appropriate title. Keep the list posted as a reminder of the importance of the research process and the role it plays in our profession.

2. Develop six questions that might be answerable through a research study. Generate your questions from your experience as a student in the clinical or educational setting.

   a.

   b.

   c.

   d.

   e.

   f.

3. Select one of the six questions in Activity 2 and determine the available related literature on the topic in the following computer databases. Identify the related search terms from the thesaurus of that source and list at least three sources of information from each database. Obtain a printout of the abstracts of the literature available. Summarize the information contained in the abstracts of your three sources.

SOURCE		SEARCH TERMS	SUMMARY OF INFORMATION
OT BibSys	1.		
	2.		
	3.		
CINAHL	1.		
	2.		
	3.		
MEDLINE	1.		
	2.		
	3.		
ERIC	1.		
	2.		
	3.		
PsychLit	1.		
	2.		
	3.		

4. Select one journal article from the above sources. Obtain a copy of the article and prepare to share with your classmates how the information contained therein relates to your identified question. Be sure to include the following components:
   a. Summarize the information contained in the article.
   b. Identify strengths and possible limitations of the study.
   c. Share how the information relates to your researchable question.
   d. Detail how the information can be applied to the OT process at your fieldwork or in your educational setting.
   e. Describe what additional information you would need to begin to prepare a literature review for your researchable question.
5. Share information gained from your journal article with your classmates. Use the space below to record the information they share with you.
   a. Topic:

   b. Source:

   c. Information summary:

   d. Application:

FOLLOW-UP

✔ Complete the Application of Competencies at the end of this chapter.

Exercise 34

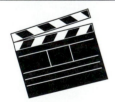

"For I might misunderstand you and the high advice you give, but there's no misunderstanding how you act and how you live."

EDGAR A. GUEST

LICENSURE

OBJECTIVES

✔ Dissect your state's licensure laws and regulations for essential information
✔ Test your knowledge regarding your state license laws and regulations
✔ Identify the expectations of a student and a practitioner as outlined in your state licensure laws and regulations

DESCRIPTION

This exercise will acquaint you with your state licensure laws. Each state has laws and rules governing the practice of occupational therapy (OT). These regulations must be adhered to in addition to the code of ethics and standards of practice as defined by the American Occupational Therapy Association. Your state laws ensure that your services protect your consumers. It is essential that you become familiar with your state laws and regulations. Adherence to the laws and regulations is imperative to practice as an OT practitioner.

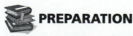 **PREPARATION**

Suggested Readings

AOTA (latest edition)
The laws and rules governing the practice of occupational therapy in your state

Study Questions

1. Fill in the following information found in your state license laws and regulations. Include information to help identify where it can be found, such as Section 1, Article 2. State the page number where the information can be found.

    State_____

    Title of Document: _____

QUESTION	ANSWER	IDENTIFYING INFORMATION	PAGE NUMBER
State the requirements to become licensed as an occupational therapy assistant (OTA) and an occupational therapist (OT).			
Define limited permit and conditions of the same.			
Describe the purpose of the licensure board.			
Describe the conditions under which a practitioner could lose his/her license.			
State the supervision requirements of COTAs.			
Describe the possible consequences of a practitioner found in violation of the licensure laws.			
Describe escrow.			
Describe the rules for displaying your license.			
Describe the continuing education requirements.			
How often are fees due?			
Describe the information given regarding limited permits.			
Describe the law as it relates to student practitioners: OT & OTA.			

2. Identify the specific principle from the Code of Ethics directing OT practitioners to follow the state licensure laws, regulations, and guidelines.

ACTIVITY
Materials

Trivial Pursuit™ game board, game pieces, dice, stop watch or one-minute egg timer. The questions you will be asked have to do with information in your state license.

GAME
Instructions

1. Play a modified game of Trivial Pursuit™. Divide into small groups of no more than four people. Take turns as a group team answering a question from the instructor about the information contained in your state licensure laws. If your team answers the question correctly within 60 seconds, roll the dice and move a game piece on the Trivial Pursuit™ game board. If your team is unable to answer the question correctly in 60 seconds, the question goes back into the instructor's stack of questions to be used later. The first team to reach the end of the board or the team that has moved the farthest wins. Record below information you learned while playing this game.

FOLLOW-UP

✔ Complete the Application of Competencies at the end of this chapter.

Exercise 35

"Whether you think you can or think you can't—you are right."

HENRY FORD

AMERICANS WITH DISABILITIES ACT

OBJECTIVES

✔ Describe the components of the Americans with Disabilities Act (ADA)
✔ Discuss "reasonable accommodations" as applicable to a variety of scenarios
✔ Define disclosure rights and responsibilities as outlined by the ADA

DESCRIPTION

This exercise will help you to understand the ramifications of the Americans with Disabilities Act (ADA). This legislative intent allows people with disabilities, through reasonable accommodations, to gain access to public buildings, transportation, recreational facilities, and places of employment. You will need to have a working knowledge of "reasonable accommodations" as an occupational therapy (OT) practitioner, for you may play a critical role in delivering the same for your clients and in training your client how to advocate for himself or herself. Additionally, as an OT practitioner, you may be evaluating and providing assistance to worksites so that their personnel can be functional in the work setting. The effects of the ADA are experienced across the life span. You will need to be well acquainted with this legislative's far reaching influences, as it is a great asset to the clients whom you will be serving.

PREPARATION
Suggested Readings

AOTA (latest edition)
Americans with Disabilities Act of 1990 (Public Law 101-336)
Equal Employment Opportunity Commission (1997)

Study Questions

1. Describe the AOTA's position on occupational therapy's role in each of the five areas of the ADA:

   a. Employment

   b. Public accommodations

   c. State and local government

   d. Public transportation

   e. Telecommunications

2. List the four parts given under the purpose of the ADA.

   a.

   b.

   c.

   d.

3. Record here the auxiliary aids and services listed in the ADA.

4. Define the term *disability* as presented in the ADA.

5. Describe what is meant by a reasonable accommodation.

6. List the factors to be considered when an accommodation may be an undue hardship.

7. Describe what constitutes a mental impairment and list the diagnoses it includes.

8. What DSM-IV diagnoses are not covered by the ADA?

9. List several life activities that may be limited for a person with a mental impairment and describe how they may be limited.

10. Describe the disclosure, rights, and responsibilities of the employer and the job applicant.
    a. Employer

    b. Applicant

11. Describe what may be included under the following accommodations:
    a. Work schedule

    b. Workplace or equipment

    c. Supervisory methods

    d. Job coach

    e. Reassignment

    f. A phone number available to employers

12. What regulations may protect an employer from an individual who may be dangerous?

13. What unique aspects of an OT's training and skills enable them to play a key role in educating the individual and the public about the ADA implications?

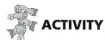 **ACTIVITY**

Materials

ADA Public Law 101-336.

Instructions

1. With a partner, determine accommodations you might suggest to clients with the following problems who are covered under the ADA. Also record whether an accommodation would be unreasonable or not as defined by the ADA. Designate this by an R for reasonable and U for unreasonable. Share your findings with the class.
   a. Tires after standing at cash register for two hours

b. Groggy from medication until 8:00 A.M.—job starts at 7:00

c. Weak hands make holding the phone impossible

d. Violent outbursts are frequent when under stress with customers

e. In the board meeting can hear only members who are sitting right next to them

f. Unable to complete writing necessary for filling out certain forms

g. Feels unsafe walking through dangerous part of plant because of vision loss

h. Absent most Mondays owing to hangover from binge drinking

i. Traveling out of town to business meetings is a great hardship because of physical condition

j. Not able to see to read computer screen to obtain e-mail messages from all employees

k. Pace of work is too rapid

l. Able to walk short distances, but job requires walking long distances.

m. Job site not on public transportation route; client unable to drive

n. Unable to climb stairs necessary to come into building at work

o. Unable to hear communication via phone necessary to follow up on customer's complaints

p. Back pain becomes unbearable after typing for two hours

q. Able to see only very large printed material

r. Steals money from other employees when not taking his or her medication

FOLLOW-UP
✔ Complete the Application of Competencies at the end of this chapter.

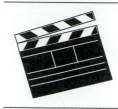

Exercise 36

"Grant that we may not so much seek to be understood as to understand."

St. Francis of Assisi

ROLE DELINEATION

OBJECTIVES

✔ Compare and contrast the role delineation of the occupational therapist (OT) and the occupational therapy assistant (OTA)
✔ Detail the supervisory relationship of the OT and the OTA
✔ Collaborate as part of an OT/OTA team to determine ongoing care for a client

DESCRIPTION

The occupational therapist (OT) and occupational therapy assistant (OTA) will work together as a team in delivering services to the client. This exercise is intended to give you practice in developing a team and collaborative relationship between the OT and the OTA. Supervision of the OTA by an OT is a must, and it is important that the role delineations are clear and that supervision involves much communication and collaboration. Establishing service competency is also a needed and vital component of the OT/OTA relationship. The stronger the relationship between the OT and the OTA, the more effective the service delivery will be. Collaboration takes initiation and persistence. The payoffs of effective collaboration are seen in client responses and positive outcome measures.

 PREPARATION

Suggested Readings

AOTA (2000)
Neidstadt and Crepeau (1998)

Study Questions

1. Who has the ethical responsibility to ensure that the amount, degree, and pattern of OT/OTA supervision is consistent with the level of their role performance?

2. Fill in the information in the following chart below describing the practitioner roles and the supervision requirements.

PERSONNEL	DESCRIPTION	SUPERVISION REQUIRED
Entry-level OT		
Intermediate-level OT		
Advanced-level OT		
Entry-level OTA		
Intermediate-level OTA		
Advanced-level OTA		

3. Summarize the four levels of supervision.

    a. Close

    b. Routine

    c. General

    d. Minimal

4. Detail the level of supervision that must occur between the OT/OTA.

5. Describe service competency.

6. Is an OTA able to initiate occupational therapy services for a new client in the absence of an OT? Is this acceptable if it occurs for only a brief period of time? Cite the source of your answers.

7. List the five factors that should be considered by the OT in determining the type of supervision required for the OTA.

    a.

    b.

    c.

    d.

    e.

8. What factor(s) may change the intensity of required supervision between the OT and the OTA?

9. Describe several methods used in providing supervision to the OTA by the OT. Align the description with the type of supervision it denotes.

ACTIVITY

Materials

Case studies 53, 43, and 46 located at the end of this chapter.

Instructions

1a. Using one of the assigned case studies and using the following guidelines as taken from the "Standards of Practice" (AOTA, 1998), work with a partner and decide which of the following specific services in the OT process can be done by the OT and which could be done by the OTA. It is understood that the OTA and OT will collaborate on all services. For this scenario the OTA is entry-level.

	OTA	OT
REFERRAL		
Accepts and responds to referral		
Refers clients		
Educates referral sources		
SCREENING		
Screens client		
Selects screening methods		
Communicates screening results		
EVALUATION		
Evaluates client		
Educates about evaluation		
Selects assessments		
Follows protocols		
Analyzes, interprets, and summarizes data		
Documents evaluation results		
Communicates evaluation results		
Recommends consultation if necessary		
INTERVENTION PLAN		
Develops intervention plan		
Prepares and documents intervention plan		
Prepares intervention goals		
Includes service provision		
Reviews intervention plan		
INTERVENTION		
Implements intervention		
Informs of benefits and risks of intervention		
Maintain current information		
Reevaluate during intervention		
Modifies intervention		
Documents services provided		
TRANSITION SERVICES		
Prepares transition plan		
Facilitates transition process		
DISCONTINUATION		
Discontinues services		
Prepares and implements discontinuation plan		
Documents changes in clients status		
Documents follow-up		

1b. Which assessments will you select to administer?

1c. How often will you reassess this client?

1d. Which supervision level is required for the OTA?

1e. Share the information with the different case studies with your class members. Record below any information you would like to remember. Go to Appendix C and discuss how the Supervision Log for OTA/OT Collaboration might be used in future practice.

2. With a paired student from either an OT or an OTA program (if you are an OTA student, pair with an OT student and vice versa), follow the directions below on the collaborative role delineation project. Assume that the OTA is a new graduate for this project and that both are working full-time in a state mental hospital. As the OT student, obtain a referral from your instructor that contains the basic information about the client. Follow the directions in a collaborative manner.

   a. *OT student:* Determine the assessment to be performed and the long- and short-term goals as indicated. Use the following space to begin your work. Once it is completed, type the information along with the basic client information you were given in the referral and send this all to the OTA student. Include your phone number and instruct the OTA student to call you on receipt of the information. (If possible, meet with each other in person to discuss the information.) Use the Supervision Log (found in the appendix) each time collaboration is initiated.

ASSESSMENTS PERFORMED	RESULTS (BUILD YOUR OWN AS YOU PROCEED)

Long-term goal 1:
Short-term goal 1a:
Short-term goal 1b:
Long-term goal 2:
Short-term goal 2a:
Short-term goal 2b:

b. *OTA student:* Review goals with the OT student and make any necessary revisions. Determine the activities appropriate for treatment by completing the treatment plan listed below. Include the activities you will use, the setup needed to complete the activities, and the estimated amount of time to completion of the activities. Note the goal that is being addressed by placing a check mark in the appropriate box. Once the plan is completed, type the information and send it to the OT student and discuss it by phone or in person to determine whether you are in agreement or revisions need to be made. Note your contact in the Supervision Log (located in the appendix). Continue to log your ensuing contacts.

| ACTIVITIES | SETUP | TIME | CHECK GOAL BEING ADDRESSED | | | | | |
			LTG 1	STG 1A	STG 1B	LTG 2	STG 2A	STG 2B

c. *OT student:* Collaborate with the OTA student to determine whether you are in agreement with the activities selected to address the goals. If you are in agreement, sign the treatment plan and return it to the OTA student.

d. *OTA student:* Write a progress note using the S.O.A.P. (subjective, objective, assessment, plan) format. Type the note and send two copies to the OT student (one of which will be returned with a countersignature).

e. *OT student:* Read and countersign the progress note. If changes need to be made, note those and return the progress note to the OTA student.

f. *OTA student:* Determine some hypothetical problem or complication that has come up in treatment that you will need assistance from the OT to help solve. Call the OT student to assist.

g. *OT student:* Assist in solving a problem that has developed in treatment. Be sure to write about this in your supervision log.

h. *OTA student:* Assume that the client has been treated and is now being discharged to another level of care. Determine the discharge setting and write a discharge summary. Type it and send it to the OT student.

i. *OT student:* Read and countersign the discharge summary. Write a discharge plan that includes recommendations to the client and possible caregivers. Send a copy of this to the OTA student along with the signed discharge summary.

j. *Both students:* After completing the above directions, type the answer to the following questions and bring them to class with your OT/OTA collaborative role delineation project for discussion.

    a. What part(s) of this exercise did you enjoy?

    b. What part(s) did you like the least?

    c. What did you learn about the OT/OTA collaborative partnership?

FOLLOW-UP

✔   Complete the Application of Competencies at the end of this chapter.
✔   Complete Performance Skill 2D on Therapeutic Use of Self.
✔   Complete Performance Skill 2E on Mock Interview.

After completing each exercise, write one thing you learned and how that learning will influence your treatment of clients.

Application of Competencies

Exercise 18 The Teaching/Learning Process
Application:

Exercise 19 Group Observation
Application:

Exercise 20 Group Leadership
Application:

Exercise 21 Group Treatment
Application:

Exercise 22 Managed Care
Application:

Exercise 23 Internet
Application:

Exercise 24 Clinical Reasoning
Application:

Exercise 25 Team Members
Application:

Exercise 26 Documentation
Application:

Exercise 27 Service Competency
Application:

Exercise 28 Service Management
Application:

Exercise 29 Supervision
Application:

Exercise 30 Professionalism
Application:

Exercise 31 Public Relations/Service Learning
Application:

Exercise 32 Advocacy
Application:

Exercise 33 Research
Application:

Exercise 34 Licensure
Application:

Exercise 35 Americans with Disabilities Act
Application:

Exercise 36 Role Delineation
Application:

Performance Skill 2A

TEACHING AN OCCUPATION

Teach an activity or craft of your choice to one or more of your classmates. Formulate the following teaching process plan to assist you.

1. Activity/craft:
2. Time needed to complete the activity/craft:
3. Number of students to teach:
4. Complete the following sections of the teaching process (Ryan, 1995a) and place a check mark in the designated column as each section is completed.

STEPS	COMPLETE
Learning objectives	
Content	
Modifications	
Steps to activity	
Materials assembly	
Workspace arrangement	
Patient or group preparation	
Instruction presentation	
Trial run of task	
Performance assessment	

5. Review your strengths and areas of concern from the activities in this section to help prepare you to teach your activity or craft. What do you need to remember to do?

6. Complete the following final check before teaching your activity or craft.
   a. Will it help to have a copy of directions for you to follow?
   b. Will it help to have a sample completed?
   c. Will it help to have diagrams?
   d. Will it help to have a sample completed in different stages?
   e. Will your learners be able to complete the entire project in the time allowed? If not, have you given all the instructions necessary for them to complete it on their own? Have you checked their performance?
   f. What could go wrong? What will you do to prevent it?
   g. What will you do if things go wrong anyway?
   h. Will your activity take the entire time? What will you do if your learners finish early?
   i. Have you selected an activity that meets the abilities and interests of your learners?
   j. Are there any adaptations that may be needed?

LEADING A GROUP

Performance Skill 2B

With a small group, plan and lead a group for the rest of your classmates. Determine the needs of your classmates, then select a topic and activity. Identified needs may be related to stress management, study skills, or time management, for example. Use this worksheet to brainstorm and begin your planning.

Members in your planning group:

Members to whom your group will present:

Time frame:

1. Needs of classmates:
   a.

   b.

   c.

   d.

   e.

   f.

2. Select one need from above that your small group will address.
3. Write three objectives that your group will accomplish:

    a.

    b.

    c.

4. Which frame of reference will you use?

5. Brainstorm and list possible activities to use to meet your stated objectives.

    a.

    b.

    c.

    d.

    e.

    f.

    g.

    h.

    i.

    j.

6. Complete a teaching process plan on the activity or activities you selected (see Performance Skill 2A).
7. Divide the tasks of the lesson plan among your small group. Determine who will carry out each step.
8. What outcome criteria will you use to measure progress?

PUBLIC RELATIONS/SERVICE LEARNING

Performance Skill 2C

Work in your small group as designated in Exercise 31. Participate in the public relations or service learning project to promote occupational therapy as determined in the exercise. Discuss with your group how to proceed. Follow the steps and directions below to develop your plan for this.

1. Name of selected agency, organization, or individual:

2. Selected plan of action/project:

3. Establish long-term and short-term goals for completion of your project.

   a. Long-term goals: _____

   _____

   _____

   b. Short-term goals: _____

   _____

   _____

4. Establish a plan to meet the goals. Begin to carry out the activities as indicated by the target dates.

ACTIVITIES	STUDENT(S) RESPONSIBLE	TARGET DATE

5. Decide on your next meeting date: _____

    Time: _____

    Place: _____

6. Record progress of members here, note whether goals have been met or not and to what degree:

7. Discuss and establish activities that remain to be completed. Continue to complete the following plan, carrying out the activities in a timely manner.

ACTIVITIES	STUDENT(S) RESPONSIBLE	TARGET DATE

8. Decide on your next meeting date: _____

    Time: _____

    Place: _____

9. Record progress toward your goals and finalize your plans below. Bring your public relations or service learning project to closure.

10. As a group, develop an evaluation form to be completed by the individuals to whom you provided the public relations or service learning project. Develop an additional form that will summarize your assessment of your group member's par-

ticipation and performance. Provide opportunity for the evaluation forms to be completed by the designated parties. Turn these evaluation forms in to your instructor. Use the space below to draft your work. Prepare a final product that is neatly typed and professional in content and appearance.

a. Community evaluation:

b. Peer evaluation:

11. Reflect upon your groups' contribution. Discuss as a class, the growth, learning, insights, and rewards that were realized.

THERAPEUTIC USE OF SELF

Performance Skill 2D

Take a look to see how much you incorporate your therapeutic use of self. Reflect on the feedback you have received from your peers, supervisors, and instructors during your course of study. Now step back and summarize the effect of this. Think about yourself in a focused way so that you become more aware of the personal resources that you bring to the therapeutic relationship. Write a paper describing your skill at using your therapeutic use of self. Follow the directions developed by Neistadt (1996).

Analysis of Therapeutic Self

In an 8- to 10-page paper:
1. Describe your personal style, referencing the following qualities. In your descriptions, include examples of illustrative behaviors that you have demonstrated in clinical helping relationships. (You may want to reflect on your level I experiences.) The following qualities are in alphabetical order—you do not have to follow this order in your paper. Rather, we would like you to choose whatever organization works best for you. The comments after each quality are meant simply to give you some ideas or to clarify the concepts.
   a. Affect, emotional tone (enthusiastic, energetic, serious, low key)
   b. Attending and listening (including your ability to reflect back on and add to what the speaker has said)
   c. Cognitive style (detail or gestalt oriented, abstract or concrete, ability to understand diverse points of view)
   d. Confidence (not only what you feel, but also what you think you show to other)
   e. Confrontation (can you do it with whom?)
   f. Empathy (for what emotions, in what situations?)
   g. Humor (do you use it, and if so, how?)
   h. Leadership style (directive, facilitative, follower)
   i. Nonverbal communication (facial expressiveness, eye contact, voice tone and volume, gestures)
   j. Power sharing (need to control, comfortable with chaos)
   k. Probing (when are you comfortable doing it, with whom, and about what?)
   l. Touch (do you use it automatically or consciously, when, where, and with whom?)
   m. Verbal communication (vocabulary, use of vernacular, ease of speaking)
2. Summarize what you see as your strengths and weaknesses relative to establishing therapeutic relationships.

3. In anticipation of your upcoming Level II fieldwork experience, delineate areas or skills that you would like to improve and suggest strategies for doing so.

You will be graded on your organization, the clarity of your writing (including how well your examples illustrate your descriptions), and your thoroughness in completing the assignment. Content here is personal and, therefore, not gradeable.

Note: Developed by Maureen E. Neistadt, ScD, OTR/L, FAOTA, for the Interactive Reasoning Seminar at Tufts University, Medford, Massachusetts, 1989.

Taken from: Neidstadt, M.E. (1996). Teaching strategies for the development of clinical reasoning. American Journal of Occupational Therapy, 50 (8), 676–684. [Used with permission.]

Performance Skill 2E

MOCK INTERVIEW

Participate in a mock job interview. Contact a local facility to set up an interview with the director of an occupational therapy department. Prepare a resume and cover letter to bring with you to the interview. On completion of the interview, obtain feedback on your performance. Use the following guide to help you prepare. Note that your interview begins the minute you make contact with the facility.

1. Become knowledgeable about the facility before your interview. Obtain the following information through the human resources or public relations office of the facility.

   Facility: _____

   Owned by: _____

   Affiliated with: _____

   Number of OTs: _____

   Number of OTAs: _____

   Other departments on the treatment team: _____

   Number of beds: _____

   Accredited by: _____

   Mission of the facility: _____

   Population served: _____

   Philosophy, theory base, and/or frame of reference used: _____

   Support provided for research: _____

   What else?_____

2. Prepare your questions ahead of time. What do you want to know about this facility as a potential future employment site?

   a.

   b.

   c.

d.

e.

f.

g.

h.

i.

j.

3. Update and proofread your resumé. What changes need to be made?

4. Prepare your cover letter specific to your interview site. Prepare an outline of the letter here.

5. Obtain written feedback on your performance from the department director with whom you interviewed, using a copy of the following form:

INTERVIEW FEEDBACK FORM					
COMPONENTS	RATE THE STUDENT (1–5)				
Initial telephone contact impression	1	2	3	4	5
Promptness to the interview	1	2	3	4	5
Physical appearance during interview	1	2	3	4	5
Cover letter introducing self	1	2	3	4	5
Resumé of employment and education history	1	2	3	4	5
Communication skills:					
Via telephone and during interview	1	2	3	4	5
Questions asked	1	2	3	4	5
Questions answered	1	2	3	4	5
Nonverbal communication and presentation	1	2	3	4	5
Preparedness and beforehand knowledge of facility	1	2	3	4	5

Rating scale
1 — poor
2 — fair
3 — good
4 — very good
5 — excellent

Strengths:

Areas of concern:

Additional comments:

CASE STUDY 8

ADULT PHYSICAL REHABILITATION

Type:
Acute Care

Age:
76 years old

Sex:
Female

Culture/Religion:

Insurance Information:

Diagnosis:
Left occipital craniotomy, duroplasty, cranioplasty

Social History:
Diane lives alone, but her daughter is visiting from out of town now. Diane has no other children. She lives in her own home and has two cats. Before admission she was independent in all homemaking tasks, including yard work and flower gardening, which are her favorite hobbies.

Diane's husband died six years ago after a heart attack. She continues to be very active with their friends at church and those with whom they played cards.

Medical History:
Diane requires moderate assistance of one to transfer and to come to sitting in bed. She complains of back pain when sitting and dizziness when coming from supine to sit. She also complains of pressure on her scalp lesion.

Diane is dependent for all self-care at this time. She attempts to feed herself but appears to be having motor planning difficulties.

She also seems to be neglecting objects on her right side. Diane is being seen by Speech Therapy due to exhibiting expressive communication problems, using inappropriate words. She is also being seen by PT, where she is learning to use the walker.

Diane has ROM WNL in all extremities. Her strength is WNL on the left side and fair overall on her right side. She displays fine motor problems on her right side and frequently drops items that are placed in her hand. Diane has intact sharp/dull; impaired localization, proprioception, and stereognosis.

CASE STUDY 9

ADULT PSYCHOSOCIAL

Type:
Acute Care

Age:
35 years old

Sex:
Female

Culture/Religion:

Insurance Information:

Diagnosis:
Bipolar affective disorder, schizophrenia

Social History:

Shirley lives alone in a one-bedroom apartment. She works as a secretary for a small business. She has a boyfriend of three years who has a diagnosis of obsessive-compulsive disorder. He has required hospitalization twice in the past two years. Shirley reports being unsure of this relationship. They enjoy going to movies and nightclubs on the weekends.

Medical History:

Shirley was admitted complaining of inability to function at home or work. She has been suffering from insomnia for the past several weeks which seems to be getting worse. She reports getting upset with her coworkers and losing her temper frequently. Shirley reports that her thoughts are confused, her mind is racing, and she cannot focus. She feels she is getting paranoid and has been obsessing about religion.

Shirley's case manager feels that she has been decompensating. Shirley is also experiencing financial difficulties because of missed work from being ill.

Shirley was diagnosed with schizophrenia at the age of 20. She has a history of smoking and drinking excessively by the age of 14. At age 17 she used LSD and cocaine. She has been hospitalized in two institutions, once for more than one year.

Shirley is oriented x3, her memory is satisfactory, and judgment and insight are partial.

CASE STUDY 10

ADULT PHYSICAL REHABILITATION

Type:
Acute Care

Age:
81 years old

Sex:
Male

Culture/Religion:

Insurance Information:

Diagnosis:
Left hemiplegia, HTN, emphysema, cerebral atherosclerosis

Social History:

Craig lives with his brother in their home. Both men are widowers with no children. Craig did the cooking and gardening; his brother did the cleaning. Both men enjoy playing cards and watching TV.

Medical History:

Craig suffered a stroke three days ago. He is oriented x3 and can follow three-step commands, and his memory is WFL. He hopes to return to his previous living arrangement.

Craig has left UE 20° shoulder flexion, 5° abduction, 10° shoulder extension, and 10° wrist extension and flexion. He has trace mass grasp and 0° finger extension. He has left shoulder subluxation with sharp pain with PROM past 95° flexion and abduction.

Craig requires moderate assistance to roll side to side and maximal assistance to bridge and scoot. He requires maximal assistance to come to sit and maximum assistance in unsupported sitting. He transfers with maximum assistance and requires maximum assistance with all of his self-care needs.

REFERENCES

Acquaviva, Jane D. 1998. *Effective Documentation for Occupational Therapy.* Bethesda, MD: *American Occupational Therapy Association.*

American Occupational Therapy Association. 1991. *S.P.I.C.E.S.: Self-Paced Introduction for Clinical Education and Supervision.* Bethesda, MD: Author.

American Occupational Therapy Association. 2000. *COTA Information Packet: 2000.* Bethesda, MD: Author.

American Occupational Therapy Association. 1996. *Managed Care: An Occupational Therapy Source Book.* Bethesda, MD: Author.

American Occupational Therapy Association. 1998. *Elements of Clinical Documentation (revision) in Reference Manual of the Official Documents of the American Occupational Therapy Association.* 7th ed. Bethesda, MD: Author.

American Occupational Therapy Association. 1998. *Standards of Practice in Reference Manual of the Official Documents of the American Occupational Therapy Association.* 7th ed. Bethesda, MD: Author.

American Occupational Therapy Association. latest edition. *Reference Manual of the Official Documents of the American Occupational Therapy Association.* Bethesda, MD: Author.

Americans with Disabilities Act of 1990. P.L. 101–336, 42 U.S.C., 12101, Federal Register, vol. 56: 144, 35543–35691.

Bailey, D. M. 1997. *Research for the Health Professional: A Practical Guide.* 2d ed. Philadelphia: F. A. Davis.

Christiansen, C., and C. Baum. 1997. *Occupational Therapy: Enabling Function and Well-Being.* 2d ed. Thorofare, NJ: Slack.

Cole, M. B. 1998. *Group Dynamics in Occupational Therapy: The Theoretical Basis and Practice Application of Group Treatment.* Thorofare, NJ: Slack.

Equal Employment Opportunity Commission. 1997. *EEOC Enforcement Guidance: The Americans with Disabilities Act and Psychiatric Disabilities.* 915.002.

Gibbs, S., M. Sullivan-Fowler, and N. W. Rowe. 1996. *Mosby's Medical Surfari: A Guide to Exploring the Internet and Discovering the Top Health Care Resources.* Chicago: Mosby.

Howe, M. C., and S. L. Schwartzberg. 1995. *A Functional Approach to Group Work in Occupational Therapy.* Philadelphia: J. B. Lippincott.

Korb, K. L., S. D. Azok, and E. A. Leutenberg. 1989. *Life Management Skills: Reproducible Activity Handouts Created for Facilitators.* Beechwood, OH: Wellness Reproduction.

Korb-Khalsa, K. L., S. D. Azok, and E. A. Leutenberg. 1993. *Life Management Skills II: Reproducible Activity Handouts Created for Facilitators.* Beechwood, OH: Wellness Reproduction.

Korb-Khalsa, K. L., S. D. Azok, and E. A. Leutenberg. 1995a. *Life Management Skills III: Reproducible Activity Handouts Created for Facilitators.* Beechwood, OH: Wellness Reproduction.

Korb-Khalsa, K. L., S. D. Azok, and E. A. Leutenberg. 1995b. *S.E.A.L.S. +Plus.* Beechwood, OH: Wellness Reproduction.

Mattingly, C., and M. H. Fleming. 1994. *Clinical Reasoning: Focus of Inquiry in a Therapeutic Practice.* Philadelphia: F. A. Davis.

Mosey, A. C. 1986. *Psychosocial Components of Occupational Therapy.* New York: Raven Press.

Neidstadt, M. E. 1996. "Teaching Strategies for the Development of Clinical Reasoning." *American Journal of Occupational Therapy,* 50(8): 676–684.

Neidstadt, M. E., and E. B. Crepeau. 1998. *Willard and Spackman's Occupational Therapy.* 9th ed. Philadelphia: J. B. Lippincott.

Pomeroy, B. 1997. *Beginnernet in Rehabilitation: A Beginner's Guide to the Internet—the World Wide Web.* Thorofare, NJ: Slack.

Purtilo, R., and A. Haddad. 1996. *Health Professional and Patient Interaction.* Philadelphia: W. B. Saunders.

Reed K. L., and S. N. Sanderson. 1999. *Concepts of Occupational Therapy.* 4th ed. Philadelphia: Lippincott Williams & Wilkins.

Rider, B. B., and J. S. Rider. 1999. *Book of Activity Cards for Mental Health.* Kalamazoo, MI: Authors.

Ryan, S. E. ed. 1995a. *The Certified Occupational Therapy Assistant: Principles, Concepts and Techniques.* 2d ed. Thorofare, NJ: Slack.

Ryan, S. E. ed. 1995b. *Practice Issues in Occupational Therapy: Intraprofessional Team Building.* Thorofare, NJ: Slack.

Thomson, L. K., D. Lieberman, R. Murphy, E. Wendt, J. Poole, and S. D. Hertfelder. 1995. *Developing, Maintaining, and Updating Competency in Occupational Therapy: A Guide to Self-Appraisal.* Bethesda, MD: American Occupational Therapy Association.

Competencies in Pediatric Practice

Exercise 37

"Look for strength in people, not weaknesses, good, not evil. Most of us find what we search for."

ANONYMOUS

OBSERVATION

OBJECTIVES

✔ Identify significant components of the clinical observation process
✔ Describe the use of skilled clinical observations in the evaluation process
✔ Differentiate behaviors that are considered typical and atypical of a child

DESCRIPTION

This exercise is designed to improve your observation skills. Observation is a critical component of the evaluation process. As an occupational therapy practitioner you need to have acute, accurate, and context-related observation skills. In observing children, it is important to know typical development so that your observations can be astute in perceiving deviations from what is typical. Observation in a clinical setting is an ongoing responsibility that will provide you with valuable information. Skilled observation provides critical and unique information that other assessment tools cannot provide.

 PREPARATION

Suggested Readings

Case-Smith, Allen, and Pratt (1996)
Dunn (1991)
Parham and Fazio (1997)

Study Questions

1. Define skilled observation.

2. How does skilled observation relate to the evaluation process?

3. What are important components to include when completing a skilled observation?

4. Describe the importance of the context when doing a skilled observation.

5. Describe the importance of understanding typical development in doing a skilled observation.

6. Give three ways in which direct skilled observations may be recorded.

7. What are clinical observations?

8. Using the "Activity Observation Guide" and the "Social Behavior Observation Guide" in Parham and Fazio (1997), list the headings that may be used to document observation.

9. Write the heading from the "Checklist for Clinical Observations of Neuromotor Status" (Case-Smith, Allen, and Pratt, 1996) for each of the following clinical observations:

    a. Following an object with the eyes

    b. Rolling over

    c. Crawling

    d. Reflexes

    e. Strength

    f. Limitations in movement

    g. Hypotonia

    h. Position of standing

    i. Walk on stairs

    j. Head righting

    k. Crossing midline

    l. Response to being held

    m. Hand dominance

10. Describe the following terms as they relate to clinical observations of neuromotor status as typically used in assessment of sensory integration:

   a. Crossing body midline

   b. Equilibrium reactions

   c. Prone extension

   d. Supine flexion

11. Describe two settings and give examples of information you would gather during an informal observation of sensory integration.

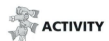 **ACTIVITY**

Materials

Children from a daycare center, a child from a clinic setting.

Instructions

1. Observe typical children in a daycare center or similar facility. Your observations will be naturalistic and informal in nature. Choose two children of different ages and record observations as listed below.

OBSERVATIONS	CHILD 1 ESTIMATED AGE _____	CHILD 2 ESTIMATED AGE _____
Describe physical appearance.		
ACTIVITY/OCCUPATION What is the child doing? Is he/she playing with others? How? Quality of eye contact? Verbal communication? Nonverbal communication? Length of attention span? Did child share? If so, How? How much space did he/she use? What senses is he/she using? Does he/she play purposefully? Does he/she put closure on activity before moving to next activity?		

MOTOR SKILLS How fluid or awkward are movements? Does he/she cross midline? Avoid crossing? How does he/she use both extremities? Keep his/her balance? Preference or avoidance for movement activities?		
HAND USE Describe grasp. Type of prehension, e.g., pincer? Evidence of tremors? Preference or avoidance of hand activities? Success experienced? Show a preferred or more skilled hand?		
MOUTH FUNCTION Does the child put objects in mouth? Hands in mouth? Position of child's mouth at rest? Any drooling noted around mouth? Describe.		

2. Discuss observations with your class and note areas you need to observe further.

3. Observe a child in a clinical setting. On completion of your observation, fill in the following observation form:

Appearance: Select a position and describe the child from head to toe. This is like a *snapshot*. Be sure to note differences in right or left side when indicated.

Position of child: ☐ Standing   ☐ Sitting   ☐ Lying   ☐ Kneeling

☐ Other: _____

Position of head: _____

Description of hair: _____

Description of eyes: _____

Description/position of mouth: _____

Any other facial features, scars, sores, saliva, nasal discharge, food, etc: _____

_____

Description and position of:

Shoulders: _____

Elbows: _____

Wrist: _____

Hands: _____

Trunk: _____

Hips: _____

Knees: _____

Feet: _____

Description of clothing: _____

Description of any splints, braces, or other equipment: _____

_____

Overall impression of appearance: _____

> **Communication:** Describe how the child communicates. Include all forms of communication.

Method of communication used most frequently: ☐ Verbal ☐ Nonverbal

Tone of voice: _____

Receptive language: _____

Initiation of conversation: _____

Expressive language: _____

Describe any unusual vocalizations: _____

Give an example of what the child says, to whom, and in what context: _____

_____

_____

_____

Describe gestures used, to whom, and in what context: _____

_____

_____

Describe sign language used, to whom, and in what context: _____

_____

Describe any other comments or types of communication used, including any argu-

mentative communication devices: _____

_____

Overall impression of communication: _____

Emotion: Describe the emotional responses of the child including how emotions are displayed and in what context. Note the changes experienced during the session. Infer the emotional state associated with the observed behavior.

BEHAVIOR	DESCRIBE SITUATION INVOLVED	RELATED EMOTIONAL STATE

Overall impression of emotional tone during session: _____

Response to Intervention: Describe how the child responded to the intervention/activity/occupation used. It may not be possible to include all of the components you are observing so focus on just one activity.

Task: _____

Attended to task _____ minutes/seconds at a time (circle one).

Ability/quality of performance: How successfully was the task accomplished? (e.g., hit the target, propelled through maze, buttoned one-inch buttons, tied shoes tight)

_____

_____

_____

_____

_____

Assistance required: _____

_____

Describe gross motor activities: Position of body, use of all extremities together:

_____

_____

_____

Describe use of hands: How are they being used; describe grasp:

Right hand: _____

_____

Left hand: _____

_____

Oral motor: Drink from cup, bottle, straw; blow; suck; close lips; move tongue; etc.: _

_____

_____

Tactile system: Describe tactile intervention and response of the child: _____

_____

_____

_____

Vestibular/proprioceptive system: Describe movement intervention and responses of

the child: _____

_____

_____

Treatment technique: Describe the intervention performed and the response of the child:

_____

_____

Adaptations/modifications made: _____

Overall impression of performance: _____

Social Involvement: Describe how the child relates to peers.

Peers present: _____

Describe environment/situation: _____

_____

Describe interaction(s): _____

_____

Describe response of child to peers: _____

_____

Describe response of peers to child: _____

_____

Overall impression of social skills: _____

> **Reaction to Authority:**   Describe how the child relates to therapists, staff members, students, teachers, and parents.

Describe separation from parent/caregiver: _____

_____

Engagement in directed activity: _____

_____

Response to redirection: _____

_____

_____

Content of conversation areas: _____

_____

Motivational techniques employed and response from child: _____

_____

_____

Acceptance of praise: _____

Overall impression of relationship to authority: _____

4. Following this second documentation, discuss your observations with the class. Fill in where you have missed information. List here *your* strengths and weaknesses in completing a skilled clinical observation and a plan to improve your skills.

STRENGTHS	AREAS OF CONCERN

FOLLOW-UP

✔ Complete the Application of Competencies at the end of this chapter.
✔ Complete a Therapeutic Use of Self Analysis found in Appendix B on your documentation of observation skills.

Exercise 38

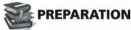

"Occupation is the very life of life."

HAROLD BELL WRIGHT

THE EVALUATION PROCESS

OBJECTIVES

✔ Describe the role of evaluation in the occupational therapy process
✔ Compare and contrast different assessment tools
✔ Administer a standardized pediatric assessment

DESCRIPTION

This exercise will help you to become familiar with the evaluation process and standardized testing in particular. The evaluation process begins after the referral is received as the screening indicates that such is needed. As part of the evaluation process, many types of tools or assessments may be used, including but not limited to interview, observation, inventories and scales, and standardized and nonstandardized tests. Becoming familiar with standardized testing is a good place to start in learning about specific assessments that will be used in the evaluation process. Standardized tests have specific procedures to follow and specific directions that are to be used each time the test is given. Both the occupational therapist (OT) and the occupational therapy assistant (OTA) can administer standardized tests.

PREPARATION

Suggested Readings

AOTA (1998)
Case-Smith, Allen, and Pratt (1996)
Frankenburg, Dodds, Archer, Bresnick, Maschka, Edelman, and Shapiro (1992)
Hinojosa and Kramer (1998)

Study Questions

1. Describe the purpose of the following types of assessments used in the evaluation process of children and give an example of each.

	PURPOSE	EXAMPLE
Interview		
Observation		
Inventories/scales/checklists		
Criterion-referenced test		
Norm-referenced test		

2. What is a standardized test?

3. What is the purpose of standardized tests in occupational therapy?

4. Define the concepts of reliability and validity.

5. Describe the inter-rater reliability of tests and how you think this may relate to service competency in test administration by an OTA.

6. Describe how to become competent in administration of test instruments.

7. Delineate the role and responsibilities of the OTA and OT in administering tests and assessments.

8. Calculate the following ages according to the specification in the Denver II Training Manual (Frankenburg et al., 1992), using the problem setup lines below. Use the test date of 6/5/00 for all of your calculations.

    a. Child's birthdate: January 6, 1999   c. Child's birthday: August 30, 1997

       Problem setup: _____   Problem setup: _____

                      _____   _____

    Age of child: _____   Age of child: _____

b. Child's birthdate: April 29, 1996   d. Child's birthday: January 7, 1998

Problem setup: _____   Problem set-up:_____

_____   _____

Age of child: _____   Age of child: _____

9. List the steps to prepare the Denver II (Frankenburg et al., 1992) form before administering the screening tool.

10. Use the child's age in Study Question 8a and list the test item you would begin with in each section of the Denver II (Frankenburg et al., 1992):

a. Personal social

b. Language

c. Fine motor-adaptive

d. Gross motor

11. Describe the criteria used to determine whether an item is failed on the Denver II (Frankenburg et al., 1992).

12. Describe the criteria used to determine whether an item is passed on the Denver II (Frankenburg et al., 1992).

13. List the five possible individual item interpretations and the criteria for each interpretation on the Denver II.

Rating: _____   Criteria: _____

_____

Rating: _____   Criteria: _____

_____

Rating: _____   Criteria: _____

_____

Rating: _____   Criteria: _____

_____

Rating: _____   Criteria: _____

_____

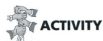 **ACTIVITY**

Materials

VCR, videotape of *Denver II: Training Video* (Frankenburg, 1990), Denver II (Frankenburg et al., 1992) test kits and forms, Bruininks-Oseretsky Test of Motor Proficiency (Bruininks, 1978) test kits and forms, Visual Motor Integration Test (VMI) (Beery, 1989) test manual and booklets, and other standardized tests as available from instructor.

Instructions

1. Take a few minutes to plan a mock situation in which you are a parent of a child who is about to receive occupational therapy services. Record your information below as you plan out your scenario. Conduct a short, semiformal interview with a peer who is assuming the role of a parent of a young client. Switch roles and allow the peer to interview you. Interview your partner and obtain information about the simulated child's reason for referral, history, diagnosis, living conditions, areas of strength, and areas of concern. Record the information from your parent interview as you go. Switch roles and allow the peer to interview you.

   YOUR SCENARIO

   a. Reason for referral

   b. History

   c. Diagnosis

   d. Living conditions

   e. Strengths

   f. Areas of concern

   YOUR "PARENT" INTERVIEW

   a. Reason for referral

b. History

c. Diagnosis

d. Living conditions

e. Strengths

f. Areas of concern

2. Watch the videotape of Denver II (Frankenburg et al., 1990) administration and record important points here.

3. Role-play with a partner how you would describe this screening tool to the child's parents. Prepare below.
   a. Introduce self.

   b. What information do you need to obtain from the parent before administering the Denver II (Frankenburg et al., 1992)?

   c. Explain the three points you need to tell the parent:

      (1)

      (2)

      (3)

4. Practice administering various items from the Denver II (Frankenburg et al., 1992) to a partner in class. Fill in the following self-evaluation on completion. To become competent in administering and interpreting the Denver II, see your instructor to take the Denver II proficiency tests and continue to practice administering the test to typical children.

ITEMS YOU ADMINISTERED	ITEMS YOU NEED TO PRACTICE	COMPONENTS OF ADMINISTRATION NEEDING CLARIFICATION

5. Watch your instructor's demonstration of the administration of the Bruininks Oseretsky Test of Motor Proficiency (Bruininks, 1978). Record important administration points here.

a. Prepare first, then find a partner and role-play how you would introduce this test to a child's caregivers and to a child.

CAREGIVER	CHILD

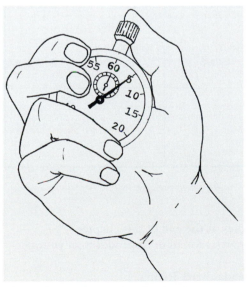

Fig. 3-1

b. Practice administering various sections of the test to a partner, and fill in the following self-evaluation on completion. Work in groups of three with one student serving as an observer. Have the observer follow along in the manual and assist in providing feedback on the accuracy of test administration.

ITEMS YOU ADMINISTERED WELL	ITEMS YOU NEED TO PRACTICE	COMPONENTS OF ADMINISTRATION NEEDING CLARIFICATION

6. Continue the above process of administering standardized tests for each new test available in your lab. Start with the VMI (Beery, 1989). Record the tests you use here along with an overview of your performances.

NAME OF TEST	STRENGTHS IN ADMINISTRATION	PREPARATION NEEDED FOR COMPETENCY IN ADMINISTRATION

FOLLOW-UP

✔ Complete the Application of Competency at the end of this chapter.
✔ Complete a Therapeutic Use of Self Analysis found in Appendix B on your performance of standardized testing.
✔ Complete Performance Skill 3D on Standardized Testing.

PEDIATRIC INTERVENTION AREAS

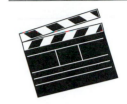

Exercise 39

OBJECTIVES

✔ List general pediatric intervention areas
✔ Align occupational therapy performance deficits with choice of intervention activities
✔ Identify diagnoses that typically exhibit deficits in the occupational therapy performance components

"For children is there any happiness which is not also noise?"

FREDERICK W. FABER

DESCRIPTION

This exercise is designed to acquaint you with a variety of general intervention areas that are addressed in pediatric settings. A variety of techniques and activities can be used to remediate deficits that children may have in the occupational therapy performance areas and components. It will be important for you to align the activities with the occupational therapy performance areas and components with the child's diagnosis, goals, and interests. It is also important to incorporate the chosen activities in a climate of play. A playful environment will capture a child's interest and motivate him or her to engage in the activity. Making the activity fun or "gamelike" will hold the child's interest and encourage participation.

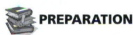 **PREPARATION**

Suggested Readings

Case-Smith, Allen, and Pratt (1996)
Scheerer (1997)

Study Questions

1. Divide into small groups to obtain information on treatment techniques. Your group will be assigned one or two of the occupational therapy (OT) performance areas related to pediatrics as outlined below. Search the OT literature for treatment techniques in the area(s) you have been assigned. Give examples of the type of child (including diagnosis) that may benefit from the treatment technique(s) you describe. Prepare a presentation to be given to your classmates. Plan to bring materials with you that may demonstrate the treatment technique(s). Prepare a handout for distribution to all students. Circle the area(s) you have been given, along with listing your partner or group member's names.

   AREAS OF INTERVENTION:
   a. Fine motor/hand grasp
   b. Handwriting
   c. Gross motor
   d. Postural control
   e. Muscle tone
   f. Visual-motor integration
   g. Oral motor
   h. Activities of daily living
   i. Psychosocial/emotional/behavioral

Group: _____
Use the space below to plan your handout and presentation.
Area of intervention:

Resources used to find information:

Diagnoses of children who may require intervention in this area:

Description of treatment interventions:

Materials for demonstration:

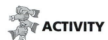 **ACTIVITY**

Materials

Materials brought by the students for their demonstration of treatment technique(s).

Instructions

1. Present your group's treatment ideas, allowing time for classmates to experiment with the treatment method and activities. Include a handout with basic information for each member of your class. Record below any additional information you want to remember about your classmate's treatment ideas as well as ideas added by your instructor:

    a. Fine motor/hand grasp:

    b. Handwriting:

    c. Gross motor:

    d. Postural control:

    e. Muscle tone:

    f. Visual-motor integration:

    g. Oral motor:

    h. Activities of daily living:

    i. Psychosocial/emotional/behavioral:

FOLLOW-UP

✔ Complete the Application of Competency at the end of this chapter.
✔ Complete Performance Skill 3A on Adding to Your Files.

RANGE OF MOTION

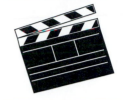

OBJECTIVES

✔ Differentiate between active and passive range of motion
✔ Delineate the purpose and use of range of motion as an assessment and as an intervention
✔ Memorize the potential range of each body joint

DESCRIPTION

Range of motion (ROM) is the arc of motion through which a joint moves. Different joints move in different directions, including flexion, extension, abduction, adduction, supination, pronation, external rotation, and internal rotation. ROM measurements are often obtained as part of the initial assessment and collected again as part of the interim and final assessments. Additionally, ROM can be used as an enabling treatment technique. It is important to understand its use and role in both assessment and intervention. ROM is presented in more depth in Chapter 5 of this manual.

"When you are dealing with a child keep all your wits about you, and sit on the floor."

AUSTIN O'MALLEY

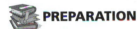 **PREPARATION**

Suggested Readings

Case-Smith, Allen, and Pratt (1996)
Pierson (1999)

Study Questions

1. Define ROM.

2. Differentiate between active and passive ROM.

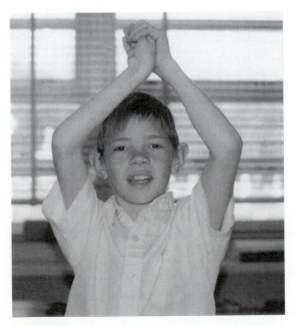

Fig. 3-2 Child self-ranging his right shoulder.
Photo courtesy of Danny Callahan.

3. When do passive and active ROM exercises need to be considered and included?

4. When might ROM assessment be indicated?

5. Fill in the following chart.

MOVEMENT	DESCRIBE STARTING POSITION	HAND PLACEMENT	MOTION
SHOULDER Flexion			
Extension			
Horizontal adduction			
Horizontal abduction			
Rotation			
Adduction			
Abduction			
ELBOW Flexion			
Extension			
FOREARM Supination			
Pronation			
WRIST Flexion			
Extension			
Ulnar deviation			
Radial deviation			
FINGER Flexion			
Extension			

Abduction			
Adduction			
Metacarpophalangeal (MP) flexion and interphalangeal (IP) extension			
THUMB Opposition			
Flexion			
Extension			
Abduction			
Adduction			

ACTIVITY

Materials

Various children's items such as stacking rings, blocks, balls, busy box, beanbags, bubbles, balloons, and large, soft-textured positioning dolls.

Instructions

1. Your instructor will demonstrate proper ROM techniques and discuss precautions. List precautions here.

2a. Perform the following passive ranges with a doll, then with your partner. Write the feedback given to you by your peers and instructor. Your instructor may initial each motion as you demonstrate competence in performing it. Practice with your partner (as if he or she were a child), performing ranges in different positions such as standing, supine, prone, sitting, and side lying. List the equipment and activities that can be used to promote ROM. Obtain some of your ideas from the children's activities available in the lab.

MOVEMENT	FEEDBACK ON STARTING POSITION	FEEDBACK ON HAND PLACEMENT	FEEDBACK ON MOTION
SHOULDER Flexion			
Extension			
Horizontal adduction			

Horizontal adduction			
Rotation			
Adduction			
Abduction			
ELBOW Flexion			
Extension			
FOREARM Supination			
Pronation			
WRIST Flexion			
Extension			
Ulnar deviation			
Radial deviation			
FINGER Flexion			
Extension			
Abduction			
Adduction			
MP flexion and IP extension			
THUMB Opposition			
Flexion			
Extension			
Abduction			
Adduction			
Equipment to promote ROM			
Activities to promote ROM			

2b. Summarize feedback you received from instructors and peers:

2c. How might you improve your skills at ROM?

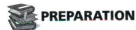 **GAME**

3. As a review, play a game of Simon Says using range of motion. Take turns being Simon. Have Simon stand before the class identifying and demonstrating the range of motion movements you just learned. Periodically have Simon say one motion but demonstrate another to confuse you. List below any movements you were unable to recall:

FOLLOW-UP

✔ Complete the Application of Competency at the end of this chapter.
✔ Complete a Therapeutic Use of Self Analysis found in Appendix B on your skill in performing range of motion.

POSITIONING AND HANDLING

Exercise 41

OBJECTIVES

✔ Identify and justify a variety of therapeutic positions
✔ Demonstrate proper body mechanics and lifting technique
✔ Incorporate positioning and handling in a therapeutic context

DESCRIPTION

The purpose of this exercise is to help you understand how handling and positioning affect a child. Proper handling is important to protect the integrity of the nervous system of the child as well as prevent injuries to the caregiver. Positioning is critical, as it can directly influence the child's muscle tone as well as skill development and function. Handling and positioning need to be team efforts. All caretakers and educators of the child need to understand and practice correct handling and positioning to facilitate function and independence in the child. Additionally, all caretakers of the child need to practice proper lifting techniques to prevent injury to themselves and the child.

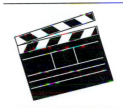

"A virtue and a muscle are alike. If neither of them is exercised they get weak and flabby."

RICHARD L. ROONEY

PREPARATION

Suggested Readings

Case-Smith, Allen, and Pratt (1996)
Kramer and Hinojosa (1999)

Study Questions

1. Define and differentiate handling and positioning. Indicate the use of both.

2. Discuss the necessary components to provide central stability in the following positions.

a. Supine

    b. Prone

    c. Sidelying

    d. Sitting

    e. Standing

3. List positioning devices that can be used with children for feeding or other activities.

4. Explain why positioning and handling with the handicapped child is important.

5. Describe when you may need to use positioning and handling techniques and devices.

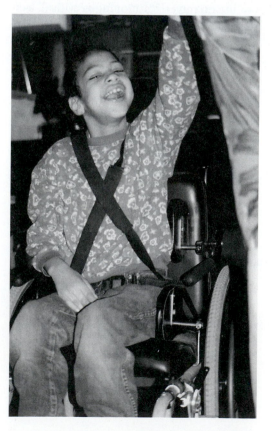

Fig. 3-3 Note the special positioning devices needed for optimal functioning.
Photo courtesy of Erica Day.

6. Describe various positions that can be used in working on hand function and why they are used.

7. Describe how muscle tone dictates the positioning and handling needs of a child.

8. Describe some of the strategies that can be used with the child with increased muscle tone to normalize that tone when handling the child (including carrying and lifting).

9. Describe strategies that can be used with the child with low muscle tone when handling the child (including carrying and lifting).

10. List the sequence of development of postural control as described by the theorist Margaret Rood.

11. Compare and contrast the neurodevelopmental and motor learning frames of reference.

12. Identify and define the key points of control as identified in the neurodevelopmental approach.

13. How can a ball or wedge be used to improve range of motion and function?

14. Describe the influence of weight bearing and weight shifting in the following positions:

    a. Prone

    b. Sitting

    c. Quadruped/creeping

    d. Kneeling

    e. Standing

15. Explain the importance of proximal joint stability and postural adjustments.

16. Detail the sequence and relationship of stability and mobility as outlined by the theorist Margaret Rood.

17. Complete the following chart. List a variety of positions, techniques, and activities that can be used to facilitate antigravity movement and/or postural reactions. Describe the purpose of each position, technique, or activity; the desired response; and the undesired response. One example has been done for you.

POSITION/TECHNIQUE/ ACTIVITY	PURPOSE	DESIRED RESPONSE	UNDESIRED RESPONSE
Child lying prone on a wedge	To improve neck extension	Child actively extending neck while engaged in an activity	Child passively laying head on the wedge

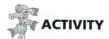

ACTIVITY
Materials

Scooterboard, large ball, wedge, prone board, sidelyer, roll, corner chair, mats, wheelchairs, large and small mannequins; various children's toys such as stacking rings, blocks, pop'n play, beanbags, small balls, hammer and pounding board; Case Study 14 located at the end of this chapter.

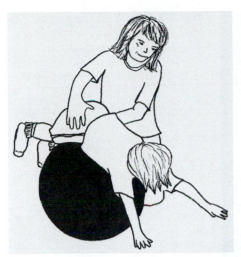

Fig. 3-4 Child positioned prone on a ball.

Instructions

1. Review proper body mechanics. Report and demonstrate proper body mechanic techniques before continuing with the other activities in this exercise. Practice lifting a large box, having your partner check off the techniques as you are observed. While lifting the box, verbally state the technique(s) you are using and have your partner check them off as they are reported.

	REPORT	OBSERVED
Make a clear path and surface. Position yourself in a comfortable position as close to the object as possible.		
Stand with your feet apart.		
Bend your knees and lift with your legs.		
Tighten your stomach muscles and tilt your pelvis.		
Keep the object as close to your body as possible.		
Lift with both hands.		
Don't lift higher than your waist.		
Turn your feet, not your back.		
When setting the object down, be sure to bend your knees.		
If you are getting help, make sure to count together.		
If you start to drop your load, go with it gently to the floor.		

2. Watch a demonstration by your instructor using the various pieces of equipment listed below and observe handling, lifting, and positioning techniques. Write your comments on the techniques.

   a. Scooter board

   b. Large ball

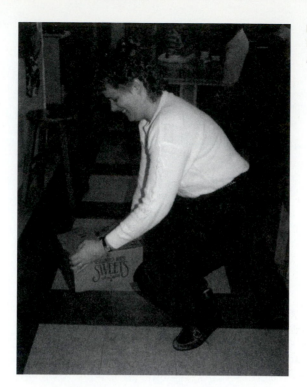

Fig. 3-5 Lifting box using proper body mechanics.
Photo courtesy of Marita Hensley.

c. Wedge

d. Prone board

e. Sidelyer

f. Roll

g. Corner chair

h. Prone stander

i. Pony chair

j. Other

k. Other

3. Observe a demonstration of proper technique for lifting and carrying a child using the one-person and two-person methods. Note the proper handling of the hypotonic and hypertonic child when lifting. Practice these techniques with a partner or use a manikin if available. Include comments on your performance generated by yourself, as well as the peer(s) with whom you are working.

	ONE-PERSON LIFT	TWO-PERSON LIFT
Describe technique		
Comments on your performance		

4. Practice putting each other in the following positions on the equipment specified. Place a check mark after successful completion of each position. Plan treatment activities for a child who could benefit from using the equipment and positions. Approximate a therapy situation and select an activity for a child to perform in the designated position. Demonstrate this to the class. Describe the setup so that the child's hands might be placed to engage in the activity. Include your rationale for activity selection.

POSITION	COMPLETED	ACTIVITY AND SETUP	RATIONALE
Sidelying on mat			
Prone on wedge			
Sidelying with sidelyer			
Sitting on ball			
Prone on ball			
Supine on ball			
Sitting on scooter			
Supine on scooter			
Prone on scooter			

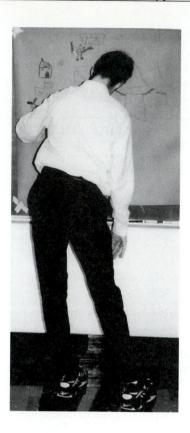

Fig. 3-6 What positions might facilitate proper trunk/hip alignment for this child? Trunk rotation?
Photo courtesy of Andy Dragan.

FOLLOW-UP

✔ Complete the Application of Competencies at the end of this chapter.

Exercise 42

"Character building begins in our infancy and continues until death."

ELEANOR ROOSEVELT

REFLEXES

OBJECTIVES

✔ Identify the emergence of and the inhibition of primitive postural and oral reflexes
✔ Describe the relationship between righting/equilibrium reactions and postural control
✔ Analyze the functional interference of delayed reflex maturation

DESCRIPTION

This exercise is designed to acquaint you with reflexes that are seen in both typical and atypical development. The emergence of and integration or inhibition of a reflex are normal parts of the developmental process. As reflexes are inhibited, the movement patterns of the same transition into controlled and voluntary movement. The delay in maturation of a reflex can result in functional problems in children. A delay is most often considered pathological and can interfere with a child's postural stability and mobility as well as oral functions. You will need to note the interferences caused by delayed reflex maturation and plan your intervention accordingly.

PREPARATION

Suggested Readings

Case-Smith, Allen, and Pratt (1996)
Neidstadt and Crepeau (1998)

Study Questions

1. What are primitive reflexes?

2. When might you see the continued presence of or reemergence of primitive reflexes?

3. With what conditions has the persistence of reflexes been associated?

4. Give the complete name for each of the following reflexes, including their emergence and integration, and draw a stick figure to represent what they look like.

REFLEX	NAME	EMERGENCE	INTEGRATION	STICK FIGURE
ATNR				
STNR				
TLR-P				
TLR-S				

5. Describe the following reflexes and give their timeline of emergence and inhibition.

REFLEX	DESCRIBE	EMERGENCE	INTEGRATION
Rooting			
Sucking			
Moro			
Grasp			
Stepping			
Protective extension			
Positive supporting			
Landau			

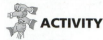 **ACTIVITY**

Materials

Floor spaces with mats.

Instructions

1. With a partner, practice assessing each other for the presence of primitive postural reflexes. Role play the typical response and the atypical response. Fill in the following chart as you perform the assessment describing the testing position, test stimulus, desired response, undesired response, and timeline of emergence to integration. The first one has been done for you.

REFLEXES AND REACTIONS	TEST POSITION	TEST STIMULUS	DESIRED RESPONSE	UNDESIRED RESPONSE	TIMELINE
PRIMITIVE REFLEXES					
Rooting	Prone or sitting	Tactile stimuli to the side of the cheek	Head turns toward the stimulus	Head does not turn	0–2 months
Moro					
Flexor withdrawal					
Plantar grasp					
Tonic labyrinthine					
Asymmetric tonic neck					
Symmetric tonic neck					
Palmar grasp					
Associated movements					
RIGHTING REACTIONS					
Labyrinthine head righting					
Optical righting					
Body righting acting on the head					

Neck righting acting on the body					
Body righting acting on the body					
Landau					
POSITIVE SUPPORTING REACTION					
Lower extremity					
Upper extremity					
EQUILIBRIUM REACTIONS AND PROTECTIVE REACTIONS					
Visual placing					
Tilting reactions					
Postural fixation reactions					
Protective: upper extremity					
Protective: lower extremity					

2. For the following ages, list the reflexes and reactions that should be present.

a. 3 months

b. 9 months

c. 20 months

d. 10 years

3. Describe a compensatory technique and a facilitative or inhibitory technique that may be used in treatment for a child with either a reflex that has persisted or a reaction that has not yet emerged. Fill in the boxes as they apply. The first one has been done for you. Note: Not all boxes will be filled in for each reflex.

	FUNCTIONAL INTEGRATION	COMPENSATORY TECHNIQUE	FACILITATIVE TECHNIQUE	INHIBITORY TECHNIQUE
Asymmetric tonic neck	Hands and head move independently	Adaptive positioning equipment and devices	N/A	Use of reflex inhibiting postures
Tonic labyrinthine in prone				
Tonic labyrinthine in supine				
Symmetric tonic neck				
Neck righting				
Upper extremity supporting				
Protective extension				
Tilting reactions				

FOLLOW-UP

✔ Complete the Application of Competencies at the end of this chapter.

Exercise 43

"It is a happy talent to know how to play."

RALPH WALDO EMERSON

PLAY

OBJECTIVES

✔ Define play and how it is used as a modality and/or a goal in treatment
✔ Develop a play activity that requires the use of inexpensive and/or recyclable materials
✔ Describe the appropriate incorporation of play in a treatment setting

DESCRIPTION

The purpose of this exercise is to help you understand the role of play in working with children. Play is often described as the most important work a child can do. In occupational therapy play can be used as a therapeutic modality and/or as a treatment goal. When used as a modality, it is done so to facilitate the completion of the established treatment goals. It is used to capture the child's interest and to provide motivation to participate in activities in which the child might not otherwise engage. When used as a goal, play becomes the end product for children who do not know how to play. For such children the goal might be to improve their skills or to facilitate playfulness. Accomplishing these milestones promotes development in the social, emotional, physical, and cognitive aspects of a child's growth.

PREPARATION

Suggested Readings

Case-Smith, Allen, and Pratt (1996)
Parham and Fazio (1997)
Labels on toys in a toy store
Library books for toy information

Study Questions

1. Think back to your childhood memories of play and compare your interests then to interests of children now.

	YOUR MEMORIES AND APPROXIMATE AGE	PRESENT-DAY CHILDREN AT SAME AGE
Favorite television shows		
Favorite movies		
Common toys		
Common games		
Crafts		
Creative/dramatic play		
Group play		

2. What are characteristics of and benefits of play?

3. What activities and techniques can you use to promote play?

4. Describe the classification or stages of play and/or games as defined by the following theorists:

   a. Reilly

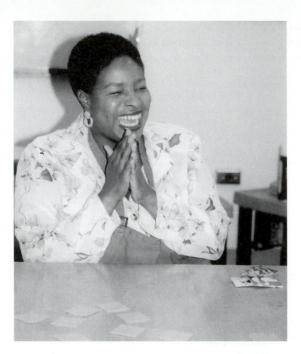

Fig. 3-7   Playfulness exhibited during a game of memory.

Photo courtesy of Tonya Jordan.

b. Takata

c. Piaget

d. Smilansky

e. Parten

5. Describe how play can be used in occupational therapy process in the following areas:

a. As assessment

b. As a modality

c. As a goal

d. For psychosocial skill development

6. List some of the developmentally appropriate toys and activities that can be used for each of the following age groups. Reading the labels and descriptions of toys at your local toy store will give you your answers.

    a. 0–2

    b. 2–4

    c. 4–7

    d. 7–12

    e. 12–18

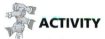 **ACTIVITY**

Materials

Book entitled *Extraordinary Play with Ordinary Things* (Sher, 1992), shoe box, tennis ball, figures of people and animals, yarn, Case Study 11 or 22 located at the end of this chapter.

Instructions

1. In a small group, take the materials presented by your instructor and devise a play activity. Let your creative juices flow and see the activity through a child's eyes. Present in a role-play situation how you would engage a child in this activity. Include the age for which this activity would be appropriate.

    a. Age of child:

    b. Materials:

    c. Activity:

2. With a partner or small group, use the case study given by your instructor to work on the following activity. Assume that the child in the case study lacks observable play skills at this time.

    a. Write two short-term goals to increase play.

b. Describe the first 60-minute treatment session with this child, including the environment, the materials you will use, and your therapeutic approach.

c. Share your plan with the class and record ideas you would like to remember.

FOLLOW-UP

✔ Complete the Application of Competencies at the end of this chapter.

Exercise 44

"The best ideas are often the results of improvisation."

CINDY KIEF

FEEDING

OBJECTIVES

✔ Demonstrate therapeutic feeding techniques
✔ Describe the importance of coordinating sucking, swallowing, and breathing
✔ Incorporate use of oral-motor toys for intervention

DESCRIPTION

This exercise is designed to help you understand the importance of the feeding techniques that need to be used in working with a child who is physically handicapped. A child who cannot independently feed himself or herself will benefit from the use of proper positioning and oral-motor activities. Such a child may also need adaptive equipment. Working toward independent feeding facilitates social acceptance by others and emotional confidence of the child. Whenever working on goals related to feeding and eating, nutritional intake also needs to be considered. Additionally the suck/swallow/breath synchrony as described by Oetter, Richter, and Frick (1995) affects many areas of nervous system functioning and needs to be considered for the child who is physically handicapped as well as the child who has sensory modulation difficulties.

PREPARATION

Suggested Readings

Case-Smith, Allen, and Pratt (1996)
Farber (1982)
Klein and Delaney (1994)
Oetter, Richter, and Frick (1995)
Reed (1991)

Study Questions

1. Differentiate between oral feeding, self-feeding, and eating.

2. Describe conditions that may interfere with oral feeding and self-feeding.

3. Describe the role of positioning in feeding.

4. List and briefly describe five strategies or techniques that OT practitioners can use for improving feeding function.

   a.

   b.

   c.

   d.

   e.

5. List three pieces of adapted feeding equipment, their use and purpose.

   a.

   b.

   c.

6. Draw the needed hand placement for jaw control on the accompanying figures. For the first picture, show the holding position if approaching the child from the front. For the second picture, show the holding position if approaching the child from the back or side.

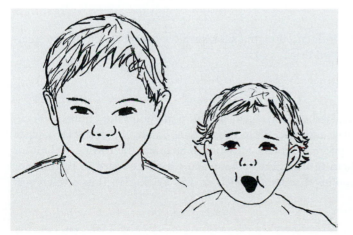

Fig. 3-8

7. When should the spoon be placed to the side of the mouth?

8. What does placement of the spoon on the center portion of the tongue promote?

9. What are the consequences of placing the food on the posterior portion of the tongue?

10. Describe several treatment techniques for the following conditions.
    a. Hypoactive gag

    b. Tongue lateralization

11. What types of food are contraindicated for use with children who have poor oral motor skills or dysphagia.

12. What delayed or pathological oral motor reflexes may be present in a child with hypertonicity?

13. Describe the suck/swallow/breath synchrony as described by Oetter, Richter, and Frick (1995).

14. Discuss how self-regulation might be influenced by oral activities, as well as by the use of one's hands and body.

15. List areas that may be influenced by the suck/swallow/breath synchrony in treatment (Oetter, Richter, and Frick, 1995).

16. Determine the anticipated outcome/goal of the oral motor functions of suck, blow, bite/crunch/chew, and lick. Write those functions in the designated space below. Identify appropriate treatment activities to facilitate these same oral motor functions and list them in the chart below placing a check mark in the box for which the activity applies. Use Oetter, Richter, and Frick (1995) as a reference.

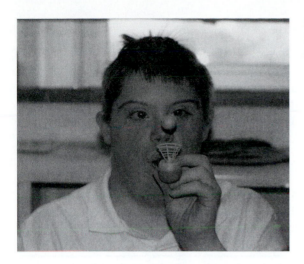

Fig. 3-9 Eyes and mouth working together.

Photo courtesy of Matthew Cavanaugh.

TREATMENT ACTIVITY	GOAL	SUCK	BLOW	BITE/ CRUNCH/ CHEW	LICK

NOTE

In preparation for the following activity, bring the following items to be utilized in class (small hand towel, liquid of your choice, soft food [e.g., pudding, applesauce] spoon, cup for drinking, finger foods [e.g., cracker, cookie] scarf or blindfold).

ACTIVITY

Materials

Scoop dishes, nosey cups, plastic-coated spoons, crazy straw, bubble soap and blower, windmill, straws, small pom-poms, Ping-Pong balls, blow instrument, blow pipe, rubber gloves, Case Study 12 located at the end of this chapter.

Instructions

1. Observe pre-feeding techniques as demonstrated by your instructor. Record a description of the techniques and their purpose. Practice the technique on a peer. Record your reaction when the technique is demonstrated on you.

TECHNIQUE/DESCRIPTION	PURPOSE	REACTION
Walking back on tongue		
Tactile stimulation using toothette		
Quick stretch around mouth		
Quick stretch under jaw		

2. Demonstrate improper feeding techniques with your partner using the four improper techniques described below. Feed each other liquids as well as solid and soft food. Experience what it is like to be fed without using proper techniques, though be sure to do so while still adhering to safety. Record your reactions in the following chart.

IMPROPER TECHNIQUES	REACTION TO LIQUIDS	REACTION TO SOLID FOODS	REACTION TO SOFT FOODS
Head extended			
Given inappropriate attention by feeder			
Feeding too fast			
Head to the side			

3. Participate in proper feeding and handling techniques after watching your instructor demonstrate the correct techniques. Write your reaction and any information you will need to help you remember these techniques.

PROPER TECHNIQUES IN POSITIONING AND HANDLING	REACTIONS AND COMMENTS		
	LIQUIDS	SOLID FOODS	SOFT FOODS
Head flexed			
Jaw control from the front			
Jaw control from the back			
Hand over hand			
Walking on tongue with spoon			
Feeding the blind client			
Assisting the blind client to eat			

4. Which position(s) and technique(s) for feeding were the most helpful and worked the best for you? Which position(s) and technique(s) were the least helpful?

MOST HELPFUL	LEAST HELPFUL

5. Experiment with various oral motor toys and/or invent oral motor games of your own. Describe what goals or skills they work toward and the degree of difficulty a child would need to successfully complete the activity.

		DEGREE OF DIFFICULTY		
ACTIVITY	GOAL/SKILL TARGETED	MILD	MOD.	MAX.
Windmill toy				
Bubbles				
Crazy straw				
Sucking pieces of paper with straw				
Blowing Ping-Pong balls				
Harmonica or flute (plastic toy)				
Blow pipe (suspend the ball)				
Other				
Other				

6. With your partner or small group, use a straw and two pom-poms to invent occupations you may use in treatment to address the feeding and oral motor skills of children. Describe the selected activity and identify the problem it addresses below.

Case description: 12 _____

ORAL MOTOR OR FEEDING PROBLEM IDENTIFIED	OCCUPATION (ACTIVITY) SELECTED

7. During lunchtime, visit a school where children with disabilities are being fed by an occupational therapy practitioner. Gather as much information as possible and record below.

   a. List commonly used equipment used at this school to assist in feeding:

   b. Describe handling techniques you observed for:
      1. Hypotonia

      2. Hypertonia

   c. Fill in the intervention and adaptive equipment used to address the problems identified below. If the problem was not observed, ask the practitioner to describe the intervention and/or equipment that would be appropriate to use.

PROBLEM	INTERVENTION	EQUIPMENT
Tongue thrust		
Bite reflex		
Hypoactive gag		
Hyperactive gag		
Oral tactile defensiveness		
Poor lip closure		
Difficulty with self-feeding		
Poor chewing		
Poor positioning		
Nutritional concerns		
Poor jaw stability		

8. Individually or with a small group, make up your own new and creative oral motor activity or game. Design the activity so that it facilitates the suck/swallow/breath synchrony as identified by Oetter, Richter, and Frick (1995) by using activities that encourage suck, blow, bite/crunch/chew, and lick functions. Include the intended goal or outcome. Discuss and demonstrate your activity with your classmates, recording all ideas below.

ACTIVITY	FUNCTION FACILITATED	GOAL/OUTCOME

FOLLOW-UP

✔ Complete the Application of Competency at the end of this chapter.
✔ Complete a Therapeutic Use of Self Analysis found in Appendix B on your skill in performing feeding and oral motor techniques.

Exercise 45

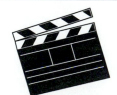

"The hand is one of the most beautifully complex and powerful machines not invented by man."

WALT WHITMAN

HAND SKILLS

OBJECTIVES

✔ Identify the sequence of grasp and hand skill development
✔ Determine intervention activities to facilitate hand skill development
✔ Relate hand skill development to a child's functional everyday activities

DESCRIPTION

This exercise will help you to understand the importance of hand skills and hand skill development. When hand skill development is lacking, the importance and the power of the hands are very noticeable. A child's hands are his or her tools of function and independence. They allow a child to interact constructively and creatively with the world. Understanding the sequence of hand skill development will enable you to design effective treatment activities to intervene when hands are not developing as expected. Engaging children in activities that promote hand skill function can often be embedded in a playful setting. At times hands need to be splinted to correct deformities and to facilitate function. Splinting is covered in Chapter 5.

PREPARATION

Suggested Readings

Asher (1996)
Case-Smith, Allen, and Pratt (1996)
Case-Smith and Pehoski (1992)

Study Questions

1. Describe the following terms as they relate to hand movements.

    a. Nonprehensile

    b. Prehensile

    c. Precision grasp

    d. Power grasp

2. Draw a picture depicting each of the following grasps. Include in your picture an item that is likely to require this type of grasp.

    a. Hook grasp

    b. Power grasp

    c. Lateral pinch

    d. Pincer grasp

    e. Tip pinch

    f. Three-jaw grasp

    g. Spherical grasp

    h. Disc grasp

    i. Cylindrical grasp

3. Draw a picture for some of the grasps that may be seen in using a writing instrument such as a pencil or crayon. Label the pictures accordingly and indicate whether or not they are efficient grasps to use.

    a.

    b.

    c.

    d.

    e.

    f.

4. Number the following sequences of grasp as they occur in development. Begin the first developmental step with number 1.

_____ Radial grasp	_____ Palmar contact
_____ Ulnar grasp	_____ Finger surface
_____ Palmar grasp	_____ Finger pad

5. Describe the following in-hand manipulation skills, an example of a functional task requiring this use, and several treatment activities to work on improving this skill.

SKILL	DESCRIPTION	TASK	TREATMENT ACTIVITIES
Finger to palm translation			
Palm to finger translation			
Shift			
Shift with stabilization			
Simple rotation			
Complex rotation			

6. List the approximate age when each of the following skills may emerge.

    a. Stabilize paper during writing

    b. Manipulate paper during scissor use

    c. Use scissors to cut complex shapes

    d. Reach across midline

    e. Use shift to separate pages

    f. Role piece of clay into a ball

    g. Use power grasp on tool

    h. Use palm to finger translation with coin

7. List several hand skill preparation activities that may be included in each of the following areas:

    a. Tactile awareness

    b. Proprioceptive input

    c. Pressure regulation

    d. Tactile discrimination

8. Briefly describe hand intervention strategies for children with hand limitations in the following categories:

    a. Severe disabilities

    b. Moderate disabilities

c. Mild disabilities

d. Muscle weakness

9. List and describe several assessments appropriate to use in evaluating hand skills and hand skill development.

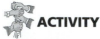 **ACTIVITY**
Instructions
 GAME

1. Take turns drawing the following hand grasps and skills on a chalkboard or demonstrate the grasp. Choose teams and choose your method to play a modified game of Pictionary™ or charades. Put a check mark in the appropriate column to keep track of your personal progress as you go.

HAND FUNCTION	KNOW	DON'T KNOW
Hook grasp		
Power grasp		
Lateral pinch		
Pincer grasp		
Tip pinch		
Three jaw grasp		
Spherical grasp		
Disc grasp		
Cylindrical grasp		
Dynamic tripod		
Static tripod		
Palm to finger translation		
Finger to palm translation		
Shift		
Simple rotation		
Complex rotation		

2. Observe a group of children and record the hand grasp or hand skills they use during play or school-related activities. If a group of children is unavailable to your class, observe an adult group. Discuss your observations as a class. Fill out the following chart as you observe the hand grasp or skill and the task the child or adult performs. An example of what you might see will get you started.

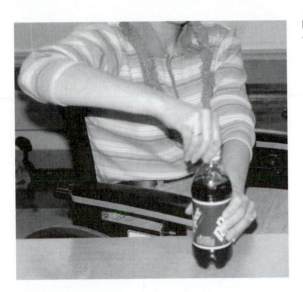

Fig. 3-10 Identify the two different types of grasp.

HAND GRASP OR SKILL OBSERVED	TASK PERFORMED
Hook grasp	Child carrying plastic pail by handle to the sand table.

GAME

3. Play the game Handagories (similar to the game Scattergories®). For each of the following hand skills, write a functional task that requires this skill. Adhere to the time limit given to you by your instructor for each item. Try to think of a unique task that requires a particular hand skill so that your answer is different from your classmates' answers. You will receive a point only if you have written a functional task that no one else in the class has identified.

a. Hook grasp

b. Power grasp

    c.   Lateral pinch

    d.   Pincer grasp

    e.   Tip pinch

    f.   Three-jaw grasp

    g.   Spherical grasp

    h.   Disc grasp

    i.   Cylindrical grasp

    j.   Palm to finger translation

    k.   Finger to palm translation

    l.   Shift

    m. Simple rotation

    n.   Complex rotation

FOLLOW-UP

✔   Complete the Application of Competencies at the end of this chapter.

HANDWRITING

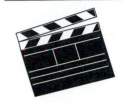

OBJECTIVES

✔ Describe developmentally appropriate readiness for handwriting
✔ Analyze the performance components of handwriting
✔ Demonstrate intervention techniques used to facilitate hand skill development

DESCRIPTION

This exercise will help you to understand handwriting and the many complexities of this highly complex skill and activity. Handwriting is one of the most frequent reasons for referral to occupational therapy among school-aged children. A child's handwriting is a critical component of his or her communication abilities. It is a skill that is needed throughout the life span. Facilitating proper postural and hand skill development, using appropriate letter formation, and using adaptive equipment can all assist a child in gaining skill in handwriting.

"Make the work interesting and the discipline will take care of itself."

E. B. WHITE

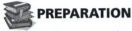 **PREPARATION**

Suggested Readings

Case-Smith, Allen, and Pratt (1996)
Case-Smith and Pehoski (1992)
Hanft and Marsh (1992)
Knight and Decker (1994)

Study Questions

1. Describe occupational therapy's role with children in regard to handwriting.

2. List the sensorimotor components that influence handwriting.

3. Explain why handwriting is so important in a school-based setting.

4. List readiness factors and skills that are needed before formal handwriting instruction is initiated.

5. Differentiate between a dynamic and a static tripod grip.

6. Discuss the relationship of pencil grip to handwriting.

7. Describe and draw a functional sitting posture needed for optimal handwriting.

8. Describe structured methods that are used to teach handwriting. Delineate whether the method was developed by educator(s) or occupational therapist(s).

9. Describe several frames of reference that would be appropriate to use in working with a child with handwriting deficiencies. Explain why.

10. List several additional remediation activities used for handwriting. Align the activities with a frame of reference and/or a theory base.

11. List and briefly describe adaptive equipment that is used in handwriting.

12. What assessments might be used to evaluate handwriting?

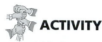 **ACTIVITY**

Materials

Evaluation Tool of Children's Handwriting (ETCH) (Amundson, 1995), Magna Doodle™, chalkboard, chalk, vibrating pen, finger paints, pennies, tweezers, spinning top, crayons and coloring book, soft therapeutic-type putty or play dough, slant board, eye-dropper, waxed sticks, sponges, letter templates from *Handwriting Without Tears* (Olsen 1998), pencil grips, olive picker, modified lined paper, computer adaptations, clipboard, fusable beads, tissues, Case Study 15, 20, or 21 located at the end of this chapter.

Instructions

1a. Observe your instructor administer the ETCH (Amundson, 1995) handwriting assessment to a member of your class who will use his/her non-dominant hand to write.
1b. Complete an Occupational Analysis (found in the Appendix A) for Handwriting. Wait to fill out the adaptation section until the end of the activity.
2. Participate in a variety of activities used in occupational therapy intervention to improve handwriting skills. Analyze these activities and equipment items and describe the hand skill required to perform the activity.
   a. Magna Doodle™

   b. Chalkboard

   c. Vibrating pen

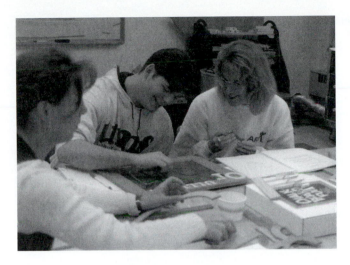

Fig. 3-11 Experiencing a variety of activities intended to improve handwriting. *Photo courtesy of Christine Tuttle, Jason Sueberling, and Melissa Bundy.*

d. Finger painting

e. Pennies in hand, moving to tip pinch

f. Tweezer games

g. Spinning top

h. Coloring

i. Putty (playdough)

j. Slant board

k. Eyedropper

l. Building letters with waxed sticks

m. Water painting

n. Practice writing letters

o. Olive picker

p. Fusable beads

q. Flipping pennies over

r. Other

3. Participate in learning/teaching letter formation skills as outlined in *Handwriting Without Tears* (Olsen, 1998).
   a. Build letters

   b. Demonstrate letter formation

   c. Draw letter in the air

   d. Trace over letter on chalkboard

   e. Erase with small sponge, dry with scrunched tissue

   f. Write on own paper

4. Try out various pieces of adapted equipment designed to assist in the writing process. Write your name using the adaptive equipment and record below how the items could be used in treatment.
   a. Pencil grips

   b. Paper

c. Computer

d. Writing surfaces/slate boards

e. Other

5. Practice writing letters as instructed in *Handwriting Without Tears* (Olsen, 1998) or another handwriting workbook. Practice both printed and cursive text. Is this how you normally write? If not, how is it different?

6. With a partner or small group analyze the following handwriting sample. List the problems you note. Speculate about the origins of those problems and what activities you may use to help the student.

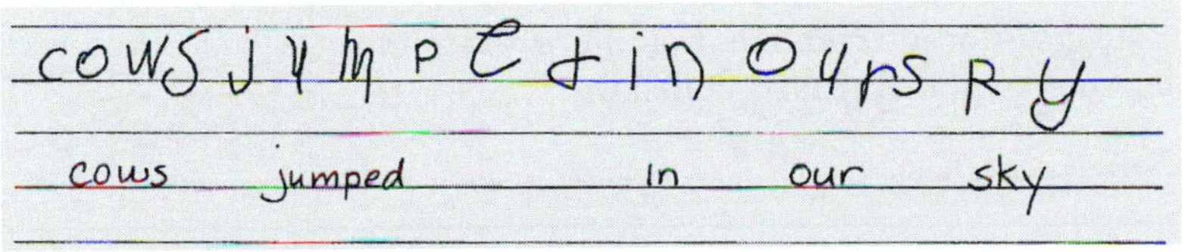

Fig. 3-12

COWS JYMPCdIN O4nSRY

cows   jumped   in   our   sky

PROBLEMS	POSSIBLE ORIGIN	INTERVENTION SUGGESTIONS

7. With a partner or small group, analyze the second handwriting sample. List the problems you note. Speculate about the origins of those problems and what activities you may use to help the student.

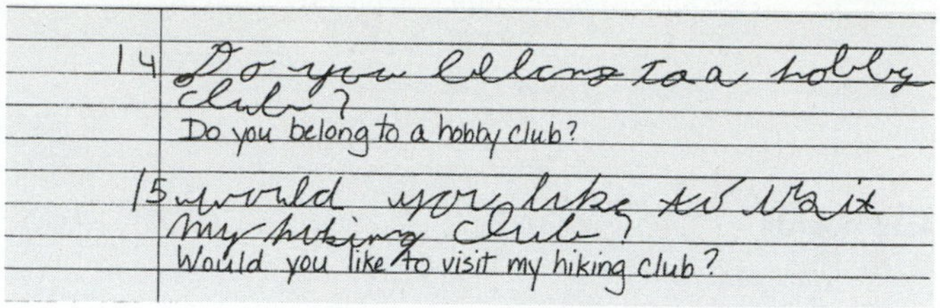

Fig. 3-13

PROBLEMS	POSSIBLE ORIGIN	INTERVENTION SUGGESTIONS

8. Use the case study provided by your instructor to develop the following treatment plan for a child with handwriting difficulties. Identify the difficulties the child has and appropriate goals for intervention. Determine the frame of reference you will use. Select appropriate therapeutic occupations.

9. Case No: _____

IDENTIFIED PROBLEMS	GOALS	FRAME OF REFERENCE	OCCUPATIONS

9. Return to your Occupational Analysis that was completed while observing the administration of the ETCH to a classmate. Fill in the section on adaptation.

FOLLOW-UP

✔   Complete the Application of Competency at the end of this chapter.

ACTIVITIES OF DAILY LIVING

Exercise 47

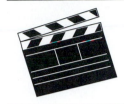

OBJECTIVES

✔ List goals targeted for gaining independence in activities of daily living (ADLs)
✔ Describe intervention approaches that are appropriate for identified deficits in ADLs
✔ Demonstrate forward and backward chaining techniques used for skill acquisition

"The object of teaching a child is to enable him to get along without his teacher."

ELBERT HUBBARD

DESCRIPTION

This exercise will improve your understanding of the importance of activity of daily living (ADL) skills in the pediatric setting. Facilitating independence in a child's ADLs is an important milestone that adds to a child's sense of accomplishment. As a child masters the ability to pull on a pair of pants or tie a shoe, his or her feelings of efficacy grow. To obtain independence, it is often necessary to break the tasks down into small learnable steps. Two methods of teaching those steps, forward chaining and backward chaining, are good techniques to learn and know. You will use them often in the pediatric setting when teaching ADLs.

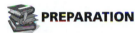 **PREPARATION**

Suggested Readings

Case-Smith, Allen and Pratt (1996)
Neidstadt and Crepeau (1998)

Study Questions

1. Differentiate between ADLs and instrumental activities of daily living (IADLs).

2. What cultural and contextual questions should be asked in planning intervention for a child with deficits in self-care?

3. When there is a problem performing self-care tasks, what are five identified ways in which a therapist can intervene?

4. Describe how the following approaches may be used in intervention to improve ADL performance:
   a. Developmental approach

   b. Remediation approach

   c. Compensatory approach

5. Describe how the following techniques can be used to increase performance in ADL:
   a. Modifying the task or task expectations

   b. Grading techniques

   c. Partial assistance

   d. Backward chaining

   e. Forward chaining

   f. Prompts or cueing

6. Briefly summarize intervention strategies used in the following areas of self-care:
   a. Toileting

   b. Dressing

   c. Bathing or showering

   d. Oral hygiene

   e. Grooming

   f. Functional communication

   g. Home management

7. What specific ADL assessments or tools are available that can be used for children?

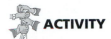 **ACTIVITY**

Materials

Shoes with laces, belts, jackets with zippers, materials for tooth brushing, front-opening shirts, slipover shirts, pants with fasteners; Case Study 2 located in Chapter One and Case Studies 13, 14, and 15 located at the end of this chapter.

Instructions

1. With your partner or in a small group, practice giving instructions using forward chaining and backward chaining techniques with the tasks below. Write a description of your techniques. Demonstrate your techniques to the class.

   a. Shoe tying

BACKWARD CHAINING	FORWARD CHAINING

   b. Donning/doffing jacket with a zipper

BACKWARD CHAINING	FORWARD CHAINING

   c. Donning/doffing front-opening shirt

BACKWARD CHAINING	FORWARD CHAINING

   d. Donning/doffing slipover shirt

BACKWARD CHAINING	FORWARD CHAINING

e. Donning/doffing pants with fasteners

BACKWARD CHAINING	FORWARD CHAINING

f. Donning/doffing belt

BACKWARD CHAINING	FORWARD CHAINING

g. Brushing teeth

BACKWARD CHAINING	FORWARD CHAINING

2. With a partner, identify ADL needs in an assigned case study. Select an approach and write a description of how it will be used in treatment addressing a child's ADL performance. Once you have finished, share your ideas with the class. Use the space below to organize your plan. Write one long-term goal for every two to four short-term goals.

a. Case 2: _____

IDENTIFIED ADL NEEDS	LONG-TERM GOAL	SHORT-TERM GOALS
Selected approach for intervention and description of how it will be used:		

b. Case 13: _____

IDENTIFIED ADL NEEDS	LONG-TERM GOAL	SHORT-TERM GOALS
Selected approach for intervention and description of how it will be used:		

c. Case 14: _____

IDENTIFIED ADL NEEDS	LONG-TERM GOAL	SHORT-TERM GOALS
Selected approach for intervention and description of how it will be used:		

d. Case 15: _____

IDENTIFIED ADL NEEDS	LONG-TERM GOAL	SHORT-TERM GOALS
Selected approach for intervention and description of how it will be used:		

FOLLOW-UP

✔ Complete the Application of Competencies at the end of this chapter.

Exercise 48

"Development of character consists solely of moving toward self-sufficiency."

QUENTIN GRISP

ADAPTATIONS

OBJECTIVES

✔ Identify adaptive equipment needed for a specific performance area
✔ Adapt an activity for the particular needs of a child
✔ Locate a source from which to obtain adaptive equipment

DESCRIPTION

This exercise is designed to help you analyze a variety of adaptive devices and equipment that may be used with a child in a pediatric setting. For each performance area a variety of assistive devices may be needed to maximize a child's abilities and facilitate independence. As a child grows and develops, new skills are gained. As new skills are gained, a child's adaptive equipment needs may vary and change. Additionally, each child has unique needs. What works for one child may or may not work for another. This is important to keep in mind in choosing adaptive equipment. Because of a child's rapid developmental changes, cost effectiveness needs to be kept in mind.

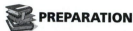 **PREPARATION**

Suggested Readings

> Case-Smith, Allen, and Pratt (1996)
> Christiansen (2000)
> Morris and Stiehl (1989)
> Various catalogues for adaptive equipment

Study Questions

1. What important qualities should an assistive device have when it is used with a child?

2. For the performance areas listed below, some of which are from "Uniform Terminology for Occupational Therapy, Third Edition" (AOTA, 1998), list and/or describe the adaptive equipment that may be used in adapting an activity or occupation that is developmentally appropriate for a child or adolescent to increase independence. For as many of the performance areas as possible, think of a method or technique that might replace a piece of adaptive equipment. Add other performance areas and descriptions as desired. Use the suggested readings and books combined with adaptive equipment catalogues to find the cost of the adaptation. Include the cost next to the name of the piece of equipment. An example is provided for you.

PERFORMANCE AREA	ADAPTATIONS	
	EQUIPMENT	METHOD/TECHNIQUE
GROOMING		
Obtaining supplies	Walker basket—$16.00	Organize needed items ahead of time; put items in pocket or apron to carry
Washing hair		
Drying hair		

Combing, styling, drying hair		
Caring for nails		
Caring for skin		
Caring for eyes		
Applying deodorant		
Using cosmetics		
ORAL HYGIENE		
Obtaining supplies		
Cleaning mouth		
Brushing teeth		
Flossing teeth		
BATHING AND SHOWERING		
Obtaining supplies		
Soaping body		
Rinsing body		
Drying body		
Maintaining bathing position		
Transferring to/from position		
TOILET HYGIENE		
Obtaining supplies		
Clothing management		
Maintaining position		
Transferring to/from position		
Cleaning body		
Caring for menstrual cycle/continence		
PERSONAL DEVICE CARE		
Cleaning and maintaining of:		
Hearing aids		
Contact lenses		
Glasses		
Orthotics		
Prosthetics		
Adaptive equipment		
DRESSING		
Selecting clothing/accessories		
Obtaining clothing from storage		
Dressing/undressing in sequence		
Fastening clothing		
Unfastening clothing		
Fastening shoes		
Unfastening shoes		
Applying/removing other devices		

FEEDING AND EATING		
Setting up food		
Selecting/using utensils/ tableware		
Bringing food to mouth		
Bringing drink to mouth		
Cleaning face, hands, clothing		
Sucking		
Masticating		
Coughing		
Swallowing		
Managing alternative methods		
MEDICATION ROUTINE		
Opening/closing containers		
Following prescribed schedules		
HEALTH MAINTENANCE		
Maintaining physical fitness		
Obtaining nutrition		
Decrease health risk factors		
SOCIALIZATION		
Interacting appropriately		
FUNCTIONAL COMMUNICATION		
Writing equipment		
Telephones		
Typewriters		
Computers		
Communication boards		
Call lights		
Emergency systems		
Braille writers		
Telecommunication devices		
Argumentative communication devices		
FUNCTIONAL MOBILITY		
In-bed mobility		
Wheelchair mobility		
Transferring to bed		
Wheelchair transfers		
Car transfers		
Ambulation		
Transporting objects		
COMMUNITY MOBILITY		
Moving self in the community		

Using public transportation		
Using private transportation		
EMERGENCY RESPONSE		
Recognizing hazardous situations		
Initiating action to decrease risk		
EDUCATIONAL ACTIVITIES		
Handwriting		
Maintaining sitting position		
Physical education class activities		
Attending to tasks		
Initiating responses		
Following directions		
Handling books		
Handling paper		
Managing classroom environment		
Using scissors		
Using glue		
Using paint brushes		
Opening packages at lunch		
Managing lunch tray		
PLAY OR LEISURE ACTIVITIES		
Identifying interests in play/leisure		
Planning play activities		
Obtaining materials for play		
Manipulating play objects		
Throwing a ball		
Catching a ball		
Hitting a ball		
Running		
Shooting basketball		
Playing board games		
Participating in unstructured play alone		
Participating in unstructured play with others		
Operating a battery operated toy or game		

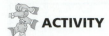 **ACTIVITY**

Materials

Case Studies 16, 17, and 18 located at the end of this chapter.

Instructions

1. Work with a partner or small group to adapt occupations for the children in the case studies assigned to you. When you are finished, share your ideas with the class. Record the ideas you would like to remember below.

a. Case 16:

PERFORMANCE AREA CONCERNS	ADAPTATIONS

b. Case 17:

PERFORMANCE AREA CONCERNS	ADAPTATIONS

c. Case 3:

PERFORMANCE AREA CONCERNS	ADAPTATIONS

d. Ideas to remember:

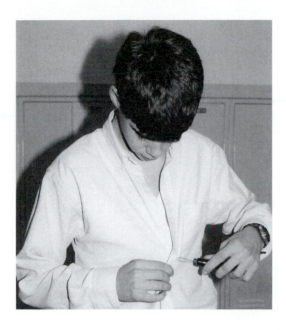

Fig. 3-14 A button hook allows this adolescent to get dressed independently.
Photo courtesy of Andy Dragan.

2. Assume the role of a future occupational therapy entrepreneur. Design a piece of adaptive equipment that is not currently available commercially. Name your piece of adaptive equipment. Indicate the purpose of your piece of adaptive equipment, draw the design, estimate the cost of construction, and indicate the manufacturer to which you might submit your design idea.

Name: _____

Purpose: _____

Design: _____

Cost: _____

Manufacturer: _____

FOLLOW-UP

✔ Complete the Application of Competencies at the end of this chapter.

BEHAVIOR MANAGEMENT

Exercise 49

OBJECTIVES

✔ Recognize constructive behavior management techniques
✔ Problem-solve alternative solutions to managing a child's behavior in a specific incident
✔ Identify cultural influences on a family's or caregiver's behavior management techniques

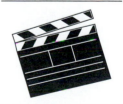

"All Children wear the sign: 'I want to be important NOW.' Many of our juvenile delinquency problems arise because nobody reads the sign."
DAN PURSUIT

DESCRIPTION

This exercise will introduce you to a variety of behavior management techniques. When working with children, you will need to learn constructive ways to manage behavior to maximize the effectiveness of the therapy sessions. Additionally, parents often need guidance in setting up programs that can work at home. Teachers in a school setting may also need strategies for a particular child who has behavioral difficulties. Children with behavior problems will be present in both physical disabilities and psychosocial settings. You will be challenged to initiate the use of proactive techniques that will structure the task, the environment, and the child to facilitate the child's cooperation and attention to task.

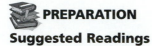

PREPARATION

Suggested Readings

Case-Smith, Allen, and Pratt (1996)
Neidstadt and Crepeau (1998)

Study Questions

1. Define the following terms:

   a. Temperament

   b. Social competence

   c. Mastery motivation

   d. Self-esteem

   e. Personal causation

   f. Learned helplessness

2. List and describe signs of emotional distress.

SIGN OF EMOTIONAL DISTRESS	DESCRIPTION

3. Briefly describe how each of the following approaches of frames of reference may
    be used in a psychosocial setting for intervention:
    a. Developmental theory

    b. Sensory integration

    c. Structured sensorimotor therapy

    d. Social learning and behavioral approaches

    e. Model of human occupation

    f. Model of social interaction

    g. Psychodynamic theory

    h. Family systems analytic theory

4. What tests and measurements are available for assessing the psychosocial-emotional
    domains of behavior?

5. Describe how the following intervention strategies can be used in pediatric treatment:
    a. Environmental adaptation

    b. Social behavior interventions

    c. Self-management and values clarification

    d. Interest groups

e. Socratic questioning

f. Social skills training

g. Child-centered intervention

h. Expressive interventions

i. Parent-focused therapy

6. Match the following behavioral strategies and related terms with their descriptions below.

Ignoring	Organization
Use of praise	Reward system
Sequence of behavioral controls	Behavior recording charts
Coordinated strategy	Punishments
Time out	Performance contracts
Overcorrection	Positive therapy environment

a. One minute of this is used for each year of a child's age.

_____

b. Therapist should convey enjoyment in being with the child.

_____

c. Therapist should identify problem behaviors and take one at a time.

_____

d. Recording behavior to earn reward.

_____

e. Mix liked and disliked activities in the session.

_____

f. All members of the team and family working together to avoid splitting and manipulation.

_____

g. Do not reveal feelings about the behavior.

_____

h. Used when other methods fail; child must know the rule and the consequences if it is broken.

_____

i. Consequence should be so unappealing that it prevents behavior.

_____

j. All parties sign and give a copy to the parents.

_____

k. Be specific about behavior that is appropriate, not just "good job."

_____

7. List characteristics of the desired treatment milieu for children and adolescents.

8. List several of the diagnoses children who benefit from psychosocial intervention may have.

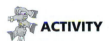 **ACTIVITY**

Materials

Markers, plain paper, Case Study 19 located at the end of this chapter.

Instructions

1. Working with a partner, plan several strategies to improve the problem behaviors identified below. Role-play these strategies, taking turns with your partner assuming the role of a child. While you are role-playing, have your classmates determine which strategy you are using and critique your choice. Record your strategy and their feedback below.

BEHAVIOR	STRATEGY TO IMPROVE PERFORMANCE
Child refuses to participate in learning shoe tying	
Critique:	
Child constantly touches everything in the environment	
Critique:	
Child goes through the motions of activities with no real effort	

Critique:	
Child initiates all tasks (usually wrong) before instructions are completed	
Critique:	
Child throws pegs when taken out of theraputty	
Critique:	
Child says negative things about self and others almost continually	
Critique:	
Child does not initiate conversation	
Critique:	
Child hits other children when involved in scooter board races that child is losing	
Critique:	
Child bites hands when upset	
Critique:	

2. Describe how each of the behaviors in the situations in question 1 may be influenced as a result of the family's social and/or cultural values.

BEHAVIOR	SOCIAL/CULTURAL VALUE THAT MAY INFLUENCE IMPROVEMENT

3. Work with a partner or small group and design a behavior recording chart and a performance contact for a child in a case study assigned to you. Work on your draft below, then use paper and markers to share and display your finished product. Make the chart and contract appealing to the child. Don't forget the reinforcement component.

a. Behavior recording chart

b. Performance contract

FOLLOW-UP

✔ Complete the Application of Competencies at the end of this chapter.

SENSORY INTEGRATION

OBJECTIVES

✔ Define sensory integration, sensorimotor, and sensory modulation disorders
✔ Analyze the sensory components of activities used in classical sensory integration treatment
✔ Design therapeutic activities using sensory integration principles

Exercise 50

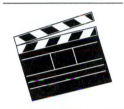

"We learn by doing."

Aristotle

DESCRIPTION

This exercise will acquaint you with the sensory integration frame of reference. This frame of reference is frequently used in working with children and is based on the original work of A. Jean Ayres. At times the sensory integration theory and frame of reference are used in their classical form in treatment: individually or in small groups with the child guiding and the therapist eliciting adaptive responses using suspended equipment. At other times the sensory integrative theory is applied to small group situations in which no suspended equipment is used. In using this format and incorporating predetermined, structured activities, it is appropriate to call such intervention *sensorimotor*. Sensory integration theory is also used as a basis for interpreting other disorders of the sensory systems, namely, sensory modulation disorders. Additionally, certification in the test administration and interpretation of the sensory integration and praxis tests is available and provides the practitioner with advanced skills and knowledge in identifying children with classical sensory integration areas of concern.

 PREPARATION

Suggested Readings

> Case-Smith, Allen, and Pratt (1996)
> Fisher, Murray, and Bundy (1991)
> Neidstadt and Crepeau (1998)
> Scheerer (1997)
> Toronto Sensory Integration Group (1987)

Study Questions

1. Define these terms:

    a. Neural plasticity

    b. Sensory registration

    c.   Sensory modulation

    d.   Hyporesponsitivity

    e.   Hyperesponsitivity

    f.   Sensory defensiveness/sensory dormancy

    g.   Sensory discrimination

    h.   Sensory nourishment

    i.   Clinical observations

    j.   Sensory integration disorders (identify and define specific types)

    k.   Classical sensory integration treatment

    l.   Adaptive responses/adaptive behavior

    m.   Expected outcomes of sensory integration treatment

    n.   Sensory integration and praxis tests

2.   Describe how the sensory integration theory and frame of reference can be applied and used in a small group setting.

3. Watch the video entitled *Sensory Integration Therapy* (Toronto Sensory Integration Group, 1987) and answer the following questions:

   a. What is sensory integration?

   b. On what is therapeutic intervention based?

   c. How might a child appear who has sensory integrative dysfunction?

   d. What are the basic sensory systems?

4. Describe how therapists can use structured free play in a treatment setting.

5. Describe how you think the process of grading and activity is used in sensory integration treatment with a child.

6. Describe some of the equipment and materials that need to be available for a child to explore a "sensory-enriched environment" (Case-Smith, Allen, and Pratt, 1996).

7. Describe the most acceptable methods in providing vestibular and tactile input.

8. Detail necessary precautions to use in providing sensory input, especially in providing vestibular and light tactile stimuli.

9. Describe the compensatory method of treatment as used in sensory integration treatment.

10. List the pros and cons of using sensory integration treatment in small groups.

PROS	CONS

11. Describe how consultative treatment may be helpful and necessary in providing treatment to a child with a disordered nervous system.

12. Differentiate sensory integration and sensorimotor.

13. List sensorimotor treatment activities that may be used to treat deficits in the following areas:
    a. Vestibular

    b. Proprioceptive

    c. Tactile

    d. Gravitational insecurity

    e. Oral motor

    f. Postural control

    g. Eye tracking

14. Summarize treatment principles and activities that are appropriate to use with a gravitationally insecure child.

15. Gather four different sensory items from your home that could be used with children and bring them to class.

ACTIVITY

Materials

Sensory integration treatment clinic, tactile materials brought by student.

Instructions

1. Visit a pediatric occupational therapy department that uses sensory integration therapy. Break into groups as designated by instructor. Participate in the following activities. After each person has an opportunity to participate in the activity at your station, proceed on to the next station. Adhere to the safety precautions detailed in your study questions. Record comments about your reaction and the primary muscles/sensory system you are using as you complete the activities below.

   a. Vestibular and proprioceptive input; heavy work and flexion pattern activities:

STATIONS	POSITION	DESIRED PERFORMANCE	COMMENTS/ SYSTEM
Platform swing	Lie supine with knees flexed.	Have person hand you five balls. Throw balls into the box.	
Scooter board	a. Sit on scooter board, on top of ramp with your legs crossed. b. Lie supine on the scooter board.	a. Go down ramp, keeping your balance. b. Carry beanbag down ramp on stomach, throw bean bag into target at end of runway. a and b. Propel back to top of ramp, pulling rope to get up the ramp.	
Disk swing	Sit on the disk, straddling rope between legs.	Pick up beanbags one at a time and throw at designated target.	
Air Pillow	Stand next to pillow.	Hold onto a rope and swing yourself over without touching the pillow.	
Whale	Sit on the whale, straddling it with your legs.	Hold onto the handles and make it go up and down.	
Bolster swing	Lie on the bolster, on your stomach. Hold on by wrapping your legs and arms around the bottom.	Have someone shake and bounce bolster trying to knock you off.	
Overall comments/reactions:			

b. Vestibular and proprioceptive input; tactile and extension pattern activities:

STATIONS	POSITION	DESIRED PERFORMANCE	COMMENTS/ SYSTEM
Platform swing	Lie prone on the swing.	Try to "catch the fish" by using the magnet. Once caught, put the fish in your "boat."	
Scooter board	Lie prone on scooter board. Go down scooter board ramp.	When reaching destination, throw beanbag into target.	
Oversized floor pillow	Lie prone at one end of pillow. Have partner hold down edges.	Slither through on your stomach until you are completely out.	
Ladder	Stand at the bottom. Have partner help secure as needed.	Climb over the top to the other side. If unable, at least climb to the top.	
Dual swing	Sit, putting one leg in each loop.	Swing in a circular motion, pushing with your feet.	
Net	Place one knee into the swing, and lie prone in the net.	Pick up the beanbags and toss them into the target by swinging in a linear direction. Stop with your hands. *Don't* stop by using your feet.	
Overall comments/reactions:			

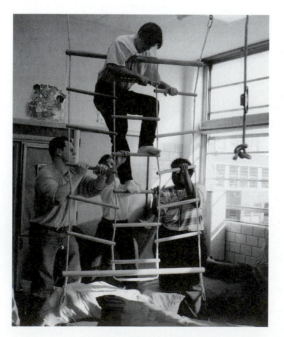

Fig. 3-15 Experiencing activities yourself before implementing them in treatment is necessary in developing clinical reasoning skills.

Photo courtesy of Rick Ernst, Carol Scheerer, Jason Sueberling, and Kim Jerdo.

c. Tactile, oral-motor, quiet time:

STATIONS	POSITION	DESIRED PERFORMANCE	COMMENTS/ SYSTEM
Box of balls	Sit, lie, play	Find the hidden toys in the box. Then hide them for the next person(s).	
Sandwich	Lie on bottom pillow.	Have partners place a pillow on top of you. Have one or two people lie on top of that pillow.	
Pastry dough	Lie prone on mat.	Have partner roll your body with the rolling pin.	
Touch and tell	Lie prone on mat.	With vision occluded, have partner rub your back and legs with various tactile objects. Try to guess what item is touching you.	
Oral	Lie prone on mat.	Use the chewies or straws and sucking motion with your mouth to pick up game pieces to play tic-tac-toe.	
Bubbles	Sit on mat with your legs to the side in a side-sit position. Position yourself so that you need to rotate your trunk to the side, opposite your feet.	Have your partner hold the basketball hoop while you try to blow bubbles into it.	
Overall comments/reactions:			

2. Divide into several groups as designated by your instructor. Participate in the various tactile, oral motor, and quiet time activities as directed. Respect your partner's preferences. Note your reactions and observations in the space provided. Identify the type of touch used: protective, discriminative, light touch and/or touch pressure.

ACTIVITY	DESCRIPTION	REACTIONS/ OBSERVATIONS	TYPE OF TOUCH
Shaving cream	Squirt and play		
Drawing on backs	Have partner sit on mat while you draw letters, shapes, messages on his/her back. Have partner identify what you have drawn.		
Tactile: box of beans and/or rice, etc.	Dig in box with hands, trying to identify what you found without looking.		
Human burrito	Have partner lie in a blanket. Slowly roll the person up as you put on desirable items. Vary the tight-ness of the roll-up.		
Seed game	Go from a tall kneel position to sitting back on your feet and putting your head on the mat. Your partner "plants" you.		
Tactile pictures	Make a picture, using macaroni, seeds, and cotton balls.		
Cornstarch	Put cornstarch in a bowl. Add a small amount of water at a time. Play with the substance.		
Body painting	Using paintbrushes or surgical brushes, paint yourself and your partner as tolerated.		

3. In groups designated by your instructor, use the materials you brought to de-vise a tactile game. Share your tactile items with other group members while creating your own game. Make sure it is a game and not just a discrimination activity. Be creative and construct a game a child would enjoy. Use the follow-ing chart to record your group's activities and those of your classmates. See the example below.

MATERIALS USED	GAME DESCRIPTION	TREATMENT IMPLICATIONS
Box, cotton balls, kidney beans, rice, harmonica	Treasure hunt: Have child remove cotton balls from top of box. Child finds harmonica buried under rice and kidney beans in box. Child plays harmonica.	Promotes tactile discrimination, stereognosis, tolerance of tactile activities, oral motor skill

4. Discuss as a class how sensory integration dysfunction might affect a child's everyday activities. Give specific examples.

FOLLOW-UP

✔ Complete the Application of Competency at the end of this chapter.

Exercise 51

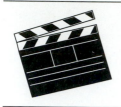

"What's done to children, they will do to society."

KARL MENNINGER

SCHOOL-BASED PRACTICE

OBJECTIVES

✔ Identify the role and function of the occupational therapy practitioner in a school-based setting

✔ Identify corrective and compensatory intervention approaches used in a school setting

✔ Discuss the roles of the individualized education plan and the transition plan in the education of a child who is handicapped

DESCRIPTION

This exercise will help you to understand the role and the functions of the occupational therapy (OT) practitioner in the school setting. Schools employ a high percentage of OT practitioners. With federal laws backing them, OT practitioners play a vital role in the education of the handicapped child. The individualized education plan (IEP) and resulting transition services are the federally granted rights of a child with an identified disability. School-based practice is both challenging and rewarding as the OT practitioner becomes a part of the child's everyday life.

PREPARATION

Suggested Readings

AOTA (latest edition)
Case-Smith, Allen, and Pratt (1996)

Study Questions

1. Identify legislation related to OT school-based services.

2. Describe the four roles of occupational therapy in the school:

   a.

   b.

   c.

   d.

3. How does the IEP process in the school differ from the OT process in other settings?

4. Describe the following corrective approaches that may be used in a school-based setting:

    a. Neurodevelopmental

    b. Sensory integration

    c. Biomechanical

5. Describe the following compensatory approaches that may be used in a school setting:

    a. Teach skill

    b. Adapt task

    c. Adapt environment

    d. Use equipment

6. Describe the differences between therapy performed in the classroom and that performed in the OT clinic.

7. Describe specific settings within the school grounds where school-based OT services may be provided.

8. Explain the role of the family and the IEP team as it relates to school-based OT services.

9. Describe three service delivery models that are used in a school setting.

10. Discuss the evaluation process and identify several assessments that would be appropriate to use in a school setting.

11. Define transition services.

12. Identify and describe the following acronyms:
    a. EHA

    b. IEP

    c. IDEA

13. At what age do transition services usually begin?

14. What are the transition services mandated by IDEA?

15. Describe the major focus of occupational therapy in the following areas of transition:
    a. Evaluation

    b. Teamwork

    c. Service planning

16. Summarize documents concerning school-based practice that are located in the *Reference Manual of the Official Documents of the American Occupational Therapy Association* (AOTA, latest edition).

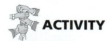 **ACTIVITY**

Materials

A neighborhood grade school, VCR, videotape entitled, "*Tools for Teachers: A Video on Practical Occupational Therapy Strategies* (Henry, n.d.)

Instructions

1a. Visit a local grade school to observe the tasks of children in a typical classroom. Go with a partner or divide into small groups so that classroom disruption is minimized. Rejoin your class at a designated time and area to share observations or meet at your next regularly scheduled class time. Fill in the information below as you observe in the classroom.

School for observation: _____

Grade observed: _____

Age of children: _____

Number of children: _____

Description of task(s) observed: _____

1b. With your partner or group, describe what performance components were used by the students during your observation of typical tasks. Fill this information in on two of the tasks you observed using the Abbreviated Occupational Analysis/Adapted (found in Appendix A) filling out the component section only.

1c. Once the abbreviated analysis is complete, work with your partner or small group to determine how the activity could be adapted for students who may be unable to perform the activity successfully owing to a disability. Use the same Abbreviated Occupational Analysis/Adapted (found in Appendix A), adding your adaptation ideas.

1d. Share your ideas from the above activity with the class and list here the adaptation ideas you would like to remember.

OCCUPATION	ADAPTATION SUGGESTIONS

2. View the video entitled, "*Tools for Teachers: A Video on Practical Occupational Therapy Strategies* (Henry, n.d.). Make a list of professionals, in addition to the OT practitioner, who may provide services to a child receiving intervention in a school setting. Divide into small groups and discuss how the information in the video might be shared with each team member. Reconvene as a class and share your ideas.

3a. Visit a department in your institution and analyze a job to determine the performance components involved in the tasks for the job required. Observe the required tasks of the job and list those on the chart below. Then assign one of the tasks to a pair or small group of students to analyze using the Abbreviated Occupational Analysis/Adapted (found in Appendix A).

Job title: _____

Location: _____

TASKS	STUDENTS RESPONSIBLE FOR ANALYZING

3b. Discuss as a class the tasks that have been analyzed.

3c. Determine as a class the suitability of this job in relation to a young adult seeking transition services. If it is determined to be suitable, describe the characteristics of the young adult who may benefit. Identify the possible barriers that may exist and the supports needed for the identified young adult student to be employed at this job site.

Job: _____

Young adult characteristics: _____

BARRIERS	SUPPORTS

3d. Discuss and record here interventions you will perform to assist the young adult student in being successful.

FOLLOW-UP

✔ Complete the Application of Competencies at the end of chapter.

Exercise 52

"Babies are such a nice way to start people."

DON HEROLD

EARLY INTERVENTION

OBJECTIVES

✔ Identify federally mandated early intervention services that are available for children with disabilities
✔ Describe the evaluation and intervention focus in early intervention
✔ Detail the role of the family and the entire team in providing early intervention services

DESCRIPTION

This exercise will help you to understand the importance of early intervention services. Early intervention services are mandated by law for children with disabilities. These services may be provided in a variety of settings. The entire early intervention team will be important in facilitating the child's development. In this context it will be critical for the occupational therapy practitioner to identify areas of concern and develop family involved intervention for the child. The family and caregivers of the child will be the child's most significant source of support.

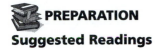 **PREPARATION**

Suggested Readings

Asher (1996)
Case-Smith, Allen, and Pratt (1996)
Kramer and Hinojosa (1998)

Study Questions

1. Define early intervention and list the settings in which it may be provided.

2. What are the services required by law that are available for children with disabilities?

3. What is an IFSP and what is included in it?

4. Describe the role of the family in the planning and implementing of early intervention services.

5. Describe the evaluation process in early intervention.

6. List areas of functioning that may be addressed in the evaluation process.

7. List and describe the three types of early intervention team approaches.

8. List some of the components of the following areas with which the occupational therapy practitioner may be concerned in treating a child in an early intervention setting. Additionally, describe assessments that might be appropriate to use for those areas as well as intervention strategies.

AREA	COMPONENT	ASSESSMENT	INTERVENTION
Fine motor			
Play			
Oral motor function and feeding			
Sensory			
Positioning			
Self-help			

 ACTIVITY

Materials

Various toys for children from birth to age 3, such as rattles, busy boxes, mobiles, balls; Case Studies 11, 16, and 18 located at the end of this chapter and Case Study 6 located in Chapter 1.

Instructions

1. Play with various available toys, briefly describe the movements/motions and skills required for a child to use that particular toy. Record your findings. An example provided below will get you started.

TOY	MOVEMENTS/MOTIONS AND SKILLS
Rattle	Grasp and release rattle; gross upper arm movements to initiate sound

2. Using the case study assigned to you by your instructor, select activities and design intervention for each identified deficit area of the child in that case study. Work in a small group or with a partner. Describe how you will involve the family in the intervention process. Once you have completed the intervention ideas, share the ideas with your classmates demonstrating with toys if possible.

CASE STUDY NO.	DEFICIT AREA	ACTIVITY/TOY	INTERVENTION	FAMILY INVOLVEMENT

FOLLOW-UP

✔   Complete the Application of Competencies at the end of chapter.

HOSPITAL SERVICES AND REHABILITATION

Exercise 53

OBJECTIVES

✔   Identify diagnostic-appropriate interventions used in a hospital and/or rehabilitation setting
✔   Develop individualized goals and intervention for a specific case study
✔   Participate in a role-play of a team meeting of members providing hospital-based service

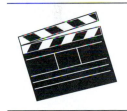

"Feel the dignity of a child. Do not feel superior to him for you are not."

ROBERT HENRI

DESCRIPTION

The purpose of this exercise is to acquaint you with hospital and rehabilitation services for children that occupational therapy practitioners may provide. The evaluation and treatment intervention provided in these settings is fairly similar to that provided in other settings; however, the diagnoses of the children seen are more often more varied and challenging. In a hospital setting, acute conditions are more frequently seen, and the needed rehabilitation may be provided to the child through the hospital and/or a separate rehabilitation facility. Hospitals and rehabilitation services may provide inpatient as well as outpatient services. As an occupational therapy practitioner in this setting you will facilitate a child's functional abilities and independence in the areas of self-care, work, and play/leisure.

PREPARATION

Suggested Readings

Case-Smith, Allen, and Platt (1996)
Christiansen (2000)

Study Questions

1. List and describe the team members you may be working with in a hospital-based program.

2. Identify the following acronyms by name:
   a. ICU

   b. CCU

   c. NICU

   d. SICU

   e. PICU

3. List four types of children who are referred to occupational therapy that need acute care.

4. Briefly describe the role of occupational therapy in each of the following conditions:
   a. Burns

   b. Bone marrow transplant

   c. Spina bifida

   d. Seizure disorder

   e. Abuse/neglect

   f. Spinal cord injury

g. Traumatic brain injury

h. Brachial plexus injuries

i. Arthrogryposis

j. Muscular dystrophy

k. Juvenile rheumatoid arthritis

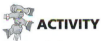 **ACTIVITY**

Materials

Case Studies 11, 16, 20, and 21 located at the end of this chapter.

Instructions

1. With an assigned case study, work with a partner or small group to plan the appropriate treatment intervention for that child in a hospital-based setting. Use the following questions to develop your treatment plan:

    a. Which assessment would be appropriate to administer?

    b. Which frame of reference will you want to use in treatment?

    c. Write two short-term goals.

    d. Identify appropriate treatment activities, the rationale for their use, and the setup needed to carry out the activities.

TREATMENT ACTIVITIES	RATIONALE	SET-UP

e. Present your case study and treatment plan to your classmates. In the space below, record ideas presented to you.

Case:

Assessments:

Frame of reference:

Goals:

Treatment activities:

Case:

Assessments:

Frame of reference:

Goals:

Treatment activities:

Case:

Assessments:

Frame of reference:

Goals:

Treatment activities:

Case:

Assessments:

Frame of reference:

Goals:

Treatment activities:

2. Participate in a role-play of a team meeting with a select number of your classmates. You will be given the case study and the role you will play and a few minutes to prepare for your participation in a team meeting. Take turns role-playing the different scenarios with your classmates. If you are not in the current role-play situation, you may assist a fellow student in preparation of his or her role.

   a. You are in a team meeting to discuss evaluation results of a child you just evaluated. Include your suggested intervention plan. Use the following chart to first plan for your contributions to the meeting and then to record the team members present and their contributions to the meeting. As an example, a dietitian may contribute the results of a nutritional assessment and the child's current body weight and mass. His or her suggestions may include recommended dietary changes and monitoring of caloric intake.

Case Description	
TEAM MEMBER	CONTRIBUTION TO TEAM MEETING

   b. Discuss the child's progress at a team meeting that has convened after you have been seeing the child for a designated amount of time. Record your role and plan for your contribution as well as those of the other team members.

Case Description	
TEAM MEMBER	CONTRIBUTION TO TEAM MEETING

c. Participate in a discharge meeting of this child. Assume that you are the one who has been treating this client since the initial evaluation.

TEAM MEMBER	CONTRIBUTION TO TEAM MEETING

d. Discuss as a class the effectiveness of the meetings.

FOLLOW-UP

✔ Complete the Application of Competencies at the end of this chapter.

Exercise 54

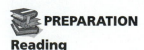

"Only a child who feels safe dares to grow forward healthily. His safety needs must be gratified."

ABRAHAM MASLOW

DURABLE MEDICAL EQUIPMENT

OBJECTIVES

✔ Identify the use and function of a variety of mobility devices
✔ Differentiate the types of features found on both manual and power wheelchairs
✔ Discuss current trends in the marketing of durable medical equipment

DESCRIPTION

This exercise will familiarize you with the mobility products that are available through a durable medical equipment supplier. Most likely, the selection of a mobility device will be made by a team of whom you will be a critical member. It is important that you are familiar with the available options when helping to select a mobility device. Mobility devices are very expensive, and insurance coverage usually pays only for periodic updates. As part of the team making the decision, you need to do so with the utmost thoroughness and care, with full understanding of the most current availability of mobility devices and their components.

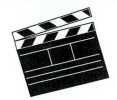 **PREPARATION**

Reading

Case-Smith, Allen, and Pratt (1996)
Trefler, Hobson, Taylor, Monahan, and Shaw (1993)

Study Questions

1. Define functional mobility.

2. Define a mobility device.

3. Give examples of durable medical equipment.

4. List at least six different types of mobility devices and their use and function.

5. Before selecting a mobility device, what questions should be answered?

6. Discuss the functional assessments that might be appropriate to use in selecting a mobility device.

7. Name the title and function of the team members who may participate in the selection process of obtaining a mobility device.

8. Identify the qualifications of a rehabilitation technology supplier.

9. A young child with cerebral palsy (spastic diplegia) uses a push walker but needs a manual wheelchair for mobility in the community and at school. He is expected to learn how to transfer into and out of the wheelchair in the future. What features do you think will be needed on his manual wheelchair for optimal independence?

10. Why is it important to consider positioning very carefully in fitting a child for a mobility device?

11. What are the benefits and the disadvantages of a manual wheelchair (including lightweight and standard weight) and/or a power wheelchair?

12. What factors promote the successful use of a mobility device?

13. List types of battery-powered mobility devices that are available for children.

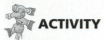 **ACTIVITY**

Materials

Pediatric wheelchairs, walkers, and other mobility devices.

Instructions

1. Visit a durable medical equipment supply store or have a supplier bring equipment to your lab. In the first chart below, record the different types of wheelchairs available and their various features or components. Use the second chart to state the purpose of each wheelchair component listed. Handle the various components and practice removing and replacing them as applicable. Check off and document your progress as you go.

TYPES OF WHEELCHAIRS	FEATURES

WHEELCHAIR COMPONENTS	PURPOSE	IDENTIFY	REMOVE	REPLACE
Lateral supports				
Lap tray				
Neck ring				
Butterfly strap/ H strap				
Seat belt				
Adductors				
Abductors				
Lumbar roll				
Other				
Other				

2. List the uses of the various available walkers.

    a. Standard walker

    b. Roller walker

    c. Cerebral palsy walker

    d. Other

3. Obtain answers to the following questions from your durable medical equipment supplier or rehabilitation technology supplier.

    a. Describe the procedure a supplier uses to custom fit children in wheelchairs. What is the cost?

    b. What is the cost for a typical (not custom built) pediatric wheelchair?

    c. How many years does the wheelchair need to last?

    d. What must be considered in regard to the child's family in ordering the wheelchair?

    e. What new mobility devices are out on the market?

    f. What are the most popular mobility devices?

    g. What are the most frustrating aspects of using a wheelchair?

    h. What type or aspects of routine maintenance need to be completed for manual wheelchairs? Power wheelchairs?

i. Who fits wheelchairs at the company represented by the durable medical equipment supplier? (position, education, title, etc.)

j. Generate additional questions and find the answers.

FOLLOW-UP

✔ Complete the Application of Competencies at the end of this chapter.

Exercise 55

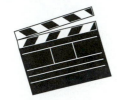

"I long to accomplish a great and noble task, but it is my chief duty to accomplish small tasks as if they were great and noble."

HELEN KELLER

VISION LOSS AND IMPAIRMENT

OBJECTIVES

✔ Define terms related to vision loss and impairment
✔ Examine experiences when vision is occluded
✔ Adapt appropriate intervention activities for a child with low vision

DESCRIPTION

This exercise is designed to acquaint you with techniques and activities that are appropriate to use with children who have visual loss and/or impairments. Infants and children with low vision need specific training and environmental adaptations. It is important to remember that a child may have multiple impairments, of which vision loss may be one. If such is the case, this will exacerbate the child's needs and impel the team to provide further support and services, especially in the incidence of deaf-blindness, and/or visual impairments secondary to another primary diagnosis, such as cerebral palsy or mental retardation. As an occupational therapy practitioner, you will play a vital role in facilitating the growth and independence of a child with a visual loss.

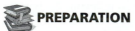 **PREPARATION**

Suggested Readings

Case-Smith, Allen, and Pratt (1996)

Study Questions

1. What is the definition of legal blindness?

2. Define the following terms:
   a. Acuity

   b. Peripheral vision

   c. Myopia

d. Hyperopia

e. Cataracts

f. Glaucoma

g. Amblyopia

h. Astigmatism

i. Cortical blindness

j. Coloboma

k. Microphthalmos

l. Nystagmus

m. Optic atrophy

n. Ptosis

o. Retinoblastoma

p. Strabismus

q. Toxoplasmosis

3. Describe how the following areas are affected in the visually impaired child.
   a. Mobility

   b. Physical environment

   c. Communication

   d. Change

   e. Concept development

4. Describe the technique used for guided walking (blind child walking with sighted guide).

5. List and describe several assessments that may be given to the child with a visual impairment.

a. Assessment			
b. Description			

6. Briefly describe goals and activities that may be used for intervention with a child who is visually impaired.
   a.

   b.

   c.

   d.

3. Pair up with a partner who is blindfolded. Teach your partner how to perform a small craft or activity. When you have finished, switch roles and use a different craft or activity. Record your observations, impressions, and feedback below as an instructor and as a learner.

	INSTRUCTOR	LEARNER
What went well?		
What didn't go well?		
What would you do another time?		
What were your feelings in this role?		

4. Pair up with a partner who is blindfolded. Use guided walking to take your partner to another room. Once there, verbally explain the layout of the room and then position your partner at the entrance to the room and direct him or her to retrieve an item located somewhere in the room. Once this has been accomplished, switch roles. Your partner will now take you to a room. Record your impressions below as you act as a guide and as you are guided. If time permits, repeat this exercise, retrieving several objects at various locations around the room.

	GUIDE	GUIDED
What went well?		
What didn't go well?		
What would you do another time?		
What were your feelings in this role?		

5. Invite a guest speaker who can demonstrate a variety of special techniques that are used with children who have low vision. Include the use of different kinds of canes, sighted guide techniques, search techniques, protective techniques, indoor trailing techniques, and demonstration of a Braillewriter. On completion of the demonstrations, with a partner, practice the different techniques. Record your observations and feelings below. Determine the performance components needed to use the techniques.

TECHNIQUE	OBSERVATIONS/ COMMENTS	FEELINGS	PERFORMANCE COMPONENTS

6a. Work with a partner or small group on a case study assigned by your instructor. Select intervention activities you will do with this child with low vision and demonstrate to the class how you will implement these activities. Briefly plan your set up and presentation below.

Case Study 13: _____

ACTIVITIES	SETUP AND PRESENTATION

6b. Record your classmates' suggestions from their presentations.

ACTIVITIES	SETUP AND PRESENTATION

FOLLOW-UP

✔   Complete the Application of Competencies at the end of this chapter.
✔   Complete a Therapeutic Use of Self Analysis found in Appendix B on your ability to give and receive assistance for vision loss.

HEARING LOSS AND IMPAIRMENT

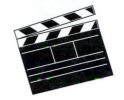

Exercise 56

OBJECTIVES

✔   Identify related terms, levels of hearing loss, and goals for children with hearing impairments
✔   Apply knowledge of basic sign language to construct sentences
✔   Synthesize total communication strategies in a role-play situation

DESCRIPTION

This exercise will introduce you to the population of children with hearing losses and impairments. A child with a hearing loss and impairment will need activities that are specifically adapted to meet his or her needs. Additionally, communication will be a major issue, and adaptations will need to be made in that area also. The use of total communication will be critical, and as a part of that, American Sign Language and/or Signing Exact English will most likely be the mode of communication. Becoming proficient in the use of fundamental signs will be important in communicating and working with children. Other populations with communication deficits such as the autistic-like child may also use sign language to communicate. You will find yourself using basic sign language in a variety of settings and with a variety of client populations.

"If a child is to keep his inborn sense of wonder . . . he needs the companionship of at least one adult who can share it, rediscovering with him the joy, excitement and mystery of the world we live in."

RACHEL CARSON

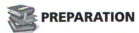 **PREPARATION**

Suggested Readings

Case-Smith, Allen, and Pratt (1996)

Study Questions

1. Describe the importance of using play and the types of sensory systems that should be emphasized in play with hearing impaired children.

2. Describe the type of sounds that are audible to a child with the following hearing loss:

    a. Mild

    b. Moderate

    c. Moderate to severe

    d. Severe

    e. Profound

3. Describe four typical goals that may be appropriate for use in occupational therapy with the hearing-impaired child. Suggest activities that might facilitate accomplishment of each goal.

    a.

    b.

    c.

    d.

4. Define the following terms:
    a. Total communication

    b. Speech reading

    c. Cued speech

    d. Sign language

    e. In-the-ear hearing aid

    f. Behind-the-ear hearing aid

    g. Body aid

    h. Phonic ear

5. Draw a single picture to represent each of the suggestions given for total communication. Title each picture. The first one is completed for you.

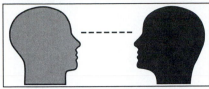

a. Face the child squarely at eye level

b.

c.

d.

e.

f.

g.

h.

i.

j.

k.

6. What assessments might be appropriate to administer to a child with a hearing loss or impairment?

7. Discuss the relationship of validity and the measurements used to test a child with a hearing loss or impairment.

 ACTIVITY

Materials

Random House American Sign Language Dictionary (Costello, 1994)

Instructions

1. Have a guest speaker who is an audiologist demonstrate different types of hearing aids and devices, explaining how they work. List below the type of device demonstrated. Describe its appearance, and record notes about its care and use.

TYPE OF HEARING AID	DESCRIPTION	CARE AND USE INSTRUCTIONS

2. Using a copy of the alphabet in American Sign Language (Costello, 1994), begin to practice learning the letters. Check off each letter as you have it memorized.

□ A □ B □ C □ D □ E □ F □ G □ H □ I
□ J □ K □ L □ M □ N □ O □ P □ Q □ R
□ S □ T □ U □ V □ W □ X □ Y □ Z

3. Have a partner finger spell words to you and see whether you can tell what is being said. Make a list of your accomplishments. Switch roles. Which letters still give you trouble?

ACCOMPLISHMENTS	LETTERS TO BE MASTERED

4. Make a list of the basic beginning signs you will need to know when working with hearing impaired children. Practice using these with a partner. If you have not already done so, decode the sign language sentence in Learning the Jargon exercise in Chapter One. Practice using these words in a sentence to your partner. Make up additional sentences with the words you know. List here the words you have mastered as well as the sentences you have constructed.

WORDS	SENTENCES

5. Divide into groups of three. Role-play teaching a hearing-impaired child to tie his or her shoes or another similar activity. The group member who is not participating should observe and document which of the eleven suggestions for total communication you are using (as found in your study questions). Switch roles until all members have had a turn. Record the feedback you received.

SUGGESTIONS FOR THE USE OF TOTAL COMMUNICATION	CHECK IF PERFORMED	COMMENTS
Face the child squarely at eye level.		
Position yourself so that the child can see your face and hands at the same time without strain.		
Make sure you have the child's attention.		
Avoid light behind you. If the child has to look into the light, he or she may be unable to clearly see your lips.		
Use a normal tone of voice. Do not exaggerate mouth movements because this practice tends to confuse the lip reader.		
Speak the word and give the sign at the same time, rather than in sequence.		
Use appropriate pauses between words, especially when finger spelling is used.		
Better results are obtained when you sit close to the child, rather than across the room.		
Keep instructions simple and to the point.		
Be consistent, especially with the young child.		
Above all, talk to the child. He or she needs to achieve the same amount of input as a hearing child, although the method may be altered.		

Used with permission from: Case-Smith, J., A. S. Allen, and P. N. Pratt. eds. 1996. *Occupational Therapy for Children.* 3d ed. St. Louis: Mosby.

FOLLOW-UP

✔ Complete the Application of Competencies at the end of this chapter.

WORKING WITH FAMILIES

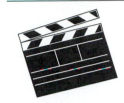

Exercise 57

OBJECTIVES

✔ Identify the role of the family/caregivers in the occupational therapy process
✔ Initiate questions directed toward family and caregivers to gather contextual information
✔ Demonstrate empathy for real-life family and caregiver situations

"Nobody's family can hang out the sign 'Nothing the matter here.'"

CHINESE PROVERB

DESCRIPTION

The purpose of this exercise is to help you understand the importance of and the role of the family and/or caregivers in the occupational therapy (OT) process. The individuals who make up the client's family may be determined by their roles, responsibilities, and life events. It is imperative that the interactions and communications of the family or caregivers be considered in all aspects of the OT process. The family or caregivers are the experts on their own child and problem solving with them about their child is critical. A child will best be served when the family or caregivers and OT practitioners work together as a cohesive team. The cultural context of each child's family will be uniquely different, and your understanding of this will be critical.

PREPARATION

Suggested Readings

Case-Smith, Allen, and Pratt (1996)

Study Questions

1. How is a family defined and what are the functions of a family?

2. Describe the following sources of diversity in families and the role these issues play in working with families:

    a. Structure

    b. Lifestyle

    c. Ethnic background

    d. Socioeconomic background

    e. Parenting style

3. Describe the impact having a child with a disability may have on the following family members:

   a. Mother

   b. Father

   c. Siblings

   d. Extended family

4. List and describe suggested methods to improve your interactions with the family.

5. Discuss specific cultural considerations in working with the families or caregivers of a child.

ACTIVITY

Materials

Guest speakers from families with a disabled child.

Instructions

1a. Invite a parent(s) or family member(s) who has a child with a disability to your class. Have each guest describe the child and the family. Immediately following the presentation, take a few minutes to formulate questions. What do you want to know about working effectively with these families? List your questions as well as the family's responses below.

DESCRIPTIONS	QUESTIONS/RESPONSES
Family 1	
Family 2	
Family 3	

1b. After the discussion, summarize the most important principles you want to remember from your guest speakers.

2a. Role-play one of the following family interactions with a partner. One of you will be the OT practitioner, and one will be the parent. Perform the scenario for your classmates, who will offer feedback. When you critique the performance of your peers, note some of the issues that are important to include in dealing with families, such as respect for family, diversity, flexibility, responsivity, accessibility, empathy, explanation for procedures and activities, suggestions of alternative resources, and use of terminology parents can understand. In your critique, describe how you observed both effective and ineffective communication.

Scenario 1: You are working with a child whose parents have just found out their son has a severe learning disability. He is 8 years old. The mother approaches you angrily before therapy one day and says, "I'm sorry, but I can't trust anything you tell me. I have done all I know for my child, and no one ever once told me he had a problem. Now how do I know what you're telling me is right?"

EFFECTIVE COMMUNICATION	HOW OBSERVED	INEFFECTIVE COMMUNICATION	HOW OBSERVED

Suggestions for improvement in handling this situation:

Scenario 2: The caregiver of a child you are working with informs you next week will be his last visit. She needs to return to work because her federal assistance will be cut off, and she will not be able to bring her child to therapy.

EFFECTIVE COMMUNICATION	HOW OBSERVED	INEFFECTIVE COMMUNICATION	HOW OBSERVED

Suggestions for improvement in handling this situation:

Scenario 3: A father of a child you have just started in treatment says to you on the phone, " Why do you always ask for my wife when you call to talk about our son? Don't you think I know anything?"

EFFECTIVE COMMUNICATION	HOW OBSERVED	INEFFECTIVE COMMUNICATION	HOW OBSERVED

Suggestions for improvement in handling this situation:

Scenario 4: You are working with a child who is one of seven children. You have made a splint for him to wear on his right hand. This splint is helping to maintain ROM and prevent contractures. It also puts his hand in a functional position, allowing some grasp to take place so that his hand may be used as an assist. He is not wearing his splint or doing any of his exercises at home. His parents both work full-time and at times seem overwhelmed with daily routines.

EFFECTIVE COMMUNICATION	HOW OBSERVED	INEFFECTIVE COMMUNICATION	HOW OBSERVED

Suggestions for improvement in handling this situation:

Scenario 5: You are working with a child and attempting to instruct his mother in activities that would be helpful at home. During the session the child is frequently distracted and requires redirection to stay away from other materials in the room. His mother screams at him and grabs his arm abruptly to bring him back to task. You believe that her interactions are inappropriate.

EFFECTIVE COMMUNICATION	HOW OBSERVED	INEFFECTIVE COMMUNICATION	HOW OBSERVED

Suggestions for improvement in handling this situation:

Scenario 6: The caregiver of a child you are treating sends a note in with her child to school. The note says that she feels she has not been kept informed of her child's progress adequately. She writes that this is just another example of how kids at this school who have problems are always given less than adequate assistance.

EFFECTIVE COMMUNICATION	HOW OBSERVED	INEFFECTIVE COMMUNICATION	HOW OBSERVED

Suggestions for improvement in handling this situation:

Other Scenarios (Make up your own):

EFFECTIVE COMMUNICATION	HOW OBSERVED	INEFFECTIVE COMMUNICATION	HOW OBSERVED

Suggestions for improvement in handling this situation:

2b. Summarize and record your own strengths and weaknesses in the role-play scenario as critiqued by yourself and your classmates.

STRENGTHS	WEAKNESSES

2c. List weaknesses in your ability to interact with families and how you plan to improve each one identified. If you are unsure how to improve, seek the assistance of your instructor or counselor.

IDENTIFIED WEAKNESSES	PLAN TO IMPROVE

FOLLOW-UP

✔ Complete the Application of Competencies at the end of this chapter.
✔ Complete a Therapeutic Use of Self Analysis found in Appendix B on your ability to communicate and interact with families.

Exercise 58

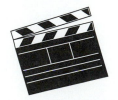

"Potential: It's all there. You've just got to work to get it out."

GLENN VAN EKEIN

CONSTRUCTING ADAPTIVE EQUIPMENT

OBJECTIVES

✔ Identify characteristics of well-constructed adaptive equipment
✔ Construct a notebook pressure switch
✔ Construct a tri-wall piece of adaptive equipment

DESCRIPTION

This exercise will give you experience in constructing adaptive equipment. In your occupational therapy practice, your clients may need adaptive equipment to facilitate their growth toward independence and function. Many pieces of adaptive equipment can be purchased commercially. However, at times the cost can be prohibitive, especially as children typically outgrow some of their adaptive equipment at a fairly rapid pace. Additionally, a commercially made piece of adaptive equipment may not suit the exact and specific needs of your client. Therefore, not infrequently, you will need to design and make your own adaptive equipment. Becoming proficient at doing so will serve you and your client well.

PREPARATION

Suggested Readings

Baker and Kilburn (1992)
Case-Smith, Allen, and Pratt (1996)
Ryan (1995a)

Study Questions

1. Briefly describe the desirable qualities of an assistive device.

2. How are single switches used to allow a child to interact with his or her environment?

3. Discuss ways to use switches and battery-operated items to meet therapeutic goals.

4. What safety precautions need to be adhered to in using a battery-operated device with a child?

5. Take a walk through a toy store. Which toys could be activated by a switch? Try to find several for each age group listed below:
   a. Early childhood

   b. Preschool

   c. School-age

   d. Adolescence

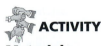 **ACTIVITY**

Materials

Items for switch construction: Plastic folders, aluminum oven liner, foam, double-sided tape, copper conduit, wire cutters, scissors, rosin care solder, soldering iron, awl, two conductor 22-gauge standard wire, battery-operated toy.
Items for tri-wall construction: Tri-wall, electric drill, saw, duct tape, dowel rods, sandpaper, glue gun, glue sticks, patterns, adhesive paper, safety goggles, *Tri-Wall Pattern Portfolio* (Baker and Kilburn, 1992).

Instructions

1. Before you begin this activity, your instructor will cover the use of the following pieces of equipment and the safety precautions that need to be used with each. Record that information here.

EQUIPMENT	USE	PRECAUTIONS
Electric drill		
Jigsaw		
Glue gun		
Electric sander		
Soldering iron		
Other		
Other		

2a. Construct a notebook pressure switch. As you follow your instructor's demonstrations, check each step as it is completed.

STEPS TO SWITCH COMPLETION (BURKHART, 1985)	✔
Cut half of the folder in half.	
Cut the oven liner to cover each piece, then tape in place with double-sided tape.	
Attach a 3-inch foam piece to each corner of one piece of the folder with double-sided tape.	
Put a hole in one corner of each folder piece with the awl.	
Cut a length of wire and strip the ends of each with wire cutters.	
Attach one end of the wire to the aluminum foil.	
Cut 1-inch square copper conduit and attach the wire with soldering iron to it.	
Insert the copper plate between the battery and the receptacle.	
Press the switch and activate the toy.	

2b. Discuss the possibilities for implementation and adaptation of your switch.

3a. Construct a piece of adaptive equipment from tri-wall patterns (e.g., stroller insert, corner seat, table, slant board and footstool) (Baker and Kilburn, 1992). Follow the steps to completion, checking each box as you go. Record comments in the space following each step. Comments may include details you would like to remember about performing this step and/or feedback you received from your instructor to improve your performance.

Adaptive equipment: _____

STEPS	✔	COMMENTS
Cut out pattern in cardboard		
Trace pattern into tri-wall		
Cut out tri-wall pieces		
Drill holes		
Cut dowel pieces needed		
Assemble		
Glue		
Tape edges		
Cover with adhesive paper		

3b. As a class, discuss and list possible items that may be constructed by using tri-wall and the new skills you have just acquired.

FOLLOW-UP

✔ Complete the Application of Competencies at the end of this chapter.
✔ For each of the completed adaptive devices fill out an Analysis of Self found in Appendix B.
✔ Complete Performance Skill 3B on Toy Adaptation.
✔ Complete Performance Skill 3C on Adaptive Equipment Construction.

INTERVENTION PLANNING

Exercise 59

OBJECTIVES

✔ Identify the components of the intervention planning process
✔ Describe the roles of the occupational therapist and the occupational therapy assistant in intervention planning
✔ Discus the relationship of problem identification, goal writing, and activity selection in the intervention planning process

DESCRIPTION

This exercise will familiarize you with the intervention planning process. Both the occupational therapist and the occupational therapy practitioner have critical roles in this process. Families and caregivers play an important role also. Problem identification, goal writing, and activity selection are all important aspects. As an OT practitioner you need to be very familiar and comfortable with the process of intervention planning. You

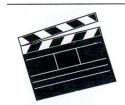

"Children need love, especially when they do not deserve it."

HAROLD S. HULBERT

also need to be able to effectively communicate the rationale for the various aspects of the treatment planning process to the child's family and/or caregivers. Your explanation will be used to promote the family's understanding and their collaborative efforts as you work together as a team. Teamwork is critical in providing effective and therapeutic intervention for children.

PREPARATION

Suggested Readings

Case-Smith, Allen, and Pratt (1996)
AOTA (latest edition)

Study Questions

1. Review and describe the intervention planning steps as outlined by the "Standards of Practice" in the *Reference Manual of the Official Documents of the American Occupational Therapy Association* (AOTA, latest edition).

2. What is critical to keep in mind in selecting activities to ensure there is a goodness-of-fit between the child and the expectations of the activity/environment?

3. What are the benefits of providing therapy in a group situation?

4. Describe child-centered activity and the philosophy behind this service delivery model.

5. Describe the advantages of team planning for intervention and how problem solving may be accomplished by a team.

6. What are the different methods occupational therapy can be delivered?

7. How might an orientation to a particular frame of reference assist in your selection of activities?

8. Describe the relationship of the evaluation process to treatment planning.

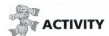 **ACTIVITY**

Materials

Case Study 6 located at the end of Chapter 1.

Instructions

1a. Work with a partner or a small group using the case study assigned by your instructor. List the areas of concern that are within the domains of occupational therapy.

1b. List below problems that are not addressed by occupational therapy, and report to what team member you would refer the client in order to address the identified problems.

AREAS OF CONCERN	TEAM MEMBER

1c. List below the assessment instruments you would like to administer.

1d. Select three priority areas of concern from your case study and use the Treatment Planning Worksheet found on the next page to plan intervention for this child. After you have selected your problems, write one long-term goal and one short-term goal for each problem. Decide on your goals and select occupations that you would use in therapy to address these problems. Include the projected time needed for this activity. Include your rationale for occupation selection and the frame of reference you might use. Describe how you would set up the occupation, the environment, yourself, and the child.

TREATMENT PLANNING WORKSHEET

PROBLEM	LONG-TERM GOAL	SHORT-TERM GOAL	OCCUPATION/ ACTIVITY/TIME	RATIONALE/ FRAME OF REFERENCE	SETUP

1e. Share your ideas with your class. Have each group member assist in presenting.

1f. Describe the roles of the occupational therapy assistant and the occupational therapist throughout Activity 1.

TASKS THAT COULD BE PERFORMED BY THE OTA	TASKS PERFORMED BY THE OT

1g. Report here how you would describe occupational therapy and the intervention plan to the child's parents.

1b. With which team members will you likely be working in treating this child? Describe what roles they will play.

FOLLOW-UP

✔ Complete the Application of Competencies at the end of this chapter.
✔ Complete Performance Skill 3E on Intervention Planning.

WELLNESS/PREVENTION FOR THE ADOLESCENT

Exercise 60

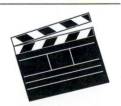

OBJECTIVES

✔ Identify the issues facing adolescents in years past as well as today
✔ Identify topics of need and interest to the adolescent
✔ Prepare a presentation on wellness and prevention that is appropriate for the adolescent population

DESCRIPTION

This exercise is intended to help you understand the issues facing adolescents and the role you as an occupational therapy practitioner might play in maintaining health and wellness in this population. Adolescence can be a very difficult period of time for some teens. With the changing times and all the issues facing adolescents, they are often prone to illness as well as faced with difficult choices and peer pressure. Dealing with wellness and prevention in this population is critical. Populations of adolescents who are already at risk are prime candidates for wellness and prevention assistance from occupational therapy practitioners.

"People have a way of becoming what we encourage them to be—not what we nag them to be."

SCUDDER N. PARKER

PREPARATION

Suggested Readings

Case-Smith, Allen, and Pratt (1996)

Study Questions

1. Find a quiet place where you will not be disturbed. Think back to your teenage years for facts and feelings on the following topics. Then reflect on present-day issues.

   a. Changes (social, emotional, physical, psychological) and your responses to them

THEN	NOW

   b. Drugs and alcohol (you may include personal accounts if you feel comfortable doing so)

THEN	NOW

   c. Deaths and/or suicides (Describe how you and others coped)

THEN	NOW

2.   Describe your fondest memory and your least favorite memory as an adolescent.

3.   What physical, cognitive, and psychosocial changes occur in adolescence?

4.   Considering the normal changes that occur in adolescence, what are some of the added challenges for the teenager with a disability?

5.   With what identity issues does an adolescent deal?

6.   What is the role of the peer group in adolescence?

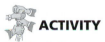 **ACTIVITY**

Materials

Resources on prevention topics found in books such as Korb-Khalsa, Azok, and Leutenberg (1995a, 1995b).

Instructions

1a.   With a small group of your colleagues, prepare a presentation that you will actually give to a group of adolescents. Include information on the subject areas listed below. You may add others as desired.

TOPIC	INFORMATION PRESENTED
Stress management	
Violence prevention	
Injury prevention	
Self-esteem	
Substance abuse prevention	
Community agencies	
Other	

1b.   Describe here the methods of presentation your group will use, including videos, posters, hands-on experiences, handouts, and the like.

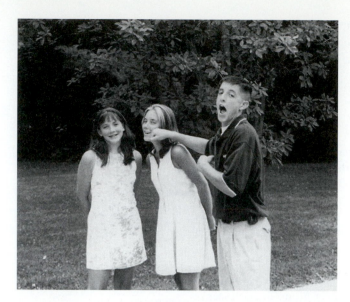

Fig. 3-17 As long as no one gets hurt, "horse-play" among siblings is a healthy part of adolescent development.

Photo courtesy of Corrie, Krista, and Rob Kief.

1c. Design a flier for inviting the students to your presentation.

1d. Assign duties and establish an outline with times specifying who will be responsible for what duty during your actual presentation.

OUTLINE OF TOPICS	TIME	STUDENT RESPONSIBLE

1e. After your actual presentation to the adolescents, discuss the strengths and weaknesses of the presentation.

STRENGTHS	WEAKNESSES

1f. What would you do differently?

1g. How was your presentation received by your audience?

1h. Were there any surprises?

FOLLOW-UP

✔ Complete an Analysis of Self on your performance of this exercise.
✔ Complete the Application of Competencies at the end of this chapter.
✔ Complete a Therapeutic Use of Self Analysis found in Appendix B on your presentation performance.

After completion of each exercise, write one concept you learned and how you anticipate that learning will influence your treatment of clients.

Application of Competencies

Exercise 37 Observation
Application:

Exercise 38 The Evaluation Process
Application:

Exercise 39 Pediatric Intervention Areas
Application:

Exercise 40 Range of Motion
Application:

Exercise 41 Positioning and Handling
Application:

Exercise 42 Reflexes
Application:

Exercise 43 Play
Application:

Exercise 44 Feeding
Application:

Exercise 45 Hand Skills
Application:

Exercise 46 Handwriting
Application:

Exercise 47 Activities of Daily Living
Application:

Exercise 48 Adaptations
Application:

Exercise 49 Behavior Management
Application:

Exercise 50 Sensory Integration
Application:

Exercise 51 School-Based Practice
Application:

Exercise 52 Early Intervention
Application:

Exercise 53 Hospital Services and Rehabilitation
Application:

Exercise 54 Durable Medical Equipment
Application:

Exercise 55 Vision Loss and Impairment
Application:

Exercise 56 Hearing Loss and Impairment
Application:

Exercise 57 Working with Families
Application:

Exercise 58 Constructing Adaptive Equipment
Application:

Exercise 59 Intervention Planning
Application:

Exercise 60 Wellness/Prevention for the Adolescent
Application:

ADDING TO YOUR FILES

Search and add occupations to your activity file for children from newborn through school age. Type a paper on each activity with the information in the following chart and assemble with a table of contents. Include in your file at least one activity that will work on the targeted areas listed below. Note on each occupation the ages for which it is intended. Be sure to have activities for a wide variety of ages. Include activities that have diverse cultural and contextual qualities. Use at least three references that you have not used previously. List the occupations and activities you have gathered. Check each box as you complete the requirements. When the chart is completed, you will have at least sixteen new activities.

TARGETED AREA	OCCUPATION	RATIONALE	PERFORMANCE CONTEXT	SUPPLIES/ MATERIALS	STEPS TO PERFORM	ADAPTATIONS	PRECAUTIONS	REFERENCES
Increase overall tone								
Decrease overall tone								
Precutting activity								
Prewriting activity								
In-hand manipulation activity								
Heavy work proprioception								
Bilateral use								
Balance								
Chalkboard activity								
Vestibular								
Tip pinch								
Hand strength								
Oral motor strength								
Tactile dis-crimination								
Tactile defen-siveness								
Visual perception								

Performance Skill 3B

TOY ADAPTATION

Adapt a toy, game, or leisure activity for a child with a disability. The child will be assigned by your instructor and should be a child you have seen or worked with on fieldwork. Make six changes to an already existing toy that you obtain and/or purchase. Two of the changes need to be structural. The other four changes can be adaptations made to the environment, social expectations, rules, and so on. Use the following worksheet to plan and record your toy adaptation.

Toy, game, or leisure activity: _____

AREAS ADAPTED	MATERIALS NEEDED	COST

Total cost: _____

Performance Skill 3C

ADAPTIVE EQUIPMENT CONSTRUCTION

Make a piece of adaptive equipment that will enable a child to be independent in an activity of daily living (ADL). In the case of a child who is multiply handicapped, assisting with ADLs may be the goal. In the case in which assistance may not be a realistic goal, the intent may be to assist the caregiver to perform the task more effectively or with less effort. Use this worksheet to plan and record.

ADL task: _____

Equipment made: _____

Describe how it is made (Include patterns where applicable):_____

_____

_____

_____

MATERIALS USED	COST

Total cost: _____

Time to construct: _____

STANDARDIZED TESTING

Administer a standardized test for which you have received instruction on in class to a child whom you select in the community. The child can be a friend's child, a relative, or a neighbor but should not be your own child. Be concerned with utilization of the skills listed below. Have a partner or instructor observe your performance and give feedback by commenting on the skills below.

TEST ADMINISTERED	SKILLS COMPLETE
Correct calculation of age	
Pertinent information to identify child	
Materials arranged appropriately	
Directions given according to manual	
Scores recorded accurately	
Scores compared to norms	
Time recorded if needed	
Attention of child was maintained	
Items given in a timely manner	
Interpret assessment	
List additional assessments needed to complete the evaluation process	

Performance Skill 3E

INTERVENTION PLANNING

Develop an intervention plan for a child from the case study given to you by your instructor.

Case description or number: _____

1. What frame of reference will you be using: _____

2. Choose three problems that are OT concerns:

   a. _____

   b. _____

   c. _____

3. What assessments might be used to evaluate the OT areas of concern?

4. List problems that will need to be addressed by other team members:

PROBLEM	TEAM MEMBERS

5. Write one short-term goal for each OT problem:

   a. _____

   b. _____

   c. _____

6. State two activities you would perform for each problem or goal, reasons you chose each activity, how you would set it up, and one way in which the activity can be graded as the client improves. Be sure to include the frame of reference that would be appropriate to use in carrying out the treatment goals and activities described. Use the worksheet that follows to record your plan.

TREATMENT PLANNING WORKSHEET

	GOAL	ACTIVITY	RATIONALE	SET UP	GRADED	FRAME OF REFERENCE
5a.						
5b.						
5c.						

CASE STUDY 11

PEDIATRICS

Type:
Hospital-based, Outpatient

Age:
2 years, 7 months

Sex:
Male

Culture/Religion:

Insurance Information:

Diagnosis:
Down's syndrome with gastroesophageal reflux

Family Situation:
Jerry is currently in foster care because of an abusive/neglectful home situation. It is believed that he will eventually rejoin his family. Jerry appears to have a close relationship with his foster mother of two months.

Strengths:
Jerry has full ROM in all extremities. On observation he is curious and interactive with people and objects. He is able to turn one page at a time in a book on an inconsistent basis. Jerry is walking when holding on to someone's hand or furniture.

Problems:
Jerry's hand use is at a 15-month level according to the Peabody Scales of Infant Motor Development. He is not participating in any self-help activities. He has made attempts at self-feeding using a primitive hand pattern. When observed picking up pegs, he uses an inferior pincer grasp with thumb and index finger or his thumb and middle finger.

Jerry tends to hold his mouth in an open position with his tongue protruding. His chin and shirt are wet from saliva.

CASE STUDY 12

PEDIATRICS

Type:
School-based

Age:
7 years old

Sex:
Male

Culture/Religion:

Insurance Information:

Diagnosis:
Developmental delay

Family Situation:
Interested, capable, two-parent family with one other child, who is a girl, age 3. There appears to be good follow-through with therapy goals at home.

Strengths:
Jerrod is curious and active and loves music. He is able to sign several words. He has full

passive ROM in UEs. Jerrod will attempt simple puzzles and walks with a walker. He will attempt to use both UEs together at times. He cooperates in dressing and undressing and is beginning to remove loose clothing and pull on some clothes. Jerrod feeds himself with a spoon and manages a cup with minimal spilling.

Problem List:
Jerrod has a short attention span and an IQ between 30 and 50. His expressive language is limited to whines and vowel sounds. He is nonfunctional with the communication board at this time. Jerrod can pull to standing but is unable to balance or walk without support. He neglects use of his right UE. His grasp in both hands is a gross palmar and a lateral pinch.

Jerrod frequently drools and swallows with difficulty. He is unable to suck on a straw and his blow is weak.

He has fluctuating tone with mild spasticity affecting UEs and LEs. Tonic (primitive) reflexes mildly affecting active movements.

PEDIATRICS

CASE STUDY 13

Type:
School-based

Age:
16 years old

Sex:
Male

Culture/Religion:

Insurance Information:

Diagnosis:
CP (spastic quadriplegia), seizures, scoliosis with rods, legally blind

Family Situation:
Ken lives with his grandmother, who has raised him since he was 3. There are no other family members that have contact.

Strengths:
Ken can swallow pureed and ground foods. He swallows best when in a J-seat. He has a "foam in place" wheelchair. Ken appears to have the ability to wash his face. He wipes his hand across his mouth when an undesired food is offered.

Problem List:
Ken requires total assistance to eat, requiring jaw control to swallow liquids that are thickened. He is dependent in all self-care. Ken participates in almost constant self-stimulatory behavior. He inconsistently shakes his head to indicate no. UE active ROM limited in all joints. He is inconsistent with activating a switch.

PEDIATRICS

CASE STUDY 14

Type:
School-based

Age:
7 years old

Sex:
Male

Culture/Religion:

Insurance Information:

Diagnosis:
Seizures, CVA at birth, CP, blind, microcephaly

Family Situation:
Jason is currently placed in a foster home. His mother was 16 when she gave birth to Jason and was unable to cope with the seriousness of his condition. She has since given up her rights as parent. No other family members are involved.

Strengths:
Jason is able to suck baby food from a spoon placed to his lips. He has normal passive ROM in all extremities.

Problem List:
Jason often displays a bite reflex when the spoon is placed in his mouth. There is some suggestion of hearing loss due to his being unresponsive to many sounds. When presented with sensory experiences, Jason demonstrates an increased flexor tone. His posture is poor, and he is unable to maintain sitting position for even brief periods of time. He doesn't use his hands for functional activities and requires total care. He has a wheelchair.

He is new to school, and the foster mother reports that he received minimal interaction at his previous foster home. She is unsure of previous occupational therapy intervention.

CASE STUDY 15

PEDIATRICS

Type:
Hospital-based, Outpatient

Age:
8 years old

Sex:
Female

Culture/Religion:

Insurance Information:

Diagnosis:
Neurofibromatosis type 1 and fine motor delay

Family Situation:
Tammy is the fifth of seven children; both parents live in the home. She attends second grade in the public school system, where she receives speech therapy.

Strengths:
Tammy enjoys playing soccer and riding her bicycle with training wheels. She appears very social and talkative. At times she is difficult to understand. Tammy is working academically at grade level. Her hand dominance has been established in her right hand.

Problem List:
Tammy has decreased muscle tone throughout, especially in her hands. She has poor coordination and speed of movements. She demonstrates poor handwriting and tires quickly when doing schoolwork. Tammy also has difficulty with buttons and snaps and is often sloppy when eating.

PEDIATRICS

Type:
Hospital-based, Outpatient

Age:
6 months, 8 days

Sex:
Female

Culture/Religion:

Insurance Information:

Diagnosis:
29 weeks premature; pregnancy complicated by history of cocaine abuse; cerebral infarction

Family Situation:
Tommy is currently in foster care. His foster mother reports being very willing to bring him in and follow through with exercises. She brings two other foster children with her to the appointment.

Strengths:
In supported sitting, Tommy demonstrates relatively stable head support and straight spine. He is alerting appropriately and tracking toys. Tommy is reportedly eating well and continues to gain a small amount of weight at a time.

Problem List:
Foster mother reports an increase in stiffness in all extremities. Tommy is noted in clinical observations to maintain his elbows in flexion, and his shoulders are held retracted into the supporting surface. He did keep his hands open most of the time during the evaluation and briefly maintained grasp on toys placed in his hands.

In the supine position he has difficulty stabilizing his trunk. He is unable to raise his head more than 30° and cannot sustain it in the midline.

PEDIATRICS

Type:
School-based

Age:
5 years old

Sex:
Female

Culture/Religion:

Insurance Information:

Diagnosis:
Spina bifida

Family Situation:
Kerri is the older of two children, both living with their parents. Kerri's younger brother is 2 years old.

Strengths:

Kerri is currently attending a half-day kindergarten program at a school for children with special needs. She is currently receiving physical and occupational therapy. Kerri enjoys vestibular input and likes to play with computer activities. She is independent in use of her walker while wearing her braces and independent in propelling her wheelchair, which she uses for most of her mobility. Kerri is a talkative young lady who appears to be learning quickly. Her ROM is WNL. She can sit independently on the floor.

Problem List:

Kerri is fearful in upright position owing to decrease in balance. She is on an NG tube at this time, refusing to eat most foods. She eats baby food and prefers to drink only water. She is sensory defensive in her mouth and oral area and frequently gags with various input and food. She also has a hyperactive gag reflex. Kerri's muscle tone is low throughout. Her legs are windswept, and her trunk tilts to the right. In observing Kerri in the classroom, there are many activities she does not participate in owing to her avoidance of various textures.

CASE STUDY 18

PEDIATRICS

Type:
Early Intervention

Age:
2 years

Sex:
Female

Culture/Religion:

Insurance Information:

Diagnosis:
Hydrocephalus, occipital encephalocele

Family Situation:
Lauren lives with her mother and five older children. There is no mention of a father figure.

Strengths:
Lauren's passive ROM and muscle tone are grossly WNL. She uses neat princer grasp to obtain a Cheerio™ with her right hand. She was observed to transfer a 1-inch block from one hand to the other.

Problems:
Lauren wears glasses and brings objects close to her eyes to manipulate them. She requires minimum assistance to transition from supine to prone to quadruped to sitting. She sits with a widely abducted and externally rotated hips and a rounded back with posterior pelvic tilt. She pivots in sitting using trunk rotation but appears very unsteady. Lauren uses a radial digital grasp to obtain 1-inch blocks with both hands. She is not able to hold a crayon adaptively and has not been observed to isolate her index finger. She also has not been observed using wrist extension or forearm supination. She can randomly drop objects but not in a controlled fashion.

Lauren eats some ground food by mouth and takes the rest via a NG tube. She is noted to have extremely weak oral musculature with excessive drooling from her mouth which is held in an open position with tongue protruding.

ADOLESCENT PSYCHIATRY

Type:
Hospital-based, Inpatient

Age:
16 years old

Sex:
Female

Culture/Religion:

Insurance Information:

Diagnosis:
Obsessive-compulsive disorder, social phobia, and depression

Social History:
Erin lives with her parents. She is the only child. She is being educated at home because of an inability to have social contacts. She reports that her interests are in computer, listening to music, and watching TV.

Medical History:
Erin was brought to the hospital because of threats of suicide and threats to kill her parents. She has been tearful, saying that her parents overreacted and that she didn't mean the threats.

Erin was admitted several years ago to a juvenile facility for problems with AD/HD that were unsuccessfully treated. She complained of stomachaches and stopped the program. Her parents report constant problems. Erin doesn't comb or bathe for weeks because she doesn't feel like it. She has a very short attention span.

PEDIATRICS

Type:
Hospital-based, Outpatient

Age:
9 years old

Sex:
Female

Culture/Religion:

Insurance Information:

Diagnosis:
Puncture wound to right palm, partially torn tendon

Family Situation:
Laura lives with both parents on a rotating basis. She lives with her mother and two brothers from Monday to Thursday and with her father and his wife from Friday to Sunday.

Strengths:
Laura is one month post injury, and her skin is healed. She is very active in sports and wishes to return to playing soccer and volleyball. She is of average intelligence and does well in school. Laura is right handed.

Problem List:

Laura's scar is approximately two-thirds of the entire surface of her hand. Her scar is very tender, and she is unable to tolerate much touch to her palm. She holds her right arm and hand in a guarded fashion, usually with her shoulder and elbow to her side.

Laura is about 1 inch from full flexion of all fingers. She lacks sensation only in the scar area. She reports some difficulty with handwriting in school and with small buttons on her shirt. When observed in an activity, such as catching a large ball, she uses right UE reluctantly and tends to keep her palm off of the surface, using her fingers instead.

CASE STUDY 21

PEDIATRICS

Type:
Hospital-based, Outpatient

Age:
9 years, 1 month

Sex:
Male

Culture/Religion:

Insurance Information:

Diagnosis:
AD/HD, meningitis

Family Situation:
Joshua lives with his mother during the week and with his father on the weekends. There are three younger children in the family, ages 6, 4, and 1. Joshua's mother reports that he had meningitis when he was two weeks old. He is in the third grade and attends special classes.

Strengths:
Joshua separated from his mother easily and was very cooperative during testing. He displayed no tactile defensiveness. During writing tasks he stabilized his paper with his right hand.

Problems:
Joshua's teacher asked for the evaluation because of increasing difficulty at school. She reports that he is unable to learn cursive handwriting, he is unable to tie his shoes, and has difficulty with snaps and buttons.

On evaluation Joshua was noted to have decreased muscle tone throughout, with decreased proximal stability. His hands were noted to have joint laxity. During writing tasks he was noted to sit left of center and used limited wrist extension and displayed hypermobility in his fingers. To hold a pencil, he used a static quadruped grasp with overlapping thumb and index hyperextension. He was noted to have a left hand preference, but it does not appear that dominance has been established.

Joshua appears to have right/left confusion and difficulty in planning sequential movements. Several times during testing he was distracted by visual stimulation.

When Joshua was placed on the ball, he immediately asked to get down. He held the prone extension pattern for 3 seconds and supine flexion for 8 seconds. He had difficulty with all movement tasks involving motor planning.

PEDIATRICS

Type:
School-based

Age:
6 years old

Sex:
Female

Culture/Religion:

Insurance Information:

Diagnosis:
Autism

Family Situation:
Kendra is one of three children who all live with their parents. She has a 10-year-old sister and a 3-year-old brother. Her parents are very supportive of all services provided.

Strength:
Kendra has normal muscle tone, ROM, posture, and balance. She demonstrates a positive response to brushing using the Wilbarger Protocol, and she craves bouncing and deep pressure input. She is independent in toileting and eating. She is very good with puzzles and does well on the playground equipment.

Problem List:
Kendra demonstrates no hand dominance. She does not seem to know how to interact with other children; she plays alone. She is unable to communicate her needs in an appropriate manner. When approached by an adult, she stares with no response.

Kendra is currently attending a school for disabled children. Kendra has a primitive grasp on a crayon or pencil and is unable to imitate any lines or shapes, only scribbles randomly.

REFERENCES

American Occupational Therapy Associations. latest edition. *Reference Manual of the Official Documents of the American Occupational Therapy Association*. Bethesda, MD: Author.

American Occupational Therapy Association. 1998. *Reference Manual of the Official Documents of the American Occupational Therapy Association*. Bethesda, MD: Author.

Amundson, S. J. 1995. *Evaluation Tool of Children's Handwriting*. Homer, AK: O.T. Kids.

Asher, I. E. 1996. *Occupational Therapy Assessment Tools: An Annotated Index*. 2d ed. Bethesda, MD: American Occupational Therapy Association.

Baker, M., and J. Kilburn. 1992. *Tri-Wall Pattern Portfolio*. Tucson, AZ: Therapy Skill Builders.

Beery, K. E. 1989. *Beery Developmental Test of Visual Motor Integration*. 3d rev. Cleveland, OH: Modern Curriculum Press.

Bruininks, R. 1978. *Bruininks-Osentesky Test of Motor Proficiency*. Circle Pines, MN: American Guidance Service.

Burkhart, L. J. 1985. *More Homemade Battery Devices for Severely Handicapped with Suggested Activities*. Handout from Assistive Technologist.

Case-Smith, J., A. S. Allen, and P. N. Pratt. 1996. *Occupational Therapy for Children*. 3d ed. St. Louis: Mosby.

Case-Smith, J., and C. Pehoski. 1992. *Development of Hand Skills in the Child*. Bethesda, MD: American Occupational Therapy Association.

Christiansen, C. ed. 2000. *Ways of Living: Self-Care Strategies for Special Needs*. 2d ed. Bethesda, MD: American Occupational Therapy Association.

Costello, E. 1994. *Random House American Sign Language Dictionary*. New York: Random House.

Dunn, W. ed. 1991. *Pediatric Occupational Therapy: Facilitating Effective Service Provision*. Thorofare, NJ: Slack.

Farber, S. D. 1982. *Neurorehabilitation: A Multisensory Approach*. Philadelphia: W. B. Saunders.

Fisher, A. G., E. A. Murray, and A. C. Bundy. 1991. *Sensory Integration Theory and Practice*. Philadelphia: F. A. Davis.

Frankenburg, W. K. 1990. *Denver II: Training Video*. Denver, CO: Denver Developmental Materials.

Frankenburg, W. K., J. Dodds, P. Archer, B. Bresnick, P. Maschka, N. Edelman, and H. Shapiro. 1992. *Denver II Training Manual*. Denver, CO: Denver Developmental Materials.

Hanft, B., and D. Marsh. 1992. *Getting a Grip on Handwriting*. Bethesda, MD: American Occupational Therapy Association.

Henry, D. n.d. *Tools for Teachers: A Video on Practical Occupational Therapy Strategies*. Phoenix, AZ: Henry Occupational Therapy Services.

Hinojosa, J., and P. Kramer. 1998. *Evaluation: Obtaining and Interpreting Data*. Sterling, VA: World Composition Services.

Klein, M. D., and T. A. Delaney. 1994. *Feeding and Nutrition for the Child with Special Needs*. Tucson, AZ: Therapy Skill Builders.

Knight, J. M., and M. J. Decker. 1994. *Hands at Work and Play: Developing Fine Motor Skills at School and Home*. Tucson, AZ: Therapy Skill Builders.

Korb-Khalsa, K. L., S. D. Azok, and E. A. Leutenberg. 1995a. *Life Management Skills III*. Beechwood, OH: Wellness Reproductions.

Korb-Khalsa, K. L., S. D. Azok, and E. A. Leutenberg. 1995b. *S.E.A.L.S. + Plus*. Beechwood, OH: Wellness Reproductions.

Kramer, P., and J. Hinojosa. 1998. *Frames of Reference for Pediatric Occupational Therapy*. 2d ed. Baltimore: Lippincott Williams & Wilkins.

Morris, G. S., and D. J. Stiehl. 1989. *Changing Kid's Games*. Champaign, IL: Human Kinetics.

Neidstadt, M. E., and E. B. Crepeau. 1998. *Willard and Spackman's Occupational Therapy*. 9th ed. Philadelphia: J. B. Lippincott.

Oetter, P., E. W. Richter, and S. M. Frick. 1995. *M.O.R.E. Integrating the Mouth with Sensory and Postural Functions*. 2d ed. Hugo, MN: PDP Press.

Olsen, J. S. 1998. *Handwriting Without Tears*. 7th ed. Potomac, MD: Handwriting Without Tears.

Parham, D. L., and L. S. Fazio. 1997. *Play in Occupational Therapy*. St. Louis: Mosby.

Pierson, F. M. 1999. *Principles and Techniques of Patient Care*. 2d ed. Philadelphia: W. B. Saunders.

Reed, K. L. 1991. *Quick Reference to Occupational Therapy*. Gaithersburg, MD: Aspen Publishers.

Ryan, S. E. 1995a. *The Certified Occupational Therapy Assistant: Principles, Concepts, and Techniques*. 2d ed. Thorofare, NJ: Slack.

Scheerer, C. R. 1997. *Sensorimotor Groups: Activities for School and Home*. San Antonio, TX: Therapy Skill Builders.

Sher, B. 1992. *Extraordinary Play with Ordinary Things*. Tucson, AZ: Therapy Skill Builders.

Toronto Sensory Integration Group. 1987. *Sensory Integration Therapy*. Tucson, AZ: Therapy Skill Builders.

Trefler, E., D. A. Hobson, S. J. Taylor, L. C. Monahan, and C. G. Shaw. 1993. *Seating and Positioning for Persons with Physical Disabilities*. Tucson, AZ: Therapy Skill Builders.

Competencies in Psychosocial Practice

Exercise 61

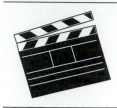

"What one hears is doubtful, what one sees with one's eyes is certain."

CHINESE SAYING

OBSERVATION SKILLS

OBJECTIVES

✔ Develop acute and accurate observation skills
✔ Record specific and measurable observations
✔ Discuss the importance of observation skills as they relate to the occupational therapy process

DESCRIPTION

This exercise is intended to sharpen our observation skills. As an occupational therapy (OT) practitioner, you will need to continually fine-tune your observation skills. You will use your observation skills during all parts of the OT process, from the first step of screening through the last step of discontinuation. Your observations will be a part of your evaluation process and will help to guide your intervention. Specific and measurable observations will guide your clinical reasoning skills as you make decisions and solve problems through the OT process for your clients. Your observations will need to encompass all the areas of your clients' life skills.

 PREPARATION

Suggested Readings

> Denton (1987)
> Early (2000)
> Mosey (1986)
> Purtillo and Haddad (1996)

Study Questions

1. List and describe several ways in which humans communicate about themselves.

2. List and describe predetermined blocks and distortions to effective listening.

3. Describe the role of observation in the evaluation process.

4. Define and describe the following types of observation:
   a. Naturalistic

   b. Analogue

   c. Participant monitoring

5. Why is it important to validate the meaning of your client's nonverbal communication to him or her?

6. Describe the importance of observation in the intervention and intervention-planning process.

7. Describe how a particular frame of reference and/or theory base may influence or bias your observations.

8. How can cultural background influence or bias observations?

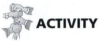 **ACTIVITY**

Materials

Bag of oranges (one orange for each student), game of Interference© (University of Missouri, 1989).

Instructions

1. Select one orange from the pile of oranges and study it carefully, as you will be asked to identify it later. Replace it in the pile. Later when you identify your orange, write in the following space your reasons for your success or failure in identifying your orange. Discuss the importance of detailed observation in clinical practice.

2. Select a partner and face each other. Have a discussion about a chosen topic for about two minutes. Observe your partner closely, taking mental note of his or her appearance. When the time is up, have your partner leave the room and change five things about his or her appearance. When your partner returns, try to find the five things he or she changed. Record comments about how accurate your observation skills were.

3. Participate in playing the game Interference© (University of Missouri, 1989). After the game, answer the following questions and then discuss the answers as a class.

   a. What was your involvement as a participant, including props and symptoms you were given?

   b. What did you observe other members demonstrating?

Fig. 4-1 The game of Interference facilitates better understanding of mental health issues.

Photo courtesy of Pam Boone, Christie Tuttle, Gina Knab, Tracy Holt, Kim Meyer, Jessica Johantges, Brenda Morris, and Paula Downey.

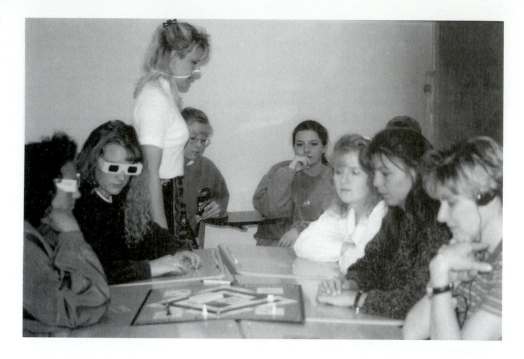

c. What were your feelings during the game? What are your feelings now?

d. What diagnoses may have represented the behaviors and symptoms demonstrated in the game?

e. Did playing this game increase your understanding of people with mental illness? If so, how?

f. How will what you learned affect your interaction of those with mental illness?

g. How did playing this game help with your observation skills?

4a. Independently read each of the following observations. Decide whether the observation recorded is measurable. Check yes if it is and no if it is not. If you check yes, write an observation using the same information that would not be measurable. If you check no, write an observation that is measurable. When you have finished, discuss this exercise as a class. The first one is completed for you.

OBSERVATION	YES	NO	OBSERVATION REVISION
The client is noted to have poor self-esteem.		X	The client said, "I am unable to do anything right."
The client is noted to be wearing soiled clothing to group.			
In group today, the client was tired.			
In talking to the client, he was angry.			
The client is definitely a loner.			
The client lost his temper by pounding his fists and throwing his project when he made a mistake.			
The client frequently cries throughout the OT session.			

4b. Take one observation that you marked as not measurable and write a problem statement and a goal for this client.

OBSERVATION	PROBLEM STATEMENT	GOAL

4c. Discuss the difficulty in writing a measurable goal from an immeasurable observation. Choose an observation that you checked as measurable and write a problem statement and goal for this client.

OBSERVATION	PROBLEM STATEMENT	GOAL

4d.   Discuss and record the difference between Activities 4b and 4c.

5.   Fill in the following observation form immediately after observing your instructor and a classmate role-playing a client/therapist interaction in a psychosocial setting.

> *Appearance:* Pick a position and describe the client from head to toe. This is like a snapshot. Be sure to note differences in right or left side when indicated.

Position of client: ☐ Standing   ☐ Sitting   ☐ Lying   ☐ Kneeling

☐ Other _____

Position of head: _____

Description of hair: _____

Description of eyes: _____

Description/position of mouth: _____

Any other facial features, scars, sores, saliva, nasal discharge, food, condition of teeth,

facial hair, make-up, jewelry, etc.: _____

_____

Description and Position of: _____

    Shoulders: _____

    Elbows: _____

    Wrists: _____

    Hands: _____

    Trunk: _____

    Hips: _____

    Knees: _____

    Feet: _____

Description of clothing: _____

Description of any splints, braces, or other equipment: _____

_____

Description of wounds, scars, dirt, etc.: _____

_____

Overall impression of appearance: _____

> *Communication:* Describe how the client communicates. Include all forms of communication.

Method of communication used most frequently: ☐ Verbal ☐ Nonverbal

Tone of voice: _____

Receptive language: _____

Initiation of conversation: _____

Expressive language: _____

Describe any unusual vocalizations: _____

Give an example of what the client says, to whom, and in what context: _____

_____

_____

_____

Describe gestures used, to whom, and in what context: _____

_____

_____

_____

Describe sign language used, to whom, and in what context: _____

_____

Describe any other comments or types of communication used, including any augmentative communication devices: _____

_____

Overall impression of communication: _____

> *Emotion:* Describe the emotional response of the client, how it is displayed and in what context. Note the changes experienced during the session. Infer emotional state associated with the observed behavior.

BEHAVIOR	DESCRIBE SITUATION INVOLVED	RELATED EMOTIONAL STATE

Overall impression of emotional tone during session: _____

> *Response to Intervention.* *Describe how the client responded to the intervention, activity, occupation utilized. It may not be possible to include all of the components you are observing, so focus on just one activity.*

Task: _____

Attended to task: _____ minutes/seconds at a time (circle one).

Ability/quality of performance: How successfully was the task accomplished? (e.g.,

craft, movement group, discussion group, ADL completion, etc.) _____

_____

_____

_____

_____

_____

Assistance required: _____

_____

Describe gross motor activities: Position of body, use of all extremities together:

_____

_____

_____

Describe use of hands: How they are being used; describe grasp:

Right hand: _____

_____

Left hand: _____

_____

Oral motor: Drink from cup, straw, blow, suck, close lips, extraneous movements of lips

and tongue, etc: _____

_____

_____

_____

Tactile system: Describe tactile intervention and response of the client: _____

_____

_____

_____

Vestibular/proprioceptive system: Describe movement intervention and responses of

the client: _____

_____

_____

Treatment technique: Describe the intervention performed response of the client:

_____

_____

Adaptations/modifications made: _____

Overall impression of performance: _____

Social Involvement: *Describe how the client relates to peers.*

Peers present: _____

Describe environment/situation: _____

_____

Describe interaction(s): _____

_____

Describe response of client to peers: _____

_____

Describe response of peers to client: _____

_____

Overall impression of social skills: _____

Reaction to Authority: *Describe how the client relates to therapists, staff members, student, practioners, and family members.*

Describe separation from family/caregiver: _____

_____

Engagement in directed activity: _____

_____

Redirection given and client response: _____

_____

_____

Content of conversation areas: _____

_____

Motivational techniques employed and response from client: _____

_____

_____

Acceptance of praise: _____

Overall impression of relationship to authority: _____

6. After completing this documentation, discuss your observations with the class. Fill in your observation pages where you have missed information. List your strengths and weaknesses in completing a skilled clinical observation, as well as your plan to improve your skills.

STRENGTHS	WEAKNESSES AND PLAN TO IMPROVE

7. Return to Activity 1. Select and identify your orange from the pile.

FOLLOW-UP

✔ Complete the Application of Competencies at the end of this chapter.

EVALUATION OF PSYCHOSOCIAL FUNCTIONING

OBJECTIVES

✔ Detail the use of observation, interview, and structured assessments in the evaluation process

✔ Identify specific assessments that are used in a psychosocial setting

✔ Administer a standardized psychosocial assessment

"To get people to understand our point of view, we must first try to understand theirs."

SIDNEY KEYES

DESCRIPTION

This exercise will acquaint you with the evaluation process that is used in psychosocial settings. As part of the evaluation process, numerous formats of collecting data are used: observation, interview, and formal assessments. Formal assessments can range from checklists to standardized tests. A variety of assessments need to be used to obtain an accurate picture of a client's functioning level, strengths, and areas of concern. It is also important to obtain information from the client's family and/or caregivers. The client's culture also needs to be taken into consideration in the evaluation process. Finally, the context of the client's current life situation needs to be considered. A total and clear picture of the client's skill and performance is critical in determining the direction of intervention.

PREPARATION

Suggested Readings

Asher (1996)
Hemphill-Pearson (1999)
Mosey (1986)
Neidstadt and Crepeau (1998)
Stein and Cutler (1998)

Study Questions

1. List the purposes of testing in a psychosocial setting.

2. Describe what is meant by a standardized test.

3. Fill out the chart on the standardized tests listed below. Give a description of the test, note the variables measured, and indicate the source from which the test can be purchased.

TYPE	DESCRIPTION	VARIABLES MEASURED	SOURCE
Allen Cognitive Level (ACL) Test Screening (Allen, 1990)			
Comprehensive Occupational Therapy Evaluation (COTE) (Brayman and Kirby, 1976)			

Bay Area Functional Performance Evaluation (BAFPE) (Williams and Bloomer, 1987)			
Kohlman Evaluation of Living Skills (KELS) (Thomson, 1992)			

4. Describe the use of the following in the psychosocial evaluation process:

   a. Clinical observation

   b. Initial interview

   c. Functional tasks

   d. Self-report inventories

   e. Standardized tests

   f. Behavioral assessments

   g. Machine monitoring

   h. Work sampling

   i. Projective testing

5. List the content of the Comprehensive Case Study Analysis (Stein, 1998) that would provide valuable information in assessing a client in a mental health setting.

6. List and briefly describe several specific assessments (in addition to those in Study Question 2) used in a psychosocial setting that incorporate the following ways of collecting data:

OBSERVATION	INTERVIEW	CHECKLIST/SURVEY/ QUESTIONNAIRE	TASKS

7. List the types of assessments that can be given in a group format.

8. What criteria can be used in selecting a particular assessment?

9. What cultural implications need to be considered in a psychosocial setting during the evaluation process?

10. How can the context influence a client's response to an assessment?

11. How do you think the following might influence a client's performance during the evaluation process?

   a. Motivation

   b. Attention span

   c. Cognitive level

   d. Interest

   e. Self-control

12. How might the client's family and/or caregivers contribute to the evaluation process?

13. List administration considerations in giving an assessment (general guidelines to follow).

14. List several functional assessments used in mental health that are mainly used with the elderly. Explain why this is the case.

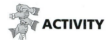 **ACTIVITY**

Materials

Several standardized and nonstandardized tests.

Instructions

1a. After observing an administration of a standardized test, practice administering that standardized test to a classmate. After the test, solicit feedback from your classmates and instructor about your performance in the areas listed below. Record your information. Practice on as many tests as time permits.

PERFORMANCE	TEST:		TEST:	
	COMMENTS		COMMENTS	
Arranged materials				
Gave verbal directions as stated				
Managed timing of items/test				
Used nonverbals appropriately				
Followed protocol				
Scored forms correctly				
Obtained results				

1b. In the space below, describe your strengths and areas of concern regarding your testing skills. How do you plan to improve in your areas of concern? If needed, solicit assistance from your instructor to determine strategies for improvement.

STRENGTHS	AREAS OF CONCERN	PLAN TO IMPROVE

1c. Discuss and record below how it will be determined whether an occupational therapy assistant (OTA) is able to administer a standardized test.

1d. Would an OTA be able to administer the tests with which you practiced? Why or why not?

2. With a partner, select one of the nonstandardized tests with which to familiarize yourself. Thoroughly review the instructor's manual. Obtain the information listed below and prepare to share your findings with the class. Record your information below and record the data from your classmates' presentations in a similar manner.

   a. Title of assessment

   b. Author

   c. Type of assessment

   d. Target population

   e. Purpose

   f. Training needed

   g. Method of administration (include setting/position, procedure, time, and equipment/materials needed)

  h. Interpretation/scoring

  i. Sample of test item

  j. Reliability

  k. Validity

  l. Strengths of assessment

  m. Limitations of assessment

FOLLOW-UP

✔ Complete the Application of Competencies at the end of this chapter.
✔ Complete a Therapeutic Use of Self Analysis found in Appendix B on your ability to listen and respond.

Exercise 63

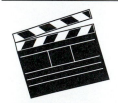

"If nobody ever said anything unless he knew what he was talking about, a ghastly hush would descend upon the earth."

Sir Alan Herbert

LISTENING AND RESPONDING

OBJECTIVES

✔ Discuss how uncovering feelings facilitates self-awareness
✔ Discuss the benefits of listening and responding with immediacy, empathy, and accuracy
✔ Practice using accurate empathy in responding to a client's communicative intent

DESCRIPTION

This exercise will help you to practice listening and responding to the communicative intent of others. You will need these skills as you interact with your clients as well as your colleagues. Asking open-ended questions can help to bring out the emotional content of one's communication. Uncovering feelings can lead a client to greater self-awareness and therefore healthier functioning. As feelings are often disguised, denied, or projected, it will be important for you as an occupational therapy practitioner to respond with immediacy and empathy to assist your clients in confronting unidentified issues. Bringing out implied meanings and facilitating accurate interpretation of the communicative intent will come with practice.

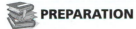 **PREPARATION**

Suggested Readings

Cole (1998)
Early (2000)
Hemphill-Pearson (1999)

Study Questions

1. Describe how uncovering feelings can lead to greater self-awareness and greater therapeutic benefits.

2. What are the benefits of asking open-ended questions?

3. Define and give an example of the use of primary accurate empathy and advanced accurate empathy.

4. Define and give an example of the use of immediacy.

5. Define confrontation as it relates to giving feedback to a client.

6. Give an example of a confrontational statement that you could say to a peer in your group who accepted a high grade on a project without contributing much information.

7. Fill in the information about how you might appropriately respond to the common psychiatric behaviors and symptoms listed below. List the diagnoses with which the symptom or behavior may be associated. Describe how you might therapeutically use yourself, how you might structure the environment, and what activities might be appropriate to use in intervention.

SYMPTOM OR BEHAVIOR	DIAGNOSIS	USE OF SELF	ENVIRONMENT	INTERVENTION ACTIVITIES
Anxiety				
Depression				

Mania				
Delusions				
Paranoia				
Hostility and aggression				
Seductive behavior				
Hallucinations				
Cognitive deficits				
Attention deficits				

8. Describe the role of using nonverbal communication in talking with or interviewing a client.

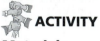 **ACTIVITY**

Materials

Index cards on which are written feeling words

Instructions

1. In a small group, start with the feeling word given on the left of the following chart and think of another feeling word that could also be used to describe that feeling. Using the new word to help you think of yet another word continue until the chart is complete. Discuss the importance of describing feelings specifically and accurately. The first one is completed for you.

At times I feel			
Frustrated	Angry	Impatient	Helpless
Afraid			
Lonely			
Angry			
Sad			

🎲 GAME

2. Divide into small groups and play the game of charades. Play the game according to the procedures and rules your group establishes. Take turns acting out a chosen feeling word previously written on an index card. Write down the behavior that is being displayed by the actor and all the different inferred emotions the behavior may represent. Use the sample below to get started.

BEHAVIOR DISPLAYED	INFERRED EMOTIONS
Student jumps up and down waving arms with a big smile on face.	Ecstatic, happy, joyful, exuberant

3. With a partner or small group practice responding using primary accurate empathy. Read each of the following comments. After reading the comment, decide what feeling you believe the person is portraying. Record the reason you believe that feeling is occurring. Formulate a response to the person, identifying a feeling and the reason you believe he or she is feeling that way. Discuss as a class the various answers. The first one is completed for you.

a. Comment: "You make me sick. Do you think you are better than the rest of us?"

FEELING	REASON	YOU WOULD RESPOND
Angry	Someone else in the group gave an example of how he or she handled a situation well.	It sounds like you are angry with him for sharing his success.

b. Comment: "I would rather just lie in bed. Leave me alone!"

FEELING	REASON	YOU WOULD RESPOND

c. Comment: "There, see I ruined another project. Are you happy? I told you I'm no good at this kind of thing."

FEELING	REASON	YOU WOULD RESPOND

d. Comment: "I'd be better off dead than to go back to that hell hole I live in."

FEELING	REASON	YOU WOULD RESPOND

e. Comment: "Talk to my parents! You have got to be kidding! That's the stupidest idea I ever heard! Do you get paid to do this job?"

FEELING	REASON	YOU WOULD RESPOND

f. Comment: "I can't sit here in this group when they are getting ready to send laughing gas through the vents."

FEELING	REASON	YOU WOULD RESPOND

g. Comments: "You expect me to talk to people like him? I can't stand to even be in the same room with him!"

FEELING	REASON	YOU WOULD RESPOND

h. Comment: "I can't believe you have the nerve to call me selfish. You are the most arrogant person I have ever met."

FEELING	REASON	YOU WOULD RESPOND

i. Comment: "When I get out of here, I plan to get good and drunk. I'll show them the mistake they made by putting me in here."

FEELING	REASON	YOU WOULD RESPOND

4a. Write about one experience that has made a significant impact on your life.

4b. Find a partner and share this experience. Take turns being the listener. While you are playing the role of the listener, identify your partner's feelings and reasons for the feelings—for example, you seem to feel _____ because _____. After each person has shared, discuss how the listener paraphrased the feelings. List the strengths and areas of concern about your performance as a communicator and a listener below.

	STRENGTHS	AREAS OF CONCERN
Communicator		
Listener		

FOLLOW-UP

✔ Complete the Application of Competencies at the end of this chapter.
✔ Complete a Therapeutic Use of Self Analysis found in Appendix B on your ability to listen and respond.

Exercise 64

"Give to other human beings every right that you claim for yourself."

ROBERT INGERSOLL

THE INTERVIEW PROCESS

OBJECTIVES

✔ Discuss the role of an interview in the occupational therapy process
✔ Identify interview techniques that are appropriate to elicit objective information
✔ Critique self and peers when obtaining information in an interview format

DESCRIPTION

This session will help you to gain specific skills that you will need in interviewing clients. An interview is especially critical in a psychosocial setting in obtaining psychosocial information. Interviews may be formal or informal and, when structured appropriately, can elicit much objective information that will be needed and helpful in the intervention process. Structuring and guiding the interview process will be a challenge as you work toward obtaining an accurate and complete picture of your client's level of performance and functioning. Critiquing your interviewing skills will help you to strengthen those skills and allow you to elicit information from a client in a timely and therapeutic manner.

PREPARATION

Suggested Readings

> Denton (1987)
> Early (2000)
> Hemphill-Pearson (1999)
> Stein and Cutler (1993)

Study Questions

1. Describe how an interview is used in the evaluation process in a psychosocial setting.

2. What is the purpose of an initial interview in a psychosocial setting?

3. Describe the difference between a structured and a semistructured interview.

4. What are some ways to prepare for an interview?

5. How might you establish rapport with your client before the interview begins?

6. What is the best way to begin an interview?

7. List the sections from the occupational history interview as outlined in Early (2000).

8. Describe the sequential steps to an interview.

9. Describe information that may be gathered from an interview.

10. Give examples of interview questions that may elicit helpful information contributing to the occupational therapy process for the age spans listed below:
    a. Adolescence

    b. Young adult

    c. Middle adulthood

    d. Late adulthood

11. Describe the difference between a direct and an indirect question, how each may be used, and what type of information might be elicited.
    a. Direct

    b. Indirect

12. Describe the difference between an open-ended and a closed-ended question, how each may be used, and what type of information might be elicited.
    a. Open

    b. Closed

13. Summarize guidelines and/or suggestions for interviewing clients in a psychosocial setting.

14. How might a particular frame of reference guide your interview questions?

15. Choose three frames of reference and write several interview questions that would be appropriate to ask using that particular model.
    a. Frame of reference:

b. Frame of reference:

c. Frame of reference:

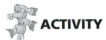 **ACTIVITY**

Materials

Videotape player and television monitor; blank tapes; camera and microphones; and Case Studies 24, 25, 26, and 27 located at the end of this chapter.

Instructions

1. Reword each of the following questions into an open-ended format as you would to gain additional in-depth information from a client. Rejoin the class and discuss your reworded questions.

    a. Do you know why you are here?

    b. So, are you feeling better since you've taken your medicine today?

    c. Do you like to play sports in your spare time?

    d. Is your sense of humor something you like about yourself?

    e. Are you always this quiet?

    f. Do you have any friends?

    g. Is your relationship with your parents good?

    h. Are you happy to get out of here soon like everyone else?

    i. Where do you work?

j. Do you have much free time?

k. Are you sad right now?

2. Discuss with the class ways in which you might establish rapport with a client before the interview. List ideas generated from your class discussion.

3. Divide into groups of three. Using an assigned case study, participate in a role-play of an interview between an occupational therapy practitioner and a client. Have the third student serve as an observer. In the interview, obtain the information indicated below and write the obtained information in the space provided. Have the observer use the Interview skills checklist found in Performance Skill 4B of this chapter as a guideline for observing the interviewer. Record feedback received from the observer when you were the interviewer. Repeat this procedure until all group members have played the roles of practitioner, client, and observer.

a. Living situation

b. Leisure time usage

c. Management of stress

d. Employment information

e. Insight into illness

INTERVIEW FEEDBACK	
STRENGTHS	AREAS OF CONCERN

4. Conduct and videotape an interview within the designated time frame suggested by your instructor. Work with a different partner from the one in Activity 3. Conduct the interview, gathering information about the performance areas of your client. Afterward, watch and critique the videotape using the Interview skills checklist found in Performance Skill 4B of this chapter. If other students are available to assist in the critique, invite them to provide feedback. Use the space below to record feedback received. Identify your responses in the interview that were not therapeutic. Record those as indicated and include a new response that would be more therapeutic.

INTERVIEW CRITIQUE	
STRENGTHS	AREAS OF CONCERN

INTERVIEW CRITIQUE OF SELF	
NONTHERAPEUTIC RESPONSE	NEW RESPONSE

FOLLOW-UP

✔ Complete the Application of Competencies at the end of this chapter.
✔ Complete a Therapeutic Use of Self Analysis found in Appendix B on your interviewing skills.
✔ Complete Performance Skill 4B on Interview.

ASSERTIVENESS

Exercise 65

OBJECTIVES

✔ Define assertive, aggressive, and passive communication and behavior
✔ Describe the DESC form of communication
✔ Outline the benefits of assertive communication and behavior

DESCRIPTION

Assertive communication and behavior are necessary skills of all occupational therapy practitioners. Communicating and acting assertively facilitates open, honest, and congruent dialogue. They are the healthiest ways of making known one's wants and needs. They facilitate cohesiveness and team building. As a practitioner, you will need to develop assertiveness skills. The more developed your skills are, the better equipped you will be to facilitate the same in your clients. Individuals with psychosocial dysfunction

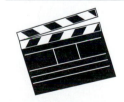

"People of character don't allow the environment to dictate their style."

LUCILLE KALLEN

often communicate and act in either a passive or an aggressive manner, both of which are destructive and unhealthy. Your role will be to work with such clients and help them to understand the unhealthiness of their ways and, at the same time, facilitate their return to health by using assertive communication and behavior.

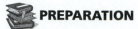 **PREPARATION**

Suggested Readings

Cara and MacRae (1998)
Davis (1998)

Study Questions

1. Describe the following communication techniques.
   a. Assertive

   b. Aggressive

   c. Passive/nonassertive behavior

2. List several of the personal rights we all have.

3. Describe how self-esteem may affect a person's use of assertive communication.

4. What are five behaviors that can help a person learn how to act assertively?

5. Describe what each of the initials represent in the DESC format of communication:
   a. D

   b. E

   c. S

   d. C

6. Describe the use of "I" statements in assertive communication behavior.

7. Describe strategies to deal with anger in an assertive manner.

8. List benefits of assertive communication and behavior.

9. Why do many clients in a mental health setting need assistance with learning assertive behavior?

10. Describe your use of assertive communication by responding to the following statements. Use the same figure below for all statements.

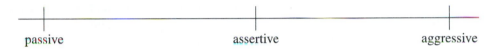

passive   assertive   aggressive

     a. Put the letter "a" on the line that best describes how you react in situations dealing with people in *authority*.

     b. Put the letter "s" on the line that best describes how you react with people whom you *supervise*.

     c. Put the letter "t" on the line that best describes how you react to people when *they* are angry.

     d. Put the letter "y" on the line that best describes how you react to people when *you* are angry.

     e. Put the letter "n" on the line that best describes how you react to a request when you really want to say *no*.

11. Describe what you would like to change about your communication style before teaching assertiveness to your clients.

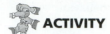 **ACTIVITY**

Materials

Blank index cards, four index cards with one of the following words written on each card: protagonist, assertive, passive, aggressive.

Instructions

1a. On each index card given to you by your instructor, write a situation in which it is difficult for you to be assertive. Describe the behavior of the person or people involved in the scenario. When you are finished, place your index cards in the center of the table.

1b. Role-play the difficult assertive situations, using randomly selected scenarios on the index cards. Four students will need to take turns participating in each situation: One person will be the protagonist in the situation, one person will be responding and acting passively, one will act assertively, and one will act aggressively. Determine these roles by drawing from the table a face-down index card with the name of each role written on the back. When you are not participating, observe the role-play and then discuss as a class whether the behavior matched the communication style being portrayed. Take turns with class members role-playing the different communication styles. Add additional comments as appropriate.

2. Describe your own strengths and areas of concern in being assertive. Additionally, develop a plan to improve your skills. Discuss your current status and plan for change with the class or a small group.

a. Strengths:

b. Areas of concern:

c. Plan:

Fig. 4-2 What grade did you receive?

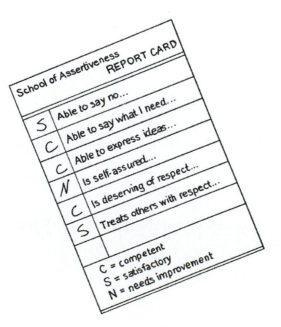

3. Discuss as a class the use of Activity 1 and how it might be used in leading an assertiveness group with clients.

FOLLOW-UP

✔ Complete a Therapeutic Use of Self Analysis found in Appendix B on your communication skills.
✔ Complete the Application of Competency at the end of this chapter.

SOCIAL SKILLS

Exercise 66

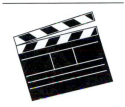

OBJECTIVES

✔ Identify the influence your family has had on your social skill development
✔ Describe constructive social conduct skills
✔ Identify appropriate intervention activities for people with social skill dysfunction

DESCRIPTION

Social skill acquisition is an important goal in working with clients who have psychosocial dysfunction. Social skills include role performance, coping skills, social conduct, interpersonal skills, self-control, and self-expression. As you work with clients who have deficits in these areas, it will be helpful for you to look at the origin of your own social skills within your family. Doing so will allow you to consider how the families of your clients may have influenced the acquisition of their social skills. Adequate and constructive social skills acquisition will enable your clients to perform in a socially acceptable manner.

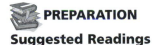 **PREPARATION**

Suggested Readings

Cara and MacRae (1998)
Cottrell (1993)
Mosey (1986)
Stein and Cutler (1998)

> "The master said, even when walking in a party of no more than three, I can always be certain of learning from those I am with. There will be good qualities that I can select for imitation and bad ones that will teach me what requires correction in myself."
>
> CONFUCIUS

Questions

1. Define role acquisition.

2. Define social skills training.

3. List ten principles of the role acquisition model. For each principle, give an illustrative example.

    a.

b.

c.

d.

e.

f.

g.

h.

i.

j.

4. Name four categories of social skills and list two illustrative examples from each category.

5. Describe the following models for social skills training:
   a. Problem-solving model

   b. Attention-focusing skills model

6. Describe how generalization and maintenance are used in social skills training.

7. What social skills might be observed during the evaluation process?

8. In the spectrum of cultural values, identify the values with which your family is most closely aligned.

9. What type of assessments might be appropriate to use to evaluate social skill functioning? Identify at least six.

10. How do you think the frame of reference used at your facility might influence your choice of social skill functioning assessment selection?

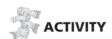 **ACTIVITY**

Materials

The Book of Activity Cards for Mental Health (Rider and Rider, 1999); *Creative Games in Group Work* (Dynes, 1993); and Case Study 19 (located at the end of Chapter 3) and case studies, 26, 27, and 28 located at the end of this chapter.

Instructions

1. Identify the social roles in your life by putting a check mark in the following chart next to the roles that apply to you. Add other social roles as appropriate for your life circumstances.

Family member		Parent			
Worker		Spouse			
Student					
Friend					
Community member					

2a. Your family is the most important social institution to which you belong. Describe here what social skills you have learned from your family. For example, what were your family's values regarding nurturing, trust, love, and communication? How might your family's culture have influenced the teaching of these values?

2b. Discuss your family's social skills with your class or small group. Record the similarities and differences in the families of your peers.

SIMILARITIES	DIFFERENCES

2c. List the social skills and/or cultural values from your family you want to keep, those you want to change, and those that would be best thrown out. An example is provided for you. Note these skills and values may differ for each person.

KEEP (PASS THESE ON TO OTHERS)	CHANGE (MODIFY THESE)	THROW OUT (DELETE THESE)
Parents displayed open and honest communication with children.	Family rules were inconsistently enforced between siblings.	Children were not allowed to even question any authority figure.

3a. Select two students who have differing views in parenting to enter into a role-play discussion on a topic related to discipline, such as the reason why or why not to spank a child. Have students who are not participating observe and take notes on the social conduct and interpersonal skills of the persons in the role-play as indicated on the following Social Skills Observation form. Once the role-play is completed, discuss your observations.

SOCIAL SKILLS OBSERVATION		
SOCIAL SKILLS	STUDENT _____ DESCRIBE USE OF SKILL	STUDENT _____ DESCRIBE USE OF SKILL
Use of words		
Tone of voice		
Facial expression		
Gestures		
Active Listening		
Listening and paraphrasing		
Expressing needs, feelings, and ideas		
Congruence between verbal and nonverbal		
Cooperation		
Negotiation		
Assertiveness		

3b. Repeat Activity 3a with larger groups of students. Each group should have a different view on a topic. Continue with the same topic if there is enough interest, or select a new topic. Designate several students as observers. Have the observers record their observations of the social skills of two selected members using the following form. Once the discussion is completed, write down observations of your own behavior. As a group, discuss the social skills observed.

SOCIAL SKILLS OBSERVATION		
SOCIAL SKILLS	STUDENT _____ DESCRIBE USE OF SKILL	STUDENT _____ DESCRIBE USE OF SKILL
Use of words		
Tone of voice		
Facial expression		
Gestures		
Active Listening		
Listening and paraphrasing		
Expressing needs, feelings, and ideas		
Congruence between verbal and nonverbal		
Cooperation		
Negotiation		
Assertiveness		
Observations of own behavior		

4a. Participate in the Knot Group. To begin, stand and form a circle with your classmates. Depending on the size of the class, more than one circle may be formed. Cross your arms in front of you and hold the hands of two other people, neither of whom may be the person next to you. Keep all hands joined for the entire group. Attempt to untie the knot without letting go of the hands in the knotted hands group that has been formed. This objective will be accomplished when all members are in one complete circle still holding hands. On completion of this activity, discuss and record the social skills involved in participating in this activity.

SOCIAL SKILLS	DESCRIBE INVOLVEMENT

4b. Discuss the method and process your group used to untie the knot by answering the following questions:

a. Who took the role of a leader?

b. Who offered the most ideas?

c. Who offered the fewest ideas?

d. Who questioned the purpose of the group or the chance to reach the goal successfully?

e. Who wanted to terminate the activity?

Fig. 4-3 Can this knot be untied?

Photo courtesy of Paula Downey, Charlene Kennedy, Kim Meyer, Leanne Pitcher, Pam Boone, and Jessica Johantges.

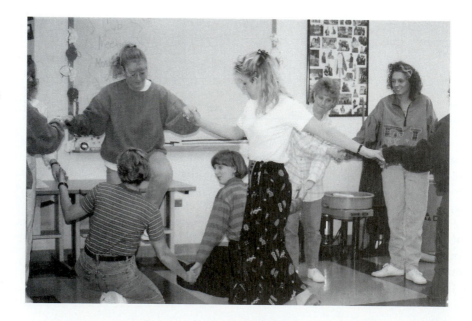

f. Describe examples of the nonverbal communication that took place.

g. Describe how differing opinions were supported.

h. How did you feel about participating during the different time segments of the group? Describe the tone of the group in each segment.
   i. Beginning

   ii. Middle

   iii. End

4c. Discuss and record the treatment implications of the Knot Group. Include populations and settings in which it might be appropriate and others in which it might not be appropriate to use.

5. Participate in several other instructor-led social activities requiring varying degrees of physical and verbal instructions. Following each activity, use the following form to write a description of the activity, the social skills required, and how each group might be used in treatment. Discuss these group activities as a class and star your favorites. An example is provided for you.

SOCIAL ACTIVITY	SOCIAL SKILLS REQUIRED	TREATMENT IMPLICATIONS
Bumper cars: Cross hands over chest and pretend you are bumper cars, gently bumping into each other	Awareness of personal space, being touched by others, self-control	Adolescent or acute adult units as part of a set of awareness activities

6. You will be given several case studies. With your partner, read each case study and write a brief description of the client in the designated area of the following chart. Choose at least two occupations you think would address the client's social skill needs and give a rationale for each choice. Discuss ideas with your class upon completion.

DESCRIPTION OF CLIENT	OCCUPATIONS	RATIONALE

FOLLOW-UP

✔ Complete the Application of Competencies at the end of this chapter.

Exercise 67

"In any project the important factor is your belief. Without belief there can be no successful outcome."

WILLIAM JAMES

COGNITIVE DISABILITY

OBJECTIVES

✔ Compare and contrast the behavioral characteristics of Allen's (Allen, Earhart, and Blue, 1992) six cognitive levels or modes
✔ Demonstrate proficiency in completing the Allen Cognitive Level Screening test (Allen, 1990)
✔ Develop an intervention plan for a stated cognitive level including the appropriate type of activities, environment, assistance, and cueing needed

DESCRIPTION

This exercise will help you to become familiar with Claudia Allen's cognitive disability model. Allen has developed an assessment technique to determine a client's level of functioning. This assessment places the functioning level of a client within one of six levels. These determined levels can then be used to guide one's choice of intervention activities, type of instruction to be used, as well as appropriate sensory cuing that a client may need. The use of Allen's cognitive levels can assist practitioners in knowing what type of external support is needed throughout the client's recovery process. This knowledge can also be useful in making plans for discharge. Although the use of this model does not advocate a change in cognition per se, an improvement in a client's functional abilities can be realized by changing and adapting the environment.

PREPARATION

Suggested Readings

Allen, Earhart, and Blue (1992)
Asher (1996)
Cara and MacRae (1998)
Early (2000)

Study Questions

1. What is the effect of a cognitive disability on a client's ability to function in everyday life?

2. State the central concept of Claudia Allen's theory of cognitive disabilities.

3. Summarize the nine propositions in Claudia Allen's theory of cognitive disabilities.

4. Describe the behavior of someone functioning at each of Claudia Allen's cognitive levels as well as interventions including activity selection, cueing, and type of assistance, which may be appropriate for someone functioning at that level.

	LEVEL 2.0	LEVEL 3.0	LEVEL 4.0	LEVEL 5.0
Behavior				
Intervention: Activity selection				
Cuing				
Type of assistance				

5. According to the model of cognitive disabilities, what happens when a person is faced with a task that is beyond his or her current cognitive level?

6. Describe how the following may be used with a client who has a cognitive deficit:
   a. Use of self

   b. Environment

   c. Occupation selections

7. Describe the following components of the Allen Cognitive Level Screening (ACL) Test (Allen, 1990):

   a. General description

   b. Purpose

   c. Supplies needed

   d. Procedure/method

   e. Administration time

8. Describe the importance of the task, task analysis, and the task environment in the cognitive disability model.

9. Detail how you think the use of the ACL might relate to a client's discharge planning.

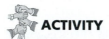 **ACTIVITY**

Materials

ACL Screening test kits (Allen, 1990), Claudia Allen's designated performance modules from 3.0 to 6.0 (Allen, Earhart and Blue, 1992) written on index cards Allen's ribbon card kits, (Allen, n.d.), Case Study 9 (located at the end of Chapter 2 and case studies), 29, 30, and 31 located at the end of this chapter.

Instructions

1. Observe your instructor administer the Allen Cognitive Level Test (Allen, 1992) to a fellow student. Document here the procedures of the test you will need to remember.

2. Learn the directions to the test then practice giving the test to another student in a client role-play situation. Have this student or a third student critique your performance. You may or may not have your "client" role-play a cognitive deficit. Critique your own performance below.

PERFORMANCE COMPONENTS	COMMENTS
Proper introduction to screening	
Materials arranged appropriately	
Directions of the protocol followed	
Standard verbal commands given	
Correct scoring obtained	

3. Select a card from the pile of cards with the different modes written on them that are placed on the table by your instructor. Role-play client behaviors using the cognitive performance level or mode on the card you selected as you complete the ribbon card project. Use characteristic verbalizations as well as actions as you role-play. Have your classmates try to determine which mode you are portraying using the *Allen Diagnostic Manual: Instruction Manual* (Earhart, Allen and Blue, 1993). The first student to report the correct mode will then take his or her turn to role-play. Use the following space to record a description of all the behaviors and the modes they represent.

BEHAVIOR	LEVEL OR MODE

4a. Work with a partner or small group on a case study provided by your instructor. Determine activity ideas for intervention, the needed environmental arrangement/materials, and therapist strategies, including cueing and assistance. Share this information with your class when complete. Record your ideas as well as your classmates' ideas.

CASE DESCRIPTION	ACTIVITY SELECTION	ENVIRONMENT/ MATERIALS	CUEING/ ASSISTANCE

4b. As a class, discuss your use of task analysis in your activity selection.

FOLLOW-UP

✔ Complete the Application of Competency at the end of this chapter.
✔ Complete Performance Skill 4E on Teaching a Basic Life Task.

Exercise 68

"Complacency is the enemy of study. We cannot really learn anything until we rid ourselves of complacency. Our attitude towards ourselves should be to be insatiable in learning and toward others to be 'timeless in teaching.'"

MAO ZEDONG

DAILY LIVING SKILLS

OBJECTIVES

✔ Define and differentiate basic activities of daily living and instrumental activities of daily living
✔ Describe symptoms of clients receiving support from mental health facilities
✔ Develop a group format that would be an appropriate modality in teaching daily living skills to a client

DESCRIPTION

This exercise is intended to introduce to you the role of daily living skills in treating clients with psychosocial problems. Individuals with mental illness often function at a level where they have difficulty attending to their daily living needs. Included in these daily living skills are not only basic self-care activities but also instrumental activities of daily living (ADLs), which include home management functions such as money management, time management, community transportation, and medication routines. The ability to care for one's self and manage one's home is frequently a concern for clients who have both chronic and acute symptoms. A group setting is often an effective way to achieve goals, as group members can benefit from the support and feedback of other group members.

PREPARATION

Suggested Readings

Cara and MacRae (1998)
Early (2000)
Neidstadt and Crepeau (1998)

Study Questions

1. Define basic daily living skills.

2. Define instrumental ADLs.

3. Describe common living skill performance area deficits that may hinder a client's successful return to the community and strategies that may be implemented to increase function.

AREA	DEFICITS	STRATEGIES
Grooming		
Clothing care		
Medication routine		

Health maintenance		
Sexual expression		
Functional communication		
Community mobility		
Money management		
Time management		
Meal preparation/cleanup		

4. Describe the role of the occupational therapy practitioner serving as a case manager in the development of daily living skills.

5. What assessments might be appropriate to use in evaluating basic ADLs?

6. What assessments might be appropriate to use in evaluating instrumental ADLs?

ACTIVITY

Materials

Index cards, *S.E.A.L. + Plus* (Korb-Khalsa, Azok, and Leutenberg, 1995), *Group Dynamics in Occupational Therapy* (Cole, 1998).

Instructions

1. With a partner or small group, determine the daily living needs of individuals who are receiving intervention in the following settings:

   a. Day treatment program for adolescents with moderate to severe deficits

b. Acute inpatient adult unit

c. Chronic institutionalized state hospital discharge unit

d. Home health with newly discharged patients living independently

2. With a partner, plan and lead an ADL group for one of the treatment settings in Activity 1. Use Cole's (1998) seven-step format as a guide for your group treatment plan (see the Group Treatment Plan form provided). Organize a role-play so that five to eight of your classmates can be active members of the group you will co-lead. Using the following Role-Play chart, develop the role for each of your group members who will role-play a client. Include the client's age, gender, diagnosis, and general directions for behavior to be displayed. Have your group members take on these roles as you and a peer co-lead the group. After the group session, critique your performance, using the Group Feedback form provided.

ROLE-PLAYS				
	AGE	GENDER	DIAGNOSIS	BEHAVIOR INFORMATION
1				
2				
3				
4				
5				
6				
7				
8				

GROUP TREATMENT PLAN

Treatment setting: _____

Session title:

Format:

Supplies:

Description of activities:

Warm-up:

Introduce activity:

Instructions for activity:

Sharing:

Discussion questions:

   Processing:

   Generalizing:

   Application:

Summary:

GROUP FEEDBACK

WHAT WENT WELL?	WHAT IMPROVEMENTS COULD BE MADE?

FOLLOW-UP

✔   Complete the Application of Competencies at the end of this chapter.

Exercise 69

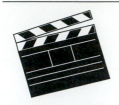

"To move the world, we must first move ourselves."

SOCRATES

MOVEMENT

OBJECTIVES

✔ Describe the benefits as well as precautions in using movement with clients in a psychosocial setting
✔ List goals that can be met in using movement as a part of intervention
✔ Plan and lead a movement group

DESCRIPTION

This exercise will help you to see the importance of movement in your everyday life as well as the lives of the clients with whom you will be working. Movement is one of the most powerful inputs that the nervous system can receive. Movement can be used during intervention to calm and quiet the nervous system and/or to alert and heighten its functioning. Movement is an integral component of a balanced life, and it needs to be used frequently and repeatedly in a treatment setting. The more you use movement, the more you will clearly see the powerful influence it exerts over your clients. Movement is an active "doing" part of occupational therapy. You will want to facilitate your clients' movements as you move them toward health and wellness.

 PREPARATION

Suggested Readings

> Bruce and Borg (1993)
> Christiansen and Baum (1997)
> Cole (1998)
> Neidstadt (1998)
> Ross (1997)

Study Questions

Fig. 4-4 Movement affects many different parts of the body.

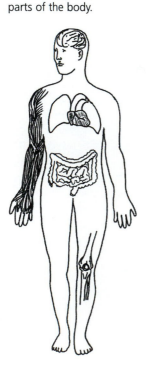

1. Define the term *movement*.

2. List and describe several movement-centered assessments.

3. Describe the chemical changes that occur in the brain during movement activities.

4. Briefly describe the following components of physical fitness:
   a. Cardiorespiratory

   b. Muscle strength

   c. Muscle endurance

   d. Flexibility

   e. Body composition

5. Describe the body's response to movement.

6. Describe reasons for inactivity or decreased fitness.

7. Describe the role of the occupational therapy practitioner in providing movement activities with clients in a psychosocial setting.

8. List several goals that may be used in movement groups.

9. Give examples of movement activities that may be used in a psychosocial setting.

10. Describe Lorna Jean King's use of movement in her sensory motor approach to individuals with schizophrenia, autism, and/or mental retardation.

11. Describe precautions you may need to adhere to in involving clients in movement activities.

12a. Estimate how many minutes or hours you spend in a typical weekday in activities involving movement. List the activities and the approximate amount of time spent in each activity.

ACTIVITY	TIME

12b. Do you think that the time you spend in movement is adequate?

12c. List one thing you could do each day to increase the amount of time and quality of movement you experience.

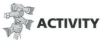 **ACTIVITY**

Materials

Parachute, lummi sticks, various-sized bouncing balls, tape player, cassette or compact disc of oldies music, beach ball, silk scarves, chairs.

Instructions

1. Participate in a movement group led by your instructor. Once completed, take a few minutes to answer the following questions regarding the group:
   a. Describe the warm-up process.

   b. List the activities performed and a description of each.

   c. Describe the cool-down process.

   d. Describe the summary, generalization, or discussion that took place after the movement activities.

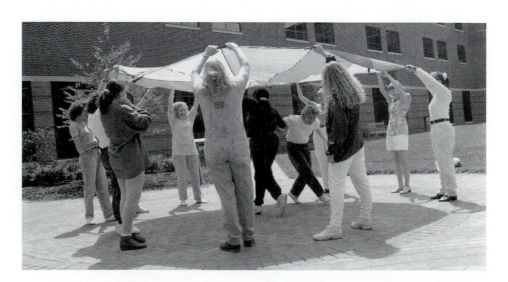

Fig. 4-5 Parachute activities are a wonderful modality to get people moving and having fun.

Photo courtesy of Paula Downey, Charlene Kennedy, Brenda Morris, and Pam Boone.

2. Participate in experiencing instructor-led movement activities that were not incorporated into the previous group. Afterward, list the activity, write a description of the activity, and state how it may be used in treatment. The first one is completed for you.

ACTIVITY	DESCRIPTION	TREATMENT IMPLICATION
Silk scarf juggle.	Each client will be given three scarves to juggle. Then they are to toss the scarves to the person next to them in the circle.	Great activity for the client in a wheelchair and for those with low strength. Good for eye-hand coordination, range of motion, and expressive movement.

3a. Divide into small groups. Plan a movement group that could be used in a psychiatric setting for one of the following populations. Circle the population for which your group will plan. Once the planning process is complete, present your group ideas or, if time permits, lead the class through your movement group. Use the space provided to plan your group and record ideas presented by other groups. Critique each group plan as it is presented.

1. Pediatric

2. Adolescence

3. Adult acute

4. Adult chronic

5. Geriatric

MOVEMENT GROUP PLAN
Describe space needed:
Equipment/materials needed:
Warm-up:
Activities:
Cool-down:
Processing/generalizing/summary:

GROUP PLAN CRITIQUE	
Population:	Population:
Population:	Population:
Your Group Population:	

3b. Discuss and record your overall impressions of the role that movement plays in providing intervention to clients in a psychosocial setting.

FOLLOW-UP

✔ Complete the Application of Competencies at the end of this chapter.

Exercise 70

"The time to relax is when you don't have time for it."

SYDNEY J. HARRIS

LEISURE PLANNING

OBJECTIVES

✔ Describe the role of leisure activities to one's overall health and wellness
✔ Describe leisure time activities appropriate for both an inpatient and outpatient setting
✔ Identify a variety of leisure time activities that are available in the community

DESCRIPTION

Leisure plays an important role in balancing one's life performance. It is considered a part of the occupational therapy triad: self-care, work, and leisure. For adults leisure activities are a means of engaging in productive activities and providing an avenue of enjoyment, relaxation, personal growth, and recreation. Recreation in its true form means to recreate, to restore, to rejuvenate. With this view in mind, leisure activities are essential in prevention and wellness of those with psychosocial dysfunction. One's involvement in leisure activities may be altered or impaired because of accident or injury. As an occupational therapy practitioner, you will be in the role of facilitating a client's return to healthy leisure time participation through leisure time planning.

PREPARATION

Suggested Readings

> Asher (1996)
> Early (2000)
> McCarthy (1993)
> Stein and Cutler (1998)
> Local newspaper
> Local telephone book

Study Questions

1. Citing several sources, define leisure.

2. What assumptions underlie leisure activities?

3. What are some of the reasons a person may have inadequate leisure skills?

4. What must be taken into account in participating in leisure planning with a client?

5. Give several examples of possible appropriate leisure time goals.

6. List several assessments that may be used in determining a client's participation and performance in leisure skills and activities.

7. List occupations that may be used for leisure interests in the areas below. Star the ones in which you currently participate.

   a. Crafts

   b. The arts

    c. Hobbies

    d. Gardening and horticulture

    e. Games

    f. Social activities

    g. Sports and exercise

8. Reflect on how you think spirituality/religion might be an important consideration in someone's leisure planning.

9. Using a local phone book and newspaper, list leisure opportunities that are available in your community that would be appropriate for mental health clients. Find several for each of the designated age groups.

ADOLESCENT	ADULT	GERIATRIC

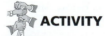 **ACTIVITY**

Materials

Leisure skill assessment, Case Studies 32 and 33 located at the end of this chapter.

Instructions

1a. Participate in a leisure skill assessment or inventory. Discuss with your class the results of your assessment. From the discussion, list ten leisure activities in which you currently do not participate. Check those that you would be interested in participating in and describe why. For the activities that you do not want to participate in, describe why not.

LEISURE ACTIVITIES	✔ to indicate interest	DESCRIBE WHY YOU WOULD OR WOULD NOT LIKE TO DO THIS

1b. As a class, determine the top ten most frequently participated in leisure time activities by your peers and list those below. Determine the components involved in those leisure activities. Put a check mark in the appropriate column indicating the components below that are involved in that leisure time activity.

LEISURE ACTIVITIES	PHYSICAL	COGNITIVE	SOCIAL	SPIRITUAL/ RELIGIOUS

1c. Identify which of the preceeding components occur the most frequently in the leisure activities you prefer.

2a. With a partner, examine the case studies given and determine leisure activities from which the client may benefit. Determine activities that would be appropriate for the client as an inpatient and activities that may be appropriate for the client as an outpatient. Give the rationale for your selection. Discuss ideas as a class when completed.

Case description:

INPATIENT LEISURE ACTIVITIES	RATIONALE	OUTPATIENT LEISURE ACTIVITIES	RATIONALE

2b. Repeat Activity 2a with another case study.

Case description:

INPATIENT LEISURE ACTIVITIES	RATIONALE	OUTPATIENT LEISURE ACTIVITIES	RATIONALE

FOLLOW-UP

✔   Complete the Application of Competencies at the end of this chapter.

TIME MANAGEMENT

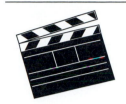

Exercise 71

OBJECTIVES

✔ Describe how time management influences the balance a person has in the areas of self-care, work, and play/leisure

✔ Critique how the use of an Activities Schedule and a Pie of Life might be used during intervention

✔ Detail a variety of time management techniques that might be used in the treatment of an individual with psychosocial dysfunction

"I must govern the clock, not be governed by it."

GOLDA MEIR

DESCRIPTION

Time management is a critical issue, especially in today's fast-paced society. Clients with psychosocial dysfunction may have difficulty with time management owing to lack of insight, low cognition, and poor problem-solving skills, among others concerns. As an occupational therapy practitioner it will be critical that you learn how to manage your own time effectively so that you can teach time management skills to your clients. It will be your challenge to promote the insight and facilitate the acquisition of problem-solving skills so that your clients can maintain a balanced life in the performance areas of self-care, work, and play/leisure. A core concept in occupational therapy—that a balanced life leads to health, wellness, and wholeness—will be your guiding premise as you help your clients to realize and understand the importance of the same.

PREPARATION

Suggested Readings

> Cara and MacRae (1998)
> Covey, Merrill, and Merrill (1994)
> Early (2000)
> Mosey (1986)

Study Questions

1. What are the skills a person must have to manage his or her time?

2. What are some of the difficulties a person may experience with time management?

3. What are several assessments that occupational therapy practitioners may administer to evaluate a person's use of time?

4. What are several strategies that occupational therapy practitioners may use in helping clients with time management?

5. What are the six steps to managing time effectively, according to Covey, Merrill, and Merrill (1994)?

6. How does the amount of time spent in the performance areas of work and play change as a person goes through the developmental stages of life?

   a. Infancy and early Childhood

   b. Middle childhood

   c. Adolescence

   d. Early adulthood

   e. Middle age

   f. Late adulthood

7. Describe the five steps as outlined by Mosey (1986) regarding intervention for individuals having difficulty with temporal adaptation.

8. Complete the following activities as adapted from the Idiosyncratic Activities Configuration (Cynkin and Robinson, 1990). Adapted with permission from: Cynkin S., and A.M. Robinson 1990. *Occupational Therapy and Activities Health: Toward Health Through Activities*. Boston: Little, Brown.

   a. Keep a small notebook and pencil with you at all times. Record everything you do every day for one week (Monday through Sunday), hour by hour.

   b. Fill in the following Activities Schedule. If you perform more than one activity at the same time (e.g., watching TV and sewing), bracket both in the same time slot. If any activity does not occupy the full hour, fill in all the activities that occupy that time slot in order of completion.

   c. Use the completed schedule to make a list of all the activities that you have done during the entire week.

   d. Classify the activities from the completed Activities Schedule and code them by color.

Activities Schedule Coding Key:

Sleep: green

Work: red

Chores: purple

Leisure alone: yellow

Leisure with others; orange

Self-care: blue

e. Complete the following Questionnaire and Addendum to Questionnaire. To do so, generate a computer-based spreadsheet with the activities from the activity box you generated as rows. Use the information from the Questionnaire to generate your columns.

ACTIVITIES SCHEDULE							
	MONDAY	TUESDAY	WEDNESDAY	THURSDAY	FRIDAY	SATURDAY	SUNDAY
12:00 Midnight to 1:00 A.M.							
1:00 A.M.– 2:00 A.M.							
2:00 A.M.– 3:00 A.M.							
3:00 A.M.– 4:00 A.M.							
4:00 A.M.– 5:00 A.M.							
5:00 A.M.– 6:00 A.M.							
6:00 A.M.– 7:00 A.M.							
7:00 A.M.– 8:00 A.M.							
8:00 A.M.– 9:00 A.M.							
9:00 A.M.– 10:00 A.M.							
10:00 A.M.– 11:00 A.M.							
11:00 A.M.– 12:00 noon							
Noon– 1:00 P.M.							
1:00 P.M.– 2:00 P.M.							
2:00 P.M.– 3:00 P.M.							
3:00 P.M.– 4:00 P.M.							

4:00 P.M.– 5:00 P.M.							
5:00 P.M.– 6:00 P.M.							
6:00 P.M.– 7:00 P.M.							
7:00 P.M.– 8:00 P.M.							
8:00 P.M.– 9:00 P.M.							
9:00 P.M.– 10:00 P.M.							
10:00 P.M.– 11:00 P.M.							
11:00 P.M.– 12:00 midnight							

QUESTIONNAIRE

I. Using the information from the completed activities schedule and activities list, record the information requested in this Questionnaire.

A. At which specific times (hour and day) is each activity done? (TIMING)

B. For how long is each activity done? (DURATION)

C. What activity comes before each activity? After each activity? (SEQUENTIAL ORDER)

D. How often during the week do you do the same activity? (FREQUENCY)

E. List the activities appearing in the completed schedule under the following headings: (FREQUENCY)

Number of times weekly:

Number of times daily:

II. Using the list of activities only:

A. For how long have you been doing each activity? (HISTORICAL DURATION)

Tabulate under the following headings:

Ever since I can remember:

More than 25 years:

15–25 years:

10–15 years:

5–10 years:

1–5 years:

Less than 1 year

B. Where do you do each activity? (SPATIAL/LOCATIONAL) Tabulate under the following headings:

Indoors:

Outdoors:

Special setting:

Same place always:

Variable (describe):

C. With whom do you do each activity? (SOCIAL 1)
   1. Tabulate as follows:
       a. With others:

           1 person:

           2–4 people:

           Small group:

           Large group:

       b. Alone (SOCIAL 2)

   2. Code each activity as follows: (SOCIAL 2)
       F = friends

       R = family

       C = colleagues (co-workers, fellow students, committee members)

       X = other (specify)

D. From whom did you learn each activity? (PERSONAL EQUATION)
   Code each activity as follows:
       P = from peers

       K = from family

       T = from teachers

       Z = from others (specify)

E. How do you feel about each activity? (PERSONAL EQUATION)

1. Use the following rating scale to indicate a number for each activity that best indicates how you feel (1 = dislike, 5 = like, with gradations in between):

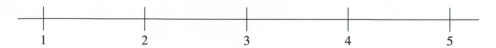

2. Tabulate under the following headings (LIKE, DISLIKE, NEUTRAL, VARI-ABLE):

Like:

Dislike:

Neutral:

Variable (explain):

3. List all your activities in order of preference (i.e., most liked first). Tabulate as follows:

Choose to do (CHOOSE TO DO):

Have to do (HAVE TO DO):

ADDENDUM TO QUESTIONNAIRE

Using the completed activities schedule, answer the following questions:

1. How many hours per week do you spend at work? _____

2. How many hours per week do you spend in sleep? _____

3. How many hours per week do you spend with leisure activities? _____

4. How many hours per week do you spend on chores (taking care of self and environment, including others in it)? _____

5. What proportion of your weekly time do you spend on each of the above categories of activities? _____

6. What proportion of your weekly time do you spend:

   a. alone? _____

   b. with others? _____

7. What proportion of your weekly time do you spend:

   a. at home? _____

   b. away from home? _____

8. What proportion of your weekly time do you spend on activities you:

   a. dislike? _____

   b. like? _____

9. What proportion of your weekly time do you spend on activities you:

   a. choose to do? _____

   b. have to do? _____

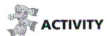 **ACTIVITY**

Materials

Blue, green, red, and yellow markers (one of each per student).

Instructions

1. Discuss with your class your experience completing Study Question #8. How did you feel about the process of completing the configuration? What did you learn about yourself? What did you learn about your computer skills?

2. Discuss as a class and record here how the activities in Study Question #8 that may be used in treatment.

3a. Participate in another time management awareness activity used in occupational therapy, called the Pie of Life. Use the following pie and four colors to indicate how much time you spend in the following areas during a 24 hour day: Leisure—blue; Individual self-care—orange; free/unscheduled time—green; school/work—yellow.

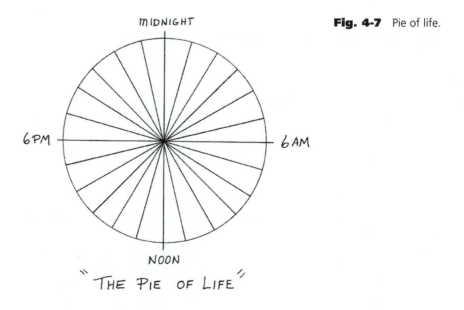

Fig. 4-6 Pie of life.

3b. Discuss your pie with the class. List and discuss possible imbalances present.

3c. Reflect on how you might correct any imbalances present in your life. Color in the following pie, making necessary but realistic changes to your schedule that would improve the balance of your life.

Fig. 4-7 Pie of life.

3d. Discuss and record how the Pie of Life may be used in treatment.

4a. As a class, discuss and record time management techniques that you and others have used successfully. Put a check by those you now use successfully, those you have tried that have not worked for you, and those you want to implement.

TIME MANAGEMENT TECHNIQUES	DO NOW	TRIED	WANT TO IMPLEMENT

4b. Discuss how the above techniques may be used in treatment.

FOLLOW-UP

✔ Complete the Application of Competencies at the end of this chapter.

STRESS MANAGEMENT

Exercise 72

OBJECTIVES

✔ Identify stressors and coping techniques used in one's personal life
✔ Describe a variety of stress management techniques that are appropriate to use with individuals who have psychosocial dysfunction
✔ Plan a series of stress management techniques to be used in a group setting

DESCRIPTION

This exercise will introduce you to the role stress plays in your personal life as well as in the lives of clients who have psychosocial dysfunction. Stress is present in everyone's life and takes its toll in unhealthy ways unless it is managed successfully. Managing one's own stress will help to encourage personal health, happiness, and success. Your effectiveness as an occupational therapy (OT) practitioner will be directly related to how well you are able to manage your own stress. Teaching stress management to your clients will also improve their performance and facilitate optional functioning in health, wellness, and wholeness. Many stress management resources are available to use with clients. You will need to familiarize yourself with these. Additionally, you will want to take advantage of courses, workshops, and seminars in which you can gain more in-depth knowledge about stress management techniques to add to your repertoire of coping skills.

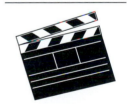

"Stress is when your mouth says yes and your body says no."

ANONYMOUS

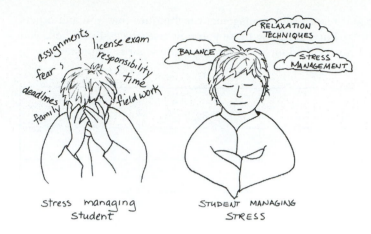

Fig. 4-8 Stress: An inevitability of life

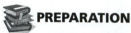

PREPARATION

Suggested Readings

AOTA (latest edition)
Cottrell (1993)
Neidstadt and Crepeau (1998)
Stein and Cutler (1998)
Tubesing and Tubesing (1994)

STUDY QUESTIONS

1. What is the percentage of medical complaints that are related to stress?

2. According to the latest edition of uniform terminology for occupational therapy (AOTA), what is the name of the performance component used to describe the ability to handle stress?

3. Differentiate between the two types of stress: eustress and distress.

4. What are some causes of stress?

5. What mediating factors can influence the effect of stress?

6. What are several general principles of stress management?

7. Describe the stress management techniques listed below and their therapeutic implications.

a. Aerobic exercise

b. Coping skills training

c. Autogenic training

d. Communication skills

e. Deep breathing

f. Laughter

g. Meditation

h. Progressive relaxation exercises

i. Verbalization/support meditation

j. Biofeedback

k. Distraction

8. What are stressors in your life and how do you cope?

STRESSORS	COPING SKILLS

9. Describe the components of the following skills that may be identified through a Stress Skills Assessment (Tubesing and Tubesing, 1994) to deal with stress:

   a. Personal management

   b. Relationship

   c. Outlook

   d. Self-care

10. What is the relationship between how you handle stress and how effectively you think you might work with clients who are under stress?

11. What do you want to accomplish or master in regard to your own stress management before working with clients on this topic?

12. Summarize strengths and areas of concern in your own current stress management status.

STRENGTHS	AREAS OF CONCERN

13. What assessments might appropriately identify stressors in an individual's life?

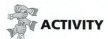 **ACTIVITY**

Materials

Stress inventory, tape player, relaxation tapes, videotape player and television monitor, relaxation video, worksheets props.

Instructions

1. Take a stress inventory (any) and summarize your results here.

2. Participate in a discussion with your class discussing stress management techniques that are used in class members' personal lives. List the techniques you and your classmates use below. Put a checkmark next to those you would like to consider including in your own life.

STRESS TECHNIQUE	✔

3. Participate in several instructor-led stress reduction activities. Use the following chart to record activities, the source where the activity can be located, and your reaction to the activity. Also include possible treatment implications. An example is completed for you.

ACTIVITY	SOURCE	REACTION	TREATMENT IMPLICATION
Get off my back	Book on stress management by Tubesing and Tubesing (1994)	I initially felt silly; it sounds great and I felt good.	This could be used at the beginning or end of an adolescent or adult group.

4a. With your partner or in a small group, plan activities for a stress management group that will meet one hour each day for one week in an acute care adult setting. Include an outline of the activities you will use, the time of day and duration in which you anticipate they will be completed, and the materials that will be needed, as well as the source of where the materials might be obtained. On completion, share your ideas with your class.

Monday		
OUTLINE OF ACTIVITIES	TIMELINE	MATERIALS NEEDED/SOURCE

Tuesday		
OUTLINE OF ACTIVITIES	TIMELINE	MATERIALS NEEDED/SOURCE

Wednesday		
OUTLINE OF ACTIVITIES	TIMELINE	MATERIALS NEEDED/SOURCE

Thursday		
OUTLINE OF ACTIVITIES	TIMELINE	MATERIALS NEEDED/SOURCE

Friday		
OUTLINE OF ACTIVITIES	TIMELINE	MATERIALS NEEDED/SOURCE

4b. Discuss the ideas with your class and record here the ideas you want to remember.

FOLLOW-UP

✔ Complete the Application of Competencies at the end of this chapter.
✔ Complete a Therapeutic Use of Self Analysis found in Appendix B on your individual and group participation in stress management activities.
✔ Complete Performance Skill 4D on Group Activity.

PSYCHOSOCIAL GROUPS

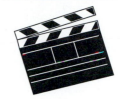

OBJECTIVES

✔ Define the use and purpose of groups in a psychosocial setting
✔ Develop content for group programming in a specific psychosocial setting
✔ Plan and co-lead a group used in a psychosocial setting

DESCRIPTION

In a psychosocial setting, a group format is often used to reach the clients' goals. Many clients in such a setting have difficulty with social relationships, and the group setting can offer practice in improving these skills. Additionally, the presence of more than one other person can provide appropriate reality-testing parameters. There are several types of group protocols that can be used to promote changes in clients with psychosocial dysfunction. As a practitioner, you will need to be familiar with these protocols so that you can use them in a variety of settings. Group treatments is used frequently in a psychosocial setting, and it is a powerful tool. As an occupational therapy practitioner you will need to be well skilled in its use.

"Great people are those who make others feel that they, too, can become great."

MARK TWAIN

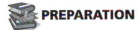 **PREPARATION**

Suggested Readings

Cara and MacRae (1998)
Cotrell (1993)
Howe and Schwartzberg (1995)
Mosey (1986)
Neidstadt and Crepeau (1998)
Stein and Cutler (1998)

Study Questions

1. List some of the most frequently used types of groups in occupational therapy in a psychosocial setting.

2. Indicate the use and prevalence of groups in a psychosocial setting.

3. What are the advantages of using groups as a modality?

4. Identify curative factors in group therapy.

5. List and describe the six major types of activity groups described by Anne Mosey (1986).

6. List the roles, communication skills, and personhood skills of an ideal group leader.

7. Describe how you think cultural relevance must be considered in choosing topics and goals for a group.

8. Explain the necessity of flexibility as a virtue of a group leader.

9. What are several guidelines for group leadership?

10. Define Anne Mosey's (1986) five developmental levels of group functioning.
    a.

    b.

    c.

    d.

    e.

11. Detail how Anne Mosey's (1986) levels can be applied with different client populations and needs.

ACTIVITY

Materials

Resources containing activity ideas for groups, *Group Dynamics in Occupational Therapy* (Cole, 1998)

Instructions

1. With a partner, plan occupational therapy groups (activity, discussion, movement, etc.) that you would like to implement on a weekly basis for one of the service areas that you have been assigned (inpatient adolescent unit, chronic institutional state hospital, adult partial hospitalization, inpatient acute adult unit,

geriatric psychiatric unit, inpatient adult substance abuse unit, inpatient eating disorder unit). Assume that you will be assigned this unit full-time and will be responsible for leading two to four groups each day. Use the space below to plan the type and topic of your group intervention. Include the times at which these groups will be offered. Share your completed plans with your classmates. Record your classmates' plans in similar charts.

Service Area:

TIME	S	M	T	W	TH	F	S

2a. With your partner and using the proposed weekly schedules, select one group from your assigned service area and write a group protocol, using Cole's (1998) seven-step format or one assigned by your instructor. Co-lead the group session with one classmate as the other classmates role-play clients from the service area you were assigned. Use the space below to plan your group session.

Group Session Outline (Cole, 1998)

Session title:

Format:

Supplies:

Description:

1. Warm-up:

2. Introduction:

3. Instructions for activity:

4. Sharing:

5. Discussion questions:

   Processing:

   Generalizing:

   Application:

   Summary:

2b. After your group session, solicit feedback from your peers about your strengths and areas of concern as a group leader. Fill out the following Leader Feedback form using their input.

LEADER FEEDBACK				
	STRENGTH ✔	COMMENT	WEAKNESS ✔	COMMENT
Thorough introduction given				
Explained purpose				
Developed body of discussion				
Involved all members				
Ended discussion appropriately				
Used appropriate tone of voice				
Maintained leadership role				
Responded to member's verbal communication				
Responded to member's nonverbal communication				
Used nonverbal communication appropriately				
Met goals of group				

FOLLOW-UP

✔   Complete a Therapeutic Use of Self Analysis found in Appendix B on your leadership abilities.

✔   Complete the Application of Competencies at the end of this chapter.

✔   Complete Performance Skill 4C on Planning a Group.

✔   Complete Performance Skill 4F on More Practice with Your Teaching.

INTERVENTION PLANNING

OBJECTIVES

✔ Describe the steps in the intervention planning process
✔ Identify how a client's strengths, areas of concern, and cultural background may influence a practitioner's choice of activities for intervention
✔ Develop a rationale for selection of treatment activities including the choice of service delivery

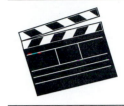

"Success is getting what you want, and happiness is wanting what you get."

IBO PROVERB

DESCRIPTION

Intervention planning is a critical component in the occupational therapy (OT) process. Intervention planning is completed in conjunction with input from the client as well as the client's family and caregivers. Numerous aspects need to be considered in the process. The frame of reference identified by the facility and/or OT practitioner will influence one's choice of occupations. The client's culture will need to be considered as occupations are selected. The client's goals will guide the intervention process, and the strengths and areas of concern of the client will assist in identifying appropriate intervention activities. Completion of intervention planning is critical to the success of client care. Desired changes and outcomes do not occur spontaneously but rather are achieved through careful deliberation and planning.

PREPARATION

Suggested Readings

AOTA (latest edition)
Cara and MacRae (1998)
Early (2000)
Neidstadt and Crepeau (1998)

Study Questions

1. Fill in the boxes according to the provision of OT services outlined in the Standards of Practice (AOTA, latest edition). Begin with the referral. Add and subtract boxes as necessary.

```
┌─────────────────────────────┐
│          Referral           │
└─────────────────────────────┘
               ⇩
┌─────────────────────────────┐
│                             │
└─────────────────────────────┘
               ⇩
┌─────────────────────────────┐
│                             │
└─────────────────────────────┘
               ⇩
┌─────────────────────────────┐
│                             │
└─────────────────────────────┘
               ⇩
┌─────────────────────────────┐
│                             │
└─────────────────────────────┘
               ⇩
┌─────────────────────────────┐
│                             │
└─────────────────────────────┘
               ⇩
┌─────────────────────────────┐
│                             │
└─────────────────────────────┘
               ⇩
┌─────────────────────────────┐
│                             │
└─────────────────────────────┘
```

2. Using the diagram completed in Study question #1, shade in red the box that indicates the standard the occupational therapist cannot delegate to the occupational therapy assistant (OTA). Shade in blue the boxes that indicate the standards for which an OTA shares partial responsibility. Shade in yellow the box that indicates the standard for which the OTA shares the majority of responsibility with the occupational therapist.

3. Describe the involvement of the client in the intervention planning process.

4. Describe the involvement of the family and/or caregiver in the intervention planning process.

5. What is the role of client motivation in the intervention planning process?

6. Explain the importance of writing specific observations to assist in goal writing.

7. What role does the OTA have in goal writing?

8. Give examples of goals for each of the performance areas that would be appropriate to address in a mental health setting.

9. Briefly summarize the use of the following response variables in selecting intervention methods.

ACTIVITY	ENVIRONMENT	USE OF SELF

10. Describe how a client's age may influence your collaboration with him/her in selection of activities to use in treatment.

   a. Adolescence

   b. Young adult

c. Middle age

d. Senior citizen

e. Late life

11. Describe the influential role of a client's culture in the intervention planning process.

12. Describe the use of crafts in the treatment of mental illness.

13. Identify crafts that are commonly used in a psychiatric setting.

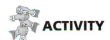 **ACTIVITY**

Materials

Case Studies 23, 27, and 33 located at the end of this chapter.

Instructions

1. Given the case study by your instructor, formulate the following intervention plan with a partner.

   a. Frame of reference to be used:

   Rationale:

   b. Identify possible cultural considerations:

   c. What assessments would be appropriate to complete on this client? Indicate whether these need to done by the occupational therapist or can be delegated to the OTA.

ASSESSMENTS	OT ONLY	OTA

d. Identify the client's strengths and areas of concern that are evident in the case description.

STRENGTHS	AREAS OF CONCERN

e. Write one long-term goal and two short-term goals:

1.

    a.

    b.

f. List seven occupations that would be appropriate to use during intervention. Include your rationale for your choice of occupations as well as service delivery model (group or individual).

OCCUPATIONS	RATIONALE	GROUP	INDIVIDUAL

2. Given another case study by your instructor, work with a different partner and formulate another intervention plan for that individual.

   a. Frame of reference to be used:

      Rationale:

   b. Identify possible cultural considerations:

   c. What assessments would be appropriate to complete on this client? Indicate whether these need to done by the occupational therapist or can be delegated to the OTA.

ASSESSMENTS	OT ONLY	OTA

   d. Identify the client's strengths and areas of concern that are evident in the case description.

STRENGTHS	AREAS OF CONCERN

   e. Write one long-term and two short-term goals:
      1.

         a.

         b.

   f. List seven occupations that would be appropriate to use during intervention. Include your rationale for your choice of occupations as well as service delivery model (group or individual).

OCCUPATIONS	RATIONALE	GROUP	INDIVIDUAL

3. Once again switch partners and proceed to outline another intervention plan for another case study.

   a. Frame of reference to be used:

   Rationale:

   b. Identify possible cultural considerations:

   c. What assessments would be appropriate to complete on this client? Indicate whether these need to done by the occupational therapist or can be delegated to the OTA.

ASSESSMENTS	OT ONLY	OTA

d. Identify the client's strengths and areas of concern that are evident in the case description.

STRENGTHS	AREAS OF CONCERN

e. Write one long-term goal and two short-term goals:

1.

   a.

   b.

f. List seven occupations that would be appropriate to use during intervention. Indicate whether group or individual intervention would be most appropriate. Include your rationale for choice of occupations as well as service delivery model (group or individual).

OCCUPATIONS	RATIONALE	GROUP	INDIVIDUAL

4. Present your plans to the class and take notes on other plans presented. Record below the ideas you would like to remember.

5. Identify your strengths and areas of concern in treatment planning.

STRENGTHS	AREAS OF CONCERN

FOLLOW-UP

✔ Complete the Application of Competencies at the end of this chapter.
✔ Complete a Therapeutic Use of Self Analysis found in Appendix B on your participation in intervention planning.
✔ Complete Performance Skill 4A on Adding to Your Files.
✔ Complete Performance Skill 4G on Intervention Planning.

Exercise 75

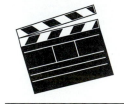

"Find the right balance in life. Man is body ... mind ... spirit. Give the right amount of attention to each."

ALFRED A. MONTAPERT

PSYCHOSOCIAL HEALTH, WELLNESS, AND PREVENTION

OBJECTIVES

✔ List local community resources that are available to promote health and wellness
✔ Describe the role of occupational therapy with the client who has an eating disorder and/or substance abuse problem
✔ Lead a group discussion using the twelve-step model

DESCRIPTION

Health/wellness treatment and prevention are critical for individuals with psychosocial dysfunction. It is not uncommon in a mental health setting for clients to have substance abuse problems and/or eating disorders in addition to other psychiatric diagnosis. Such individuals often need ongoing support. Most communities have many resources that can provide support and intervention. As an occupational therapy (OT) practitioner you will not only provide OT intervention but also be a source of referral information. Established models of group intervention can be adjusted for use in an OT setting, and you will need to be familiar with these models.

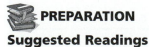 **PREPARATION**

Suggested Readings

Bruce and Borg (1993)
Cara and MacRae (1998)

Local and community publications, such as newspaper and telephone book
Neidstadt and Crepeau (1998)

Study Questions

1. Describe the role of occupational therapy in the area of health promotion and disease prevention with the psychiatric population.

2. Describe the twelve-step model and list the twelve steps.

3. List diagnostic criteria for substance-related disorders and eating disorders.

4. Describe the role of occupational therapy in the treatment of substance abuse and eating disorders, including the treatment methods used, appropriate goals, types of groups appropriate to lead, and activities that could be used.

a. Substance abuse

TREATMENT METHODS	GOALS

TYPES OF GROUPS	ACTIVITIES

b. Eating disorders

TREATMENT METHODS	GOALS

TYPES OF GROUPS	ACTIVITIES

5. Search local publications and make phone calls when necessary to locate services available in your community for the following areas. Describe these services, and include the cost of them. Gather any written materials when possible. Be prepared to share the information with your class.

a. Stress management

AGENCY/LOCATION	DESCRIPTION	COST

b. Substance abuse

AGENCY/LOCATION	DESCRIPTION	COST

c. Support/counseling for families of substance abusers

AGENCY/LOCATION	DESCRIPTION	COST

d. Support/counseling for people with mental illness

AGENCY/LOCATION	DESCRIPTION	COST

e. Support/counseling for families of people with mental illness

AGENCY/LOCATION	DESCRIPTION	COST

f. Inexpensive leisure activities

AGENCY/LOCATION	DESCRIPTION	COST

g. Support/counseling for people with eating disorders

AGENCY/LOCATION	DESCRIPTION	COST

6. What do you do to stay healthy in the following areas?

    a. Body:

    b. Mind:

    c. Spirit:

7. Interview one person you admire and ask them what they do to stay healthy in these same areas.

    a. Body:

    b. Mind:

    c. Spirit:

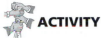 **ACTIVITY**

Materials

Materials brought by students, Case Study 7 (located at the end of Chapter 1) and Case Studies 34, and 35 located at the end of this chapter.

Instructions

1. Share the information from Study Question 5 that you found with your class-mates and record their information as well.

TOPIC	AGENCY/LOCATION	DESCRIPTION	COST

2. With the case study assigned and your small group, determine the needs of the client, the resources that are available, and what is needed for the client to access those resources. When you are finished, share the information with your class.

a. Client description:		
NEEDS	RESOURCES AVAILABLE	WHAT'S NEEDED

b. Client description:		
NEEDS	RESOURCES AVAILABLE	WHAT'S NEEDED

c. Client description:		
NEEDS	RESOURCES AVAILABLE	WHAT'S NEEDED

3a. With a small group, plan and lead a group discussion with clients with eating disorders or substance abuse problems using the twelve-step method. Plan this group for an outpatient setting that has males and females ranging from 20 to 60 years of age, with approximately twelve clients attending each week. Include in your group clients who may have a dual diagnosis of eating disorders or substance abuse and/or an additional psychiatric disorder(s).

Setting description: _____

_____

Selected discussion topic: _____

Format used (worksheets, index cards, etc.): _____

Time outline: _____

_____

_____

_____

3b. Role-play part of this discussion group as a class. Record impressions of all group presentations here as each group role-plays for the class.

FOLLOW-UP

✔   Complete the Application of Competencies at the end of this chapter.

After completing each exercise, write one concept you learned and how you anticipate that learning will influence your treatment of clients.

Application of Competencies

Exercise 61 Observation Skills
Application:

Exercise 62 Evaluation of Psychosocial Functioning
Application:

Exercise 63 Listening and Responding
Application:

Exercise 64 The Interview Process
Application:

Exercise 65 Assertiveness
Application:

Exercise 66 Social Skills
Application:

Exercise 67 Cognitive Disability
Application:

Exercise 68 Daily Living Skills
Application:

Exercise 69 Movement
Application:

Exercise 70 Leisure Planning
Application:

Exercise 71 Time Management
Application:

Exercise 72 Stress Management
Application:

Exercise 73 Psychosocial Groups
Application:

Exercise 74 Intervention Planning
Application:

Exercise 75 Psychosocial Health, Wellness, and Prevention
Application:

Performance Skill 4A

ADDING TO YOUR FILES

Search and add occupations to your activity file for individuals from adolescents to older adults. Type a paper on each activity with the information in the following chart and assemble these with a table of contents. Include in your file at least two activities that will work on each of the targeted areas listed below. Note on each occupation the ages for which it is intended. Be sure to have activities for a wide variety of ages. Include activities that have diverse cultural and contextual qualities. Use at least three references that you have not used previously. List the occupations and activities you have gathered. Check each box as you complete the requirements. When the chart is completed, you will have at least eighteen new activities.

Check box as you complete each section

TARGETED AREA	OCCUPATION	RATIONALE	PERFORMANCE CONTEXT	SUPPLIES/ MATERIALS	STEPS TO PERFORM	ADAPTATIONS	PRECAUTIONS	REFERENCES
Movement								
Cooking								
Assertiveness								
Stress Management								
Scrap Craft								
Craft								
Cognitive								
Social								
Daily Living Activities								

INTERVIEW

Given a case study, prepare and conduct an interview with someone role-playing a client. Videotape your interview and use this form to critique yourself. You may also solicit feedback from a peer and/or your instructor. Put a check mark in the box if the skill was observed. Write comments as desired.

SKILLS	✔	SELF/PEER/ INSTRUCTOR COMMENTS
Interview lasted designated amount of time		
Communicated interest and concern to the client		
Communicated respect to the client		
Communicated empathy to the client		
Stated the purpose of the interview		
Stated his or her role in the interview		
Appeared professional		
Adequately explained the principles of occupational therapy		
Observed and responded to client's nonverbal communication		
Actively listened to the client during the interview		
Used silence appropriately		
Asked open-ended questions		
Kept the interview appropriately focused		
Used the appropriate level of terminology		
Asked for clarification of vague terms		
Avoided giving advice		
Allowed the client to fully express himself or herself		
Fully obtained information required		
Appeared clear and knowledgeable in questions asked		
Appeared confident		
Terminated session appropriately		
Total:		

PLANNING A GROUP

Plan a group for clients in a psychosocial setting. These may be clients you are seeing in your fieldwork or case studies that your instructor may give you. Use the group protocol format in Cole (1998) or a similar one to document your written plans. Use the format below to prepare a rough draft of your group plan.

1. List clients, ages, and diagnosis.

CLIENT	AGE	DIAGNOSIS

2. Determine the common needs of this group of clients.

3. Prepare the group protocol, including a group treatment plan outline and a group session plan outline.
4. Prepare an occupational analysis of one of the activities you have selected.

Performance Skill 4D

GROUP ACTIVITY

Prepare a group activity for any topic such as leisure planning, time management, or stress management. Look over your previous notes and feedback from your practice sessions done earlier in this chapter. What did you learn from other practice leaders? Use that information and begin to plan here. Use the format below to prepare a rough draft of your group plan.

Topic of group:

Activities you will use (i.e., worksheets, index cards, game format):

Questions you will ask to generate discussion:

How will you begin?

What will be your rules?

How will you ensure that all members participate?

What problems may occur and how will you deal with them?

TEACHING A BASIC LIFE TASK

Teach a basic life task (such as riding a bus or doing laundry) to your classmates as if they were low-functioning psychiatric patients. Use this sheet to begin preparing.

1. Life task: _____

2. Time frame: _____

3. Number of participants: _____

4. Activities you will use: _____

    _____

    _____

5. Fill out a lesson plan for this group (see Chapter Two for lesson plan outline).

6. Ask yourself these questions in preparation:
    a. Are you organized?

    b. Will the members be *active* participants?

    c. Is your environment set up conducive to learning?

    d. What problems may you encounter? What will you do?

    e. What props will you use to facilitate hands-on learning?

    f. Have you prepared an introduction?

    g. How will you know whether your group has been effective?

Performance Skill 4F

MORE PRACTICE WITH YOUR TEACHING

Teach a group of students a craft or activity. Use this worksheet to assist you in this process.

1. Activity: _____

2. Time frame: _____

3. Number in group: _____

4. Materials necessary: _____

5. Fill out a lesson plan.

6. Ask yourself these questions in preparation:
   a. Will it help to have a sample?

   b. Am I using interesting methods to teach?

   c. How can I make sure I am well prepared?

   d. What have I learned from previous teaching sessions that I want to remember?

Performance Skill 4G

INTERVENTION PLANNING

Working in groups or with a partner, plan intervention with the case study provided by your instructor.

1. Identify problems and check which ones you will treat. Put a team member in the space if referring out.

PROBLEM	TEAM MEMEBER

PROBLEM	TEAM MEMEBER

2. Identify strengths.

3. Identify possible cultural considerations.

4. Write one long-term goal and one short-term goal for three of the identified problems to treat.

Problem: _____

Long-term goal: _____

Short-term goal: _____

Problem: _____

Long-term goal: _____

Short-term goal: _____

Problem: _____

Long-term goal: _____

Short-term goal: _____

5. Describe one occupation you will select for each of the three problems above.

PROBLEM	OCCUPATION

6. Which team members will you be working closely with on this client?

ADOLESCENT PSYCHOSOCIAL

Type:
Inpatient

Age:
14 years old

Sex:
Female

Culture/Religion:

Insurance Information:

Diagnosis:
Borderline personality disorder

Social History:
Rachel is one of three children. She lives with her family, who are extremely frustrated with her behavior. Rachel reports not having a good relationship with either parent. She attends high school and is in the ninth grade. She has recently been suspended for dysfunctional behavior. No further information is available at this time.

Medical History:
Rachel has received extensive psychiatric treatment and has been out of the hospital one month. She was readmitted because she got in a fight and cut a girl with a bottle. This happened at school and is the reason for her suspension. Rachel's parents report that she has lots of mood swings. Rachel says that she does these things to make her parents stronger. She doesn't like being touched and doesn't like people being close to her or walking behind her. It appears at this time that Rachel will need chronic care. She has depleted her insurance benefits. Plans need to be made.

ADULT PSYCHOSOCIAL

Type:
Acute Care

Age:
30 years old

Sex:
Female

Culture/Religion:

Insurance Information:

Diagnosis:
Acute psychosis

Social History:
Gloria lives alone in an apartment and works as a waitress. She reports that she has no friends or other interests besides work. When not at work, she watches TV.

Medical History:
Gloria was admitted complaining of her insides hurting and feelings of being smothered. She stopped taking medication several months ago. She has been hospitalized two times previously, approximately five years apart. Gloria is oriented and denies any hallucinations or use of alcohol or drugs. She is currently complaining of anxiety and thoughts of suicide.

ADOLESCENT PSYCHOSOCIAL

Type:
Inpatient

Age:
17 years old

Sex:
Female

Culture/Religion:

Insurance Information:

Diagnosis:
Adjustment disorder, asthma

Social History:
Sally lives with her parents and five other children: two older boys and three younger girls. She attends high school and is in the twelfth grade. Sally had a part-time job as a cashier in a grocery store, which she quit three weeks ago. She reports that she was unable to focus on her job. Sally enjoys school and is on the high school soccer team. She likes to listen to music and hang out with her friends, which she hasn't done much of recently.

Medical History:
Sally is a victim of date rape. This happened approximately four months ago. The rape resulted in pregnancy and an abortion, which she feels was forced on her by her parents. She has been crying all week. Sally has been unable to eat or sleep. She says she wishes she was dead at times but reports no suicidal plans. She has avoided social contact, especially with males.

ADULT PSYCHOSOCIAL

Type:
Acute Care

Age:
49 years old

Sex:
Female

Culture/Religion:

Insurance Information:

Diagnosis:
Dysthmic disorder

Social History:
Vera lives with her boyfriend of three years in a two-bedroom apartment. She says that he is strange but she can accept that. She is thinking of moving, but he is asking her to stay. She is not sure what to do.

Vera spends most of her free time at flea markets and garage sales. She worked at a department store in the past. She is currently receiving disability payments.

Medical History:

Vera has a panic attack disorder with failure to resolve with outpatient therapy. She complains of being unable to sleep and unable to leave her house. She has reported no suicidal ideation but says that she is unable to function and states that she can't go on like this.

Vera's history of psychiatric problems goes back to early childhood. She has been hospitalized numerous times in several hospitals.

Vera ambulates with a cane because of an injury from a car accident four years ago. Vera's cognitive function is WNL, functioning at a 5+ on Allen Cognitive Level Screening Test.

CASE STUDY 27

ADULT PSYCHOSOCIAL

Type:
Chronic Inpatient

Age:
24 years old

Sex:
Female

Culture/Religion:

Insurance Information:

Diagnosis:
Axis I: Anorexia nervosa
Axis II: Borderline personality disorder

Social History:

Margot is single and lives with her parents. She has one sister, who is three years older. Margot has attended college to become a dietician several times for a few months at a time but has then quit without obtaining a degree. She has held several part-time jobs over the years in various clerk-type positions. She has difficulty keeping friends in a relationship, owing to her intense pursuit of them once they enter the relationship.

Medical History:

Margot has been hospitalized approximately seven times since she was first diagnosed with anorexia at the age of 17. She has been transferred from an acute care setting at this time because she is unresponsive to treatment. She currently weighs 76 pounds, with a height of 5'3".

Margot has attempted suicide two times: once by staying in the car while it was left running in the garage, the other time by taking pills. She has many scars on her forearms from self-mutilating behaviors.

Margot has demonstrated intense anger at several residents who tease her for not eating.

CASE STUDY 28

ADOLESCENT PSYCHOSOCIAL

Type:
Inpatient

Age:
17 years old

Sex:
Female

Culture/Religion:

Insurance Information:

Diagnosis:
Psychotic depression

Social History:
Jessica lives with her grandparents. Her parents have been divorced for years and have been unable to cope with Jessica's problems. She has few friends and is often in trouble at school. The school personnel report that she has poor social skills.

Her favorite activities are reading mystery novels, playing video games, and listening to music.

Medical History:
Jessica has been treated for two months for her depression with medication and counseling. She has gotten worse over the past few weeks, exhibiting isolation and some mania. Jessica's father has bipolar disorder and has at times been extremely out of control.

Since her admission yesterday, Jessica has been seen tumbling down the hall in the hospital. She has also been intrusive, going into others' rooms. She has taken things that do not belong to her, and security had to be called when she refused to give them back.

Jessica says that when she is quiet, she can hear the devil talk to her.

CASE STUDY 29

ADULT PSYCHOSOCIAL

Type:
Acute Care

Age:
72 years old

Sex:
Male

Culture/Religion:

Insurance Information:

Diagnosis:
Axis I: Major depression, recurrent dementia
Axis II: None
Axis III: Hypothyroidism, parkinsonism

Social History:
George lives in a nursing home. He was put there by his wife, who was unable to care for him at home. She is 71 years old and has arthritis and walks with a cane. She is very involved in her husband's care.

Medical History:
George was admitted because of increasing depression, insomnia, agitation, impairment of concentration and memory, and occasional falls. He is reported to stop and stare for long periods of time, unable to respond to questions. George has very noticeable psychomotor retardation. He has a long history of major depression and pseudodementia.

George takes a long time to process information presented to him, and his judgment is grossly impaired. He seems to have no insight into his illness.

At this time, George uses a wheelchair with a restraint. He needs to be fed dinner and assisted with ambulation. George assists in his bathing and dressing but for the most part is dependent. He has not been eating satisfactorily.

George is able to communicate in an understandable manner but rarely initiates conversation.

CASE STUDY 30

ADULT PSYCHOSOCIAL

Type:
Acute Care

Age:
24 years old

Sex:
Male

Culture/Religion:

Insurance Information:

Diagnosis:
Axis I: Schizophrenia, paranoid type
Axis II: Schizoid personality
Axis III: CSF shunt for hydrocephalus

Social History:
Shawn lives by himself and works in a factory. His family convinced Shawn that he needed hospitalization. They report that he has acted very strangely and paranoid for over a year and is getting rapidly worse. He has garbage all over his apartment.

Shawn reports having no friends or girlfriend. He rarely engages in social interaction with peers and is often seen lifting heavy objects as if he were weight lifting.

Medical History:
Shawn was admitted with a complaint of not able to function doing everyday tasks and responsibilities. He threatens others, saying that he will break their arm or kill them. His sleep and appetite are impaired. His hygiene is unkempt: he appears to go without a bath for weeks. His family and co-workers report him seeing and hearing things that aren't there. He also forgets things very easily.

Shawn has a history of substance abuse, smoking pot, and sniffing gasoline. He is currently not receiving any mental health treatment. His family reports that when they attempt to help him, he threatens to kill them.

At this time, Shawn is disoriented and confused. He has been noted to have difficulty making decisions. He is willing to come to groups.

CASE STUDY 31

GERIATRIC PSYCHOSOCIAL

Type:
Acute Inpatient

Age:
87 years old

Sex:
Female

Culture/Religion:

Insurance Information:

Diagnosis:
Major depression

Social History:
Mildred lives in an apartment alone. She has a daughter who is involved and is very active in her neighborhood church. She has a cleaning lady come in once a week to do laundry and cleaning. She likes to cook and bake, belongs to a women's club, watches TV, and walks for exercise. Mildred is one of five children; all others have passed away. She had five children, two of whom died, one just last year.

Medical History:
Before admission, Mildred had been increasingly tearful and depressed. She had been confused, often talking about her parents in the present tense. At this time she has decreased cognitive functioning and altered thought processes in the way of delusions and has a potential for injury. Mildred also has arthritis and comes in with a broken wrist due to a fall at home.

Since admission, Mildred has required moderate assistance to complete ADLs and maximum assistance to participate in any groups. She is currently functioning at ACL 4.0.

ADULT PSYCHOSOCIAL

Type:
Outpatient Partial Day

Age:
31 years old

Sex:
Male

Culture/Religion:

Insurance Information:

Diagnosis:
Bipolar disorder

Social History:
Robert is a divorced father of two children. He has a son who is 10 years old and a daughter who is 8 years old. He has been divorced for four years. He has a degree in engineering and has been employed until recently. He quit his job to start a business of his own, spending all of his money and investments from several other people. He has lost all of his money as well as his business. Several business associates are suing him.

Robert has spent some of his leisure time running and working out at the gym. He has custody of his children one weekend per month.

Medical History:
Robert is now presenting with suicidal ideation, although he has not attempted suicide yet. He has been unable to leave his apartment and sleeps approximately sixteen hours a day. He has lost ten pounds and reports having no worth or reason for living. He takes lithium inconsistently.

CASE STUDY 33

ADULT PSYCHOSOCIAL

Type:
Acute Care

Age:
71 years old

Sex:
Male

Culture/Religion:

Insurance Information:

Diagnosis:
Depression/anxiety

Social History:
Anthony lives alone in a high-rise apartment for the elderly; he has lived there for six years. He has a son in town who checks on him. Anthony states that he has no interests and feels that he is not physically able to participate in any activities. He reports working in the past as a carpenter. He previously enjoyed building as a hobby.

Medical History:
Anthony has a history of hypertension, diabetes, anxiety, depression, and arthritis. He has a several-month history of postural lightheadedness. He was admitted after a fall today when he fractured his mandible. He had cataract surgery three years ago.

Anthony is independent in all self-care skills. He appears very quiet and keeps to himself. He scored a 4+ on the Claudia Allen test on admission. He has had previous admissions for his anxiety and depression. He seems to be admitted mostly in the winter months.

CASE STUDY 34

ADOLESCENT PSYCHOSOCIAL

Type:
Inpatient

Age:
15 years old

Sex:
Female

Culture/Religion:

Insurance Information:

Diagnosis:
Depression

Social History:
Cathy lives with her mother and younger brother. Her parents are divorced. She attends high school, is in the tenth grade, and is doing poorly. Cathy enjoys playing the piano and other instruments. She also enjoys listening to classical music. Cathy spends time reading novels, writing, doing calligraphy, and watching TV.

Medical History:
Cathy was admitted with the following problems: suicidal ideation, poor impulse control, eating disturbance, low self-esteem, ineffective coping skills, poor communication

skills, and anxiety. She has poor family relations and a history of physical abuse. Cathy recently reported her mother to 241-KIDS for abusing her. Her mother is being denied contact with Cathy at this time. Residential placement is being considered.

Cathy identifies some of her problems as decreased motivation and decreased energy. She feels that her school problems are due to decreased concentration, increased frustration, poor self-esteem, and poor coping skills. She has described her goals as wanting to stay in groups and in control of her feelings.

CASE STUDY 35

ADULT PPSYCHOSOCIALSYCHIATRY

Type:
Chronic Inpatient

Age:
29 years old

Sex:
Male

Culture/Religion:

Insurance Information:

Diagnosis:
Axis I: Chronic paranoid schizophrenic, polysubstance abuse
Axis II: Antisocial personality disorder, narcissistic personality disorder

Social History:
Harry is single and collecting disability. He was admitted from a forensic facility with the status of NGRI (not guilty by reason of insanity). He fatally stabbed his ten-year-old nephew. He was living with his girlfriend and his parents before his conviction. Harry reports that his father is into Satan worshipping and alcohol abuse. He reports enjoying going out with his friends, drinking, and playing pool and darts. At one point in his life he held a job as a construction worker.

Medical History:
On admission, Harry reported hearing voices and seeing things. He has been hospitalized many times for his mental illness. He has been known to abuse various substances, including cocaine and alcohol.

He attends few groups and requires maximum assistance to participate in any self-care.

REFERENCES

Allen, C. K. 1990. Allen Cognitive Level (ACL) Screening test. Available from Allen Conferences, Inc., Ormond Beach, FL.

Allen, C. K. n.d. Ribbon Cards. Available from Allen Conferences, Inc., Ormond Beach, FL.

Allen, C. K., C. A. Earhart, and T. Blue. 1992. *Occupational Therapy Treatment Goals for the Physically and Cognitively Disabled.* Rockville, MD: American Occupational Therapy Associaton.

American Occupational Therapy Association. latest edition. *Reference Manual of the Official Documents of the American Occupational Therapy Assocation.* Bethesda, MD: Author.

Asher, I. E. 1996. *Occupational Therapy Assessment Tools: An Annotated Index.* 2d ed. Bethesda, MD: American Occupational Therapy Association.

Brayman, S. J., and T. Kirby. 1976. Comprehensive Occupational Therapy Evaluation (COTE). *American Journal of Occupational Therapy,* 30(2): 94–100.

Bruce, M. A., and B. Borg. 1993. *Psychosocial Occupational Therapy: Frames of Reference for Intervention.* 2d ed. Thorofare, NJ: Slack.

Cara, E., and A. MacRae. 1998. *Psychosocial Occupational Therapy in Clinical Practice.* Albany: Delmar Publishers.

Christiansen, C., and C. Baum. eds. 1997. *Occupational Therapy: Enabling Function and Well-Being.* 2d ed. Thorofare, NJ: Slack.

Cole, M. B. 1998. *Group Dynamics in Occupational Therapy: The Theoretical Basis and Practice Application of Group Treatment.* 2d. ed. Thorofare, NJ: Slack.

Cottrell, R. P. F. 1993. *Psychosocial Occupational Therapy: Proactive Approaches.* Bethesda, MD: American Occupational Therapy Association.

Covey, S. R., A. R. Merrill, and R. R. Merrill. 1994. *First Things First.* New York: Simon and Schuster.

Cynkin, S., and A. M. Robinson. 1990. *Occupational Therapy and Activities Health: Toward Health Through Activities.* Boston: Little, Brown.

Davis, C. M. 1998. *Patient Practioner Interaction: An Experiential Manual for Developing the Art of Health Care* 3d ed. Thorofare, NJ: Slack.

Denton, P. L. 1987. *Psychiatric Occupational Therapy: A Workbook of Practical Skills.* Boston: Little, Brown.

Dynes, R. 1993. *Creative Games in Group Work.* Bichester, England: Winslow Press.

Earhart, C. A., C. K. Allen, and T. Blue. 1993. *Allen Diagnostic Manual: Instruction Manual.* Available from Allen Conferences, Inc., Ormond Beach, FL.

Early, M. B. 2000. *Mental Health Concepts and Techniques for the Occupational Therapy Assistant.* 3d ed. Philadelphia: Lippincott Williams & Wilkins.

Hemphill-Pearson, B. J. ed. 1999. *Assessments in Occupational Therapy Mental Health.* Thorofare, NJ: Slack.

Howe, M. C., and S. L. Schwartzberg. 1995. *A Functional Approach to Group Work in Occupational Therapy.* Philadelphia: J. B. Lippincott.

Korb-Khalsa, K. L., S. D. Azok, and E. A. Leutenberg. 1995. *S.E.A.L. + Plus.* Beechwood, OH: Wellness Reproductions.

McCarthy, K. 1993. *Activities of Daily Living: A Manual of Group Activities and Written Exercises.* Framingham, MA: Therapro.

Mosey, A. C. 1986. *Psychosocial Components of Occupational Therapy.* New York: Raven Press.

Neidstadt, M. E., and E. B. Crepeau. eds. 1998. *Willard and Spackman's Occupational Therapy.* 9th ed. Philadelphia: J. B. Lippincott.

Purtillo, R., and A. Haddad. 1996. *Health Professional and Patient Interaction.* 5th ed. Philadelphia: W. B. Saunders.

Rider, B. B., and S. J. Rider. 1999. *The Book of Activity Cards for Mental Health.* Kalamazo, MI: Authors.

Ross, M. 1997. *Integrative Group Therapy: Mobilizing Coping Abilities with the Five-Stage Group.* Bethesda, MD: American Occupational Therapy Association.

Ryan, S. E. 1995b. In *The Combined Volume: Practice Issues in Occupational Therapy: Intraprofessional Team Building.* Thorofare, NJ: Slack.

Stein, F., and S. K. Cutler. 1998. *Psychosocial Occupational Therapy: A Holistic Approach.* San Diego: Singular Publishing Group.

Thomson, L. K. 1992. *Kohlman Evaluation of Living Skills.* Bethesda, MD: American Occupational Therapy Association.

Tubesing, N. L., and D. A. Tubesing. 1994. *Structured Exercises in Stress Management: A Handbook for Trainers, Educators, and Group Leaders.* Vol. 1. Duluth, MN: Whole Person Associates.

University of Missouri. 1989. *Interference: A Simulation of the Symptoms, Systems, and Side Effects of Mental Illness.* Missouri: Author.

Williams, H. D., and J. Bloomer. 1987. *Bay Area Functional Performance Evaluation (BaFPE).* 2d ed. Pequannock, NJ: Maddak.

Competencies in Adult Physical Rehabilitation Practice

CHAPTER FIVE CONTENTS

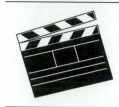

Exercise 76

"Each person's map of the world is as unique as their thumbprint."

MILTON ERICKSON

OBSERVATION SKILLS

OBJECTIVES

✔ Discuss the role of observation in the occupational therapy process
✔ Document specific observations of diagnoses encountered in a physical rehabilitation setting
✔ Record specific and detailed observations on a client seen in a physical rehabilitation setting

DESCRIPTION

Observation is an important part of the evaluation and treatment process of clients in all settings, including a physical rehabilitation one. Through both formal and informal observation, much information can be learned about a client. Once your eye is trained to pick up on the subtleties of a client's appearance, communication, and behavior, you will be surprised by the wealth of information that you had simply not been trained to attend to earlier. Observation, though, always needs to be substantiated and validated by collecting further data from your client and your client's family and/or caregivers. Observation is one of the tools used to complete the total picture of a client's functioning level and performance skills.

 PREPARATION

Suggested Readings

Early (1998)
Pedretti (1996)
Trombly (1995)

Study Questions

1. In meeting or approaching a client for the first time, what observations would be most important?

2. Describe techniques that are useful in determining asymmetries.

3. Describe the typical posture of an adult with hemiplegia.

4. Describe the visual presentation of an associated reaction.

5. Describe observations an occupational therapy (OT) practitioner might make for a client with the following conditions:
    a. Rheumatoid arthritis

    b. Cerebral vascular disease

     c. Traumatic brain injury

     d. Spinal cord injury

     e. Orthopedic injuries

     f. Cancer

     g. Pulmonary disease

     h. Chronic pain

     i. Degenerative diseases

     j. Burns

6. How is observation used during treatment?

7. How is observation used in the evaluation or reevaluation phase of treatment?

8. Differentiate between formal and informal observation.

9. Describe methods for validating one's observations of a client, including other people and instruments that might be used.

ACTIVITY
Materials

Videotape of a person or client who has a diagnosis that is often seen in a physical disabilities setting.

Instructions

1a. Fill in the following observation form for a person you observed or a video of a person you watched.

> *Appearance:* Pick a position and describe the client from head to toe. This is like a snapshot. Be sure to note differences in right or left side when indicated.

Position of person: ☐ Standing   ☐ Sitting   ☐ Lying   ☐ Kneeling

☐ Other _____

Position of head: _____

Description of hair: _____

Description of eyes: _____

Description/position of mouth: _____

Any other facial features, scars, sores, saliva, nasal discharge, food, condition of teeth,

facial hair, make-up jewelry, etc.: _____

Description and position of:

    Shoulders: _____

    Elbows: _____

    Wrists: _____

    Hands: _____

    Trunk: _____

    Hips: _____

    Knees: _____

    Feet: _____

Description of clothing: _____

Description of any splints, braces, or other equipment: _____

_____

Description of wounds, scars, dirt, etc.: _____

Description of wheelchair or other ambulatory devices: _____

> *Communication:* Describe how the client communicates. Include all forms of communication.

Method of communication used most frequently: ☐ Verbal   ☐ Nonverbal

Tone of voice: _____

Ability to understand: _____

Initiation of conversation: _____

Unusual sounds:_____

Give a description of what the person says, to whom, and in what context: _____

_____

_____

_____

Describe gestures used, to whom, and in what context:_____

_____

_____

_____

Describe sign language used, to whom, and in what context: _____

_____

Other comments or communication: _____

_____

> **Emotion:**   *Describe the emotional response of the client, how it is displayed and in what context. Note the changes experienced during the session. Infer emotional state associated with the observed behavior.*

BEHAVIOR	DESCRIBE SITUATION INVOLVED	RELATED EMOTIONAL STATE

Overall mood of session: _____

> **Response to Intervention:**   *Describe how the client responded to the intervention, activity, or occupation used. It may not be possible to include all of the components you are observing so focus on just one activity.*

Task: _____

Attended to task _____ minutes/seconds at a time (circle one).

Describe use of hands—how are they being used:

Right hand: _____

_____

Left hand: _____

_____

Ability/quality of performance: How successfully was the task accomplished?

_____

_____

_____

_____

_____

_____

Assistance required: _____

_____

Describe gross motor movements: position of body, use of all extremities together:

_____

_____

_____

_____

Vestibular system: Describe movement and responses of the person: _____

_____

_____

_____

Social Involvement: *Describe how the client relates to peers.*

Peers present: _____

Describe environment/situation: _____

_____

Describe interaction(s): _____

_____

Describe response of client to peers and peers to client: _____

_____

Overall impression of social skills: _____

> ***Authority Involvement:*** *Describe how the client relates to therapists, staff members, and student practioners.*

Engaged in directed activity: _____

_____

Redirection given and response from client: _____

_____

_____

Content of conversation areas: _____

_____

Motivational techniques employed and response from client: _____

_____

_____

Acceptance of praise: _____

_____

Overall impression of relationship to authority: _____

_____

1b. Following this activity, discuss your observations as a class. Fill in the information you may have missed. List your strengths and areas of concern regarding obtaining clinical observations, as well as your plan to improve your skills.

STRENGTHS	AREAS OF CONCERN

IMPROVEMENT PLAN:

FOLLOW-UP

✔ Complete the Application of Competencies at the end of this chapter.

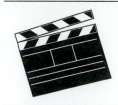

"You grow up the day you have the first real laugh-at yourself."

ETHEL BARRYMORE

STANDARDIZED ASSESSMENTS

OBJECTIVES

✔ Describe the relationship of hand function to activities of daily living, work, and leisure
✔ Administer standardized tests according to standard procedures
✔ Solicit peer and instructor critique of hand function assessment performance

DESCRIPTION

This exercise will familiarize you with some of the assessments that are used in a physical rehabilitation setting. In evaluating a client, a variety of assessments need to be given to obtain an accurate picture of that client's strengths and areas of concern. Many of the component-based assessments that are used in a physical rehabilitation setting such as sensation, range of motion, and manual muscle testing, are covered later in this chapter. This exercise concentrates on the standardized assessment of hand function and gives you ample opportunity to learn to administer a variety of instruments. Hand function is just one of the important areas that influence an individual's performance in the areas of activities of daily living, work, and leisure. To determine a cleint's interests, values, and notes, assessments other than component-based assessments will also need to be given.

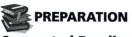

PREPARATION

Suggested Readings

Pedretti (1996)

Study Questions

1. Describe clinical reasoning and its use in the evaluation process.

2. What is the difference between a standardized test and a nonstandardized test?

3. Detail the impact the following contexts have on a client's performance:
   a. Temporal

   b. Environmental

4. Describe the role and importance of the following types of assessments when used in a physical rehabilitation setting:
   a. Medical records

   b. Interview

    c. Observation

    d. Standardized tests

    e. Nonstandardized tests

5. List the knowledge and skills an occupational therapy practitioner needs to administer standardized tests.

6. Why is there a need for standardized testing in occupational therapy?

7. From the readings as well as your own understanding, describe the role of one's hands in functioning as a tool in the following areas:
    a. Activities of daily living

    b. Work

    c. Leisure

8. Outline the following measures of hand function/dysfunction:
    a. Observation and topographical

    b. Physical (soft tissue, edema, sensibility)

    c. Grip and pinch strength

    d. Functional

9. Describe the incidence of, and the work-related risk factors associated with, cumulative trauma disorders.

10. How do you think a client's family and/or caregiver might contribute to the evaluation process?

ACTIVITY

Materials

Stopwatches, Minnesota Rate of Manipulation Test (University of Minnesota Employment Stabilization Research Institute, 1933), Pennsylvania BiManual Test (American Guidance Service, 1969), Jebsen Hand Function Test (Jebsen, Taylor, Trieschmann, Trotter, and Howard, 1969), Purdue Pegboard Test (Tiffin, 1960), Nine Hole Peg Test (Mathiowetz, Weber, Kashman, and Volland, 1985), Motor Free Visual Perception Test (Colarusso, Hammill and Merceir, 1995), and Hand Volumeter Test (Ramsammy & Brand, n.d.).

Instructions

1. Familiarize yourself with the following standardized tests. Practice giving the tests to a partner, recording the results. Compare your results to norms when they are available. Include in the comment section any aspects of your performance that were noteworthy or parts of the assessments that you need reminders to administer correctly. Discuss as a class the similarities and differences among classmates' scores.

    a. Purdue Peg Board Test (Tiffin, 1960)

	FIRST TRIAL	SECOND TRIAL	NORMS
Right hand			
Left hand			
Both hands			
Assembly			
Comments:			

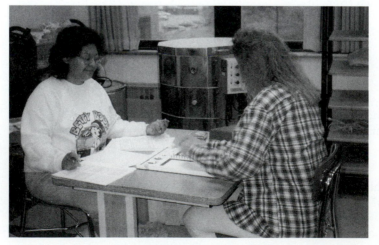

Fig. 5-1 Administering the Purdue Pegboard Test.

Photo courtesy of Renee Davis and Michelle Moore.

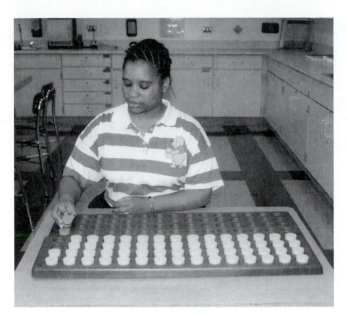

Fig. 5-2 Performing the Minnesota Rate of Manipulation Test.
Photo courtesy of Tiffany Walker.

b. Minnesota Rate of Manipulation Test (University of Minnesota Employment Stabilization Research Institute, 1933)

	TRIAL 1	TRIAL 2	NORMS
The placing test			
The one-hand turning and placing test			
The two-handed turning and placing test			
Comments:			

c. Pennsylvania BiManual Test (American Guidance Service, 1969)

	SCORE	NORMS
Right hand		
Left hand		
Comments:		

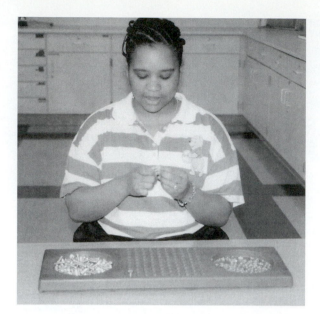

Fig. 5-3 Pennsylvania BiManual Test assembly of nuts and bolts. *Photosy of Tiffany Walker.*

d. Nine Hole Peg Test (Mathiowetz, Weber, Kashman, and Volland, 1985)

	SCORE	NORMS
Assembly		
Disassembly		
Comments:		

e. Jebson Hand Function Test (Jebsen, Taylor, Trieschmann, Trotter, and Howard, 1969)

	RIGHT	LEFT	NORMS
Writing			
Card turning			
Small common objects			
Simulated feeding			
Checkers			
Large light objects			
Large heavy objects			
Comments:			

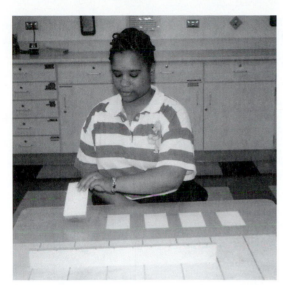

Fig. 5-4 Jebsen Hand Function Test card turning.
Photosy of Tiffany Walker.

f. Hand Volumeter Test (Ramsammy and Brand, n.d.)

Right hand	Amount of water displaced:
Left hand	Amount of water displaced:
Comments:	

g. Motor Free Visual Perception Test (Colarusso, Hammill, and Merceir, 1995)

AREA	CORRECT RESPONSES	INCORRECT RESPONSES	NORMS
Spatial relations			
Visual discrimination			
Figure-ground			
Visual closure			
Visual memory			
Comments:			

2. Administer one test that you have already practiced to a classmate, this time with another classmate or instructor observing and recording your performance in the following areas:

Identify which test you have selected: _____

	OUTSTANDING	SATISFACTORY	NEEDS IMPROVEMENT
Arranged test materials appropriately			
Instructions given accurately			
Correct demonstrations given			
Correct use of stopwatch			
Score recorded appropriately on form			
Summary of your performance:			

3. Continue to practice administering the above-mentioned tests. Have a peer observer or instructor rate your performance on the following Competency Checklist.

COMPETENCY CHECKLIST

Put a plus sign in the box if performed correctly, and a minus sign if done incorrectly. The numbers on the chart correspond to the following items:

1. Arranged test materials appropriately
2. Instructions given accurately
3. Correct demonstrations given
4. Correct use of stopwatch
5. Score recorded appropriately on form

TEST ADMINISTERED	1	2	3	4	5

FOLLOW-UP

✔ Complete the Application of Competencies at the end of this chapter.
✔ Complete a Therapeutic Use of Self Analysis found in Appendix B on your performance of standardized testing.

MUSCLE TESTING

Exercise 78

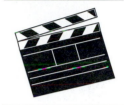

OBJECTIVES

✔ Identify instruments used to test muscle strength
✔ Identify muscle grades and assessment procedures for muscle testing
✔ Perform a manual muscle test

DESCRIPTION

This exercise will assist you in learning how to assess muscle strength. You may work with clients who have muscle weaknesses for a variety of reasons. To design an effective intervention plan and document outcomes, you will need to establish a baseline of your client's strength. At times your muscle testing will take a functional approach, and you will complete a functional muscle strength test. At other times you will complete a more formal and thorough assessment of manual muscle testing. Although different approaches and philosophies are associated with functional and manual muscle testing, the procedure and sequence followed in doing so are similar. As part of assessing muscle strength, you will also look at grasp and pinch performance.

"Worry never robs tomorrow of its sorrow, it only zaps today of its strength."

A.J. CRONIN

PREPARATION

Suggesting Readings

Kendall, McCreary, and Provance (1993)
Pedretti (1996)

Study Questions

1. List three general classifications of physical dysfunction in which muscle weakness is a primary symptom.

2. Differentiate between functional muscle testing and manual muscle testing.

3. List the purpose of manual muscle testing and functional muscle testing.

4. What criteria are used to determine muscle grades?

5. List and describe the muscle testing grades that are commonly used (include number grade and word or letter grade).

6. Given F+ muscle strength and low endurance, in what kind of activities can a client be expected to participate?

7. List three purposes for assessing muscle strength.

8. Define endurance and discuss its correlation with muscle strength.

9. Define what is meant by substitution.

10. Outline the procedural steps in performing a manual muscle test and a functional muscle test.

11. Outline the suggested sequence for positioning your client to complete a manual muscle test.

12. Describe the position of the upper extremity in testing strength using the dynamometer.

13. Draw a picture that describes the functional muscle testing position used in each of the following movements:
    a. Scapular evaluation

    b. Shoulder flexion

    c. Elbow flexion

    d. Elbow extension

    e. Wrist flexion

    f. Wrist extension

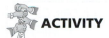
ACTIVITY

Materials

Dynamometer, pinch meter

Instructions

1. Following demonstrations by your instructor, measure and record the following grasp and pinch strengths on your partner, using the dynamometer and pinch meter, respectively. Record your results and compare them with standard norms.

	LEFT	NORM	RIGHT	NORM
Grip				
Lateral pinch				
Tip pinch				
3-jaw				

2. Perform a functional muscle test on your partner for the movements recorded below. Have your partner demonstrate a different muscle grade each time and practice scoring it correctly.

MOVEMENT	SCORE	CORRECT	INCORRECT
Scapular elevation			
Scapular abduction			
Scapular adduction			
Scapular depression			
Shoulder flexion			
Shoulder extension			
Shoulder abduction			
Shoulder external rotation			
Shoulder internal rotation			
Elbow flexion			
Elbow extension			
Forearm supination			
Forearm pronation			
Wrist flexion			

MOVEMENT	SCORE	CORRECT	INCORRECT
Finger metacarpo-phalangeal (MP) flexion and inter-phalangeal (IP) extension			
Finger MP extension			
Finger abduction			
Finger adduction			
Thumb MP and IP flexion			
Thumb palmar abduction			
Opposition of thumb to fifth finger			
Thumb MP and IP extension			

3. Observe a demonstration of a manual muscle test. Discuss and record the subjective aspects of this test.

4. Perform a manual muscle test by measuring and recording your partner's muscle strength for the movements listed in the following chart. Learn the procedure as your instructor demonstrates and/or from pictures in a book. Use the chart to record comments you receive on the accuracy of your testing position, hand placement, resistance given, and scoring while performing the test.

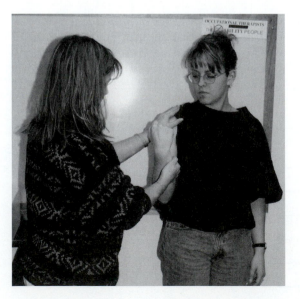

Fig. 5-5 Assessing muscle strength.
Photo courtesy of Jessica Johantges and Christie Tuttle.

	TESTING POSITION	HAND PLACEMENT	RESISTANCE GIVEN	SCORE RECORDED
SUPINE				
Scapula abduction upward rotation				
Shoulder horizontal adduction				
Shoulder adduction				
SIDELYING				
Shoulder flexion				
Shoulder extension				
PRONE				
Scapula depression				
Scapula adduction				
Scapula abduction				
Shoulder extension				
Shoulder external rotation				
Shoulder internal rotation				
Shoulder horizontal abduction				
Elbow extension				
SITTING				
Scapula elevation				
Shoulder flexion				
Shoulder abduction				
Elbow flexion				
Wrist				
Finger				
Thumb				

FOLLOW-UP

✔ Complete the Application of Competencies at the end of this chapter.

Exercise 79

"Internal balance is health and internal unbalance is sickness."

CLARENCE COOK LITTLE

VITAL SIGNS

OBJECTIVES

✔ Describe and perform vital signs procedures
✔ Discuss the relationship between cardiopulmonary function and activity
✔ Identify signs of cardiopulmonary distress

DESCRIPTION

This exercise will help you to learn how to take a client's vital signs. Vital signs are an indication of a client's physiological status and need to be monitored in working with a client with cardiopulmonary complications. One's heart rate, respiratory rate, and blood pressure—three of the most commonly monitored vital signs—change in response to one's age, health, and participation in activity. You will need to be knowledgeable about your client's vital signs at rest and monitor them as you gauge their response to your therapeutic intervention. You will also need to be able to identify signs of cardiopulmonary distress and know the appropriate safety procedures to follow.

 PREPARATION

Suggested Readings

Neidstadt and Crepeau (1998)
Pedretti (1996)
Pierson (1999)
Rothstein, Roy, and Wolf (1998)

Study Questions

1. Define the following terms:

   a. Vital signs

   b. Pulse

   c. Respiratory rate

   d. Blood pressure

   e. Tachycardia

   f. Bradycardia

    g. Hypotension

    h. Hypertension

    i. Dyspnea

    j. Arrhythmia

    k. Bradypnea

2. Why, when, and with whom it is important for an occupational therapy practitioner to monitor vital signs?

3. List the location of the pulse measurement sites that can be located on the body.

4. Describe the procedure necessary to measure pulse.

5. List words used to describe pulse.

6. Identify the normal adult pulse rate and blood pressure ranges.

7. Describe the procedure necessary to measure blood pressure by auscultation.

8. Describe the procedure necessary to measure respiration and give the normal adult respiration range.

9. Describe how pulse, blood pressure, and respiration are affected by physical activity:

   a. Pulse

   b. Blood pressure

   c. Respiration

10. Locate and cite the source and page number containing a table with established norms for pulse, blood pressure, and respiration rate.

11. Describe the signs of cardiopulmonary distress.

12. Describe the procedure to follow when a client has abnormal cardiopulmonary responses and when he or she is in acute cardiopulmonary distress.

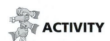 **ACTIVITY**

Materials

Blood pressure cuffs and stethoscopes.

Instructions

1. Following a demonstration from your instructor, measure your partner's pulse, blood pressure, and respiration rate in the following conditions and record the results below. Compare your results with established norms. Solicit feedback from your instructor about your technique, accuracy, and recording. Place that in the space provided.

RECORD OF VITAL SIGNS					
VITAL SIGNS	INITIAL READING AT REST	NORM	AFTER A TEN-MINUTE WALK	NORM	10 MINUTES AFTER WALK
Pulse					
Blood pressure					
Respiration					

FEEDBACK ON TECHNIQUE			
VITAL SIGN	TECHNIQUE	ACCURACY	RECORDING
Pulse			
Blood pressure			
Respiration			

2. Obtain the resting rates of blood pressure, pulse, and respiration rates of family members and friends. Obtain the data from individuals with ages throughout the life span. Record your information below and compare the results with established norms. Discuss your findings with your classmates.

SUBJECT	AGE	BLOOD PRESSURE		PULSE		RESPIRATION	
		READING	NORM	READING	NORM	RESPIRATION	NORM

FOLLOW-UP

✔ Complete the Application of Competencies at the end of this chapter.

SENSORY ASSESSMENT AND REEDUCATION

Exercise 80

OBJECTIVES

✔ Identify assessment tools useful in identifying sensory deficits
✔ Demonstrate appropriate procedures to use in identifying sensory deficits
✔ Select treatment techniques for diminishing the effects of sensory deficits

DESCRIPTION

This exercise will familiarize you with the assessment and intervention procedures that are used with individuals who have sensory deficits. Sensation plays a role in one's state of alertness. Sensation also plays an important precursory role for movement. A person's motor performance depends on both feedback and feedforward mechanisms. Evaluating and treating sensory deficits will be an integral role you will play as you work with clients having sensory deficits. Because of the nature of the deficits, specific procedures will need to be followed in testing for somatic sensation. Doing so will give you an accurate picture of your client's sensory perception.

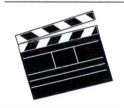

PREPARATION

Suggesting Readings

Pedretti (1996)
Trombly (1995)

"Life is a series of problems; do we want to moan about them or solve them?"

SCOTT PECK

Study Questions

1. List several of the diagnoses that may have sensory loss as a symptom.

2. Why is sensory evaluation necessary and important to occupational therapy?

3. Describe assessments and/or techniques that are used in identifying a client's strengths and areas of concerns in the following areas:
   a. Light touch

   b. Pressure sensation

   c. Thermal sensation

   d. Superficial pain

   e. Olfactory

   f. Gustatory

   g. Position and motion sense

4. Outline the procedural steps in testing for somatic sensation.

5. Describe the following terms related to treatment of sensory dysfunction:
   a. Effect sensation has on movement

   b. Compensatory technique

   c. Remedial treatment

    d. Treatment of hypersensitivity

    e. Compensatory treatment

6.   Describe the following terms as they relate to remedial treatment:
    a. Moving touch

    b. Constant touch

    c. Pressure

    d. Touch localization

    e. Tactile agnosia

    f. Sensory retraining

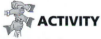 **ACTIVITY**

Materials

Safety pin, key, coins, cotton balls, cotton swabs, blindfolds; salt, sugar, lemon, vinegar; extracts of coffee, almond, chocolate, lemon, and peppermint; Case Study 36 located at the end of this chapter.

Instructions

1.   Observe a video or a demonstration of sensory testing and note the following:
    a. How is the procedure explained to the client?

    b. How is the test set up? Include how the client's vision is occluded.

    c. What deficits did you observe?

2. After the demonstration, perform the tests of light touch, deep touch, pain, stereognosis, proprioception on your partner and record your information on the following forms.

DEPARTMENT OF OCCUPATIONAL THERAPY REPORT
UPPER EXTREMITY GROSS SENSORY EVALUATION

Patient Name: _____   UH # _____

Diagnosis: _____   Date of Onset: _____

I. Sharp/Dull Discrimination

☐ Intact   ▨ Impaired   ■ Absent

Comments _____

II. Hot/Cold

☐ Intact   ▨ Impaired   ■ Absent

Comments _____

(continues)

Used with permission from Spinal Cord Injury: A Treatment Guide for Occupational Therapists. Occupational Therapy Department, Spinal Injuries Service, Ranchos Los Amigos Hospital, Downey, CA.

III. Light Touch

☐ Intact ▨ Impaired ■ Absent

Comments _____

IV. Position Sense

Int. (intact) Imp. (impaired) Abs. (Absent)

	Left			Right		
	Int.	Imp.	Abs.	Int.	Imp.	Abs.
Fingers (index, middle)						
Fingers (ring, little)						
Thumb						
Wrist						
Forearm Rotation						
Elbow						
Shoulder						

Comments _____

Comments _____

V. Stereognosis/Object Recognition

Int. (intact) Imp. (impaired) Abs. (Absent)

	Int.	Imp.	Abs.
right			
left			

_____ out of _____ objects identified correctly

_____   _____
Therapist's Signature   Date

Source: Illustrations reprinted with permission from: Spinal Cord Injury: A Treatment Guide for Occupational Therapists. Occupational Therapy Department, Spinal Injuries Service, Rancho Los Amigos Hospital, Downey, CA. Thorofare, NJ: Charles B. Slack, Inc; 1974.

Taken from: Daniel, M.S., Strickland, L.R. (1992). Occupational therapy protocol management in Adult Physical Dysfunction (gaithersburg MD: Aspen Publishers). Used with permission

Used with permission from Spinal Cord Injury: A Treatment Guide for Occupational Therapists. Occupational Therapy Department, Spinal Injuries Service, Ranchos Los Amigos Hospital, Downey, CA.

3. Test and record your partner's olfactory and gustatory sensations. Make a similar rating scale for gustation.

Key: + = Can detect and identify odor

− = Can detect odor, cannot identify odor

O = Cannot detect or identify odor

S = Can detect same odors, both nostrils

D = Can detect different odors, both nostrils

4. Work with a partner on the case you have been assigned. Describe treatment techniques you may implement for the client's sensory loss indicated as well as a rationale for each technique. Describe treatment precautions that might be necessary for a person with this deficit. Share this with your class when completed.

SENSORY DEFICIT	TREATMENT TECHNIQUE	RATIONALE	PRECAUTIONS

5. Practice administrating a variety of sensory tests with a partner who has decided ahead of time what deficits he or she will have. Find and record those deficits accurately. Solicit feedback from your partner, instructor, or a peer observer on your mastery of the procedural skills listed below.

TEST ADMINISTERED	EXPLAINED PROCEDURE TO CLIENT	OCCLUDED VISION ACCURATELY	CORRECTLY TESTED ALL DERMATOMES	RECORDED RESPONSE ON FORM

6. Practice several sensory reeducation techniques with a partner and determine the therapeutic implications for each. Record this information, along with your reaction.

TECHNIQUE	TREATMENT IMPLICATION	REACTION

FOLLOW-UP

✔ Complete the Application of Competencies at the end of this chapter.

TRANSFERS AND POSITIONING

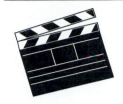

OBJECTIVES

✔ Identify proper equipment needed for both the client and the therapist to perform a safe transfer

✔ Describe correct bed positioning and maneuvering techniques for a client with hemiplegia

✔ Demonstrate a wheelchair standing pivot and sliding board transfer to various surfaces

"I'm looking forward to looking back on all this."

SANDRA KNELL

DESCRIPTION

Transfers allow a client to move from one position or surface to another. As an occupational therapy practitioner you may be assisting or supervising such a transfer, allowing the client to be as independent as possible. It is important that both you and the client remain safe in the process. Several pieces of equipment may need to be used to do so. Positioning of the client is critical after the transfer is completed. For individuals with neurological impairment, proper positioning will facilitate function and help to prevent further deformities. It is important to consider positioning at the same time you learn transfers so that you can facilitate your client's functioning and participation in appropriate occupational endeavors.

PREPARATION

Suggested Readings

Pedretti (1996)
Pierson (1999)
Trombly (1995)

Study Questions

1. List the basic principles of body mechanics.

2. Name several factors that could affect a client's ability to learn how to transfer or benefit from transfer training.

3. List and briefly describe the types of transfers.

4. Answer these questions about sliding board transfers:

    a. For whom are sliding board transfers best suited?

    b. What physical attributes are required of the client to do a sliding board transfer?

5. What piece of equipment may need to be used at the beginning of transfer training? When during the transfer training can it be eliminated?

6. What equipment is needed to ensure the safety of the therapist as well as the client?

7. What guidelines should the practitioner consider before attempting to have the client transfer?

8. Describe the steps in a standing pivot transfer.

9. What precautions must be considered in positioning a client with a
   a. Neurological impairment?

   b. Spinal cord injury?

10. When positioning a client who has had a cerebral vascular accident, describe how you would properly place the involved arm for the following resting positions:
    a. Lying on affected side

    b. Lying on unaffected side

    c. Lying on back

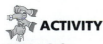 **ACTIVITY**

Materials

Mat table, commode, bath bench, hospital bed, positioning pillows, transfer board, wheelchair, transfer belt.

Instructions

1. Review the principles of body mechanics to ensure your safety as well as the safety of your client. Refer to Chapter Three (Exercise 41, Positioning and Handling) in this book if you have not already done so.

2. With your class, discuss conditions that interfere with transfers. The first one has been done for you.

IDENTIFY CONDITION	HOW IT INTERFERES WITH TRANSFERRING	INTERVENTION TECHNIQUES
Client is fearful of falling	Client may grab therapist's neck, move quickly, refuse to move, or verbally call out	Move slowly; talk client through transfer; complete the transfer in stages; reassure client; allow client to control movement as much as possible

3. Position a manikin or a partner with right- or left-sided hemiplegia in a bed. Have a peer and/or your instructor check your technique. Record how you correctly placed the upper extremities, lower extremities, and the positioning pillows for each position listed below.

POSITION	CORRECT UE PLACEMENT	CORRECT LE PLACEMENT	CORRECT PLACEMENT OF PILLOWS
On affected side			
On unaffected side			
Supine			

4. Describe and demonstrate a method for moving a client up in bed, down in bed, rolling to the side, and coming to a sitting position for the following client conditions.

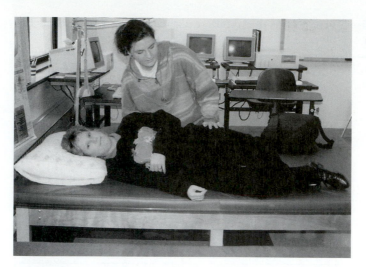

Fig. 5-6 Sidelying positioning in progress.

Photo courtesy of Charlene Kennedy and Gina Knab.

	CLIENT CONDITION			
	HEMIPLEGIA	QUADRIPLEGIA	PARAPLEGIA	OTHER
Moving up in bed				
Moving down in bed				
Rolling side to side				
Coming to a sitting position				

5. Watch your instructor perform standing pivot and sliding board transfers from a wheelchair to various surfaces as indicated on the following page. Check the boxes as you note the components of the transfer being performed. After the demonstration, perform these same transfers with a partner, checking your progress as you complete each skill.

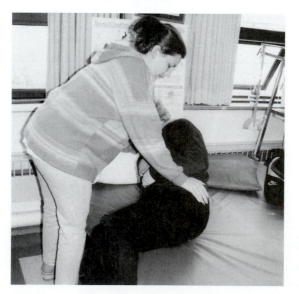

Fig. 5-7 Physical assistance provided in coming to sitting.

Photo courtesy of Gina Knab.

| COMPONENTS OF THE TRANSFER | INSTRUCTOR | | | | | | STUDENT | | | | | |
| | STANDING PIVOT | | SLIDING BOARD | | | | STANDING PIVOT | | SLIDING BOARD | | | |
	Mat	Commode	Bath Bench	Mat	Commode	Bath Bench	Mat	Commode	Bath Bench	Mat	Commode	Bath Bench
Correct placement of wheelchair												
Correct direction of transfer												
Handled wheelchair appropriately												
Proper application of transfer belt												
Correct instructions given to patient												
Proper placement of practioner's body												
Correct body mechanics used												
Proper speed in moving patient from chair to mat												
Correct placement of sliding board if used												
Comments:												

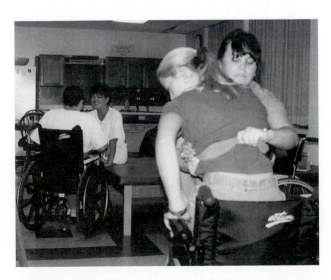

Fig. 5-8 Transfer training.

Photo courtesy of Melissa Brashear, Becky Bolin, and Anna Sharpsheir.

6. Continue practicing your transfer techniques to all surfaces available at your facility (e.g., car, bed, sofa). Document your progress below.

FOLLOW-UP

✔ Complete the Application of Competencies at the end of this chapter.

Exercise 82

"The great dividing line between success and failure can be expressed in five words: I did not have time."

ANONYMOUS

RANGE OF MOTION

OBJECTIVES

✔ Differentiate between active and passive range of motion
✔ Demonstrate correct placement of and reading from a goniometer in measuring joints of the upper body
✔ Describe functional limitations that may occur as a result of limited range of motion

DESCRIPTION

As an occupational therapy practitioner, you will measure range of motion informally at times and at other times obtain formal measurements. Measurement of range of motion may be completed as an assessment. In doing so, proficient use of a goniometer is a necessity. Unfortunately, it is easy to and rather common to make errors. You will need to guard against this. Repeated practice of obtaining measurements will help to avoid mistakes. Additionally, it is important that you thoroughly understand all the motions through which each joint passes so that you can use range of motion activities in either an active or a passive manner as part of intervention.

 PREPARATION

Suggested Readings

Daniels and Worthington (1986)
Pedretti (1996)
Trombly (1995)

Study Questions

1. Define range of motion (ROM).

2. Describe what is meant by active range of motion.

3. Describe passive range of motion.

4. What is a goniometer?

5. Using the 180° system, what row of figures do you read on the goniometer in measuring the elbow? The shoulder?

6. On what does glenohumeral joint motion depend?

7. Why is it important to assess scapula mobility?

8. List several causes of joint limitation.

9. What is the importance of looking at functional activities in doing ROM?

10. What can be done if a particular joint has a permanent ROM limitation?

11. List several purposes of completing a ROM assessment.

12. Describe the general procedures for evaluating range of motion.

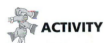

ACTIVITY

Materials

Goniometers (large and small) 180°, 360°; finger

Instructions

1. Discuss as a class the principles and precautions to use in measuring ROM and in using ROM as a treatment technique. Record your notes below.

PRINCIPLES	PRECAUTIONS

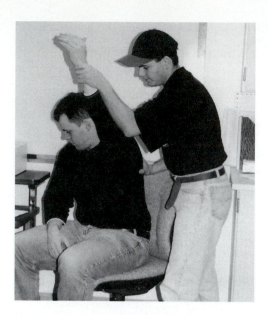

Fig. 5-9   Practicing the functional ROM check.

Photo courtesy of Rick Ernst and Jason Sueberling.

2. Perform an upper extremity functional ROM screening (Early, 1998) check by having your partner name ROM movements as you demonstrate how you would complete the motion. Place a check mark in the column below as you complete the movement successfully. Reverse roles and check off your partner's performance. Additionally, have your partner silently perform a movement as you identify the movement by name. The extra boxes give you ample room to practice this skill.

MOVEMENT	MOVEMENT PERFORMED			MOVEMENT IDENTIFIED		
Trunk forward ✓ and **/**						
Trunk lateral ✓						
Shoulder ✓ and **/**						
Shoulder external rotation						
Shoulder internal rotation						
Shoulder abduction						
Pronation and supination						
Elbow ✓ and **/**						
Finger ✓ and **/**						
Thumb opposition						
Wrist ✓ and **/**						
Wrist radial and ulnar deviation						

3. Using your goniometers, measure and record the following movements on your partner. Use all three types (180°, 360°, and finger) and both sizes (small and large) in taking the measurements. You may use a textbook for pictorial guidelines. Record the typical range and then check to see whether your partner's measurements are within the range specified. If measurements are not in the specified range, check your accuracy first, then ask your partner whether he or she has a limitation. Continue to practice until technique is mastered.

MOVEMENTS	PARTNER MEASURE					TYPICAL RANGE
SHOULDER						
Flexion						
Extension						
Abduction						
Horizontal adduction						
Horizontal abduction						
Internal rotation						
External rotation						
ELBOW AND FOREARM						
Flexion						
Supination						
Pronation						
WRIST						
Flexion						
Extension						
Radial deviation						
Ulnar deviation						
FINGERS						
Metacarpophalangeal (MP)						
Flexion						
Extension						
Proximal interphalangeal (PIP)						
Flexion						
Extension						
Distal Interphalangeal (DIP)						
Flexion						
Extension						
THUMB						
MP Flexion						
IP Flexion						
Abduction						
Adduction						

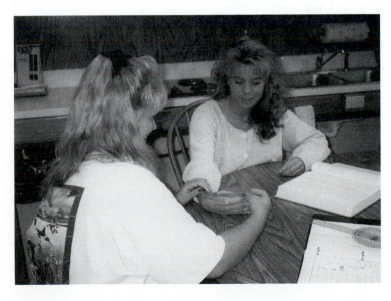

Fig. 5-10
Goniometric measurement of wrist flexion.

Photo courtesy of Lori McBreen and Angie Englert.

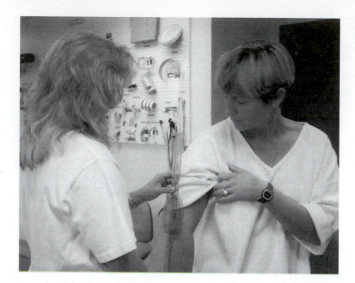

Fig. 5-11 Measuring ROM.

Photo courtesy of Michelle Kenkel.

4. With a partner or small group, determine possible functional limitations a person may have if each of the following measurements was the greatest range that individual could achieve.

JOINT/MOVEMENT	MEASUREMENT	FUNCTIONAL LIMITATION(S)
SHOULDER		
Flexion	90°	
Extension	10°	
Abduction	90°	
Internal rotation	20°	
ELBOW		
Extension	−20°	
Flexion	90°	
WRIST		
Extension	10°	
Flexion	0°	

5. Perform passive ROM on your partner and record comments on the components of your performance listed below. Solicit comments from your partner and instructor.

PERFORMED ALL MOVEMENTS OF JOINT	USED CORRECT HAND PLACEMENT	USED PROPER SPEED OF MOVEMENTS	PROPER PROCEDURE FOLLOWED

🎲 GAME

6. Play an advanced game of Simon Says. Have your instructor or student leader call out positions and ranges in the upper extremity (e.g., Simon says 110° shoulder flexion). Assume the position and range as quickly as possible. Have Simon periodically try to trick you by saying one position and/or range while doing another. Remain in the game as long as you assume the stated position and range. See how long you can stay in the game. Record below any movements that you continually missed.

7. Once your ROM measurement skills are proficient, schedule a time with your instructor for him or her to rate your performance using the following scale.

MOTION MEASURED	Instructed Client in Correct Movement	Proper Placement of Goniometer	Proper Goniometer Reading Taken	Correct Placement of Reading on Form
SHOULDER				
Flexion				
Extension				
Abduction				
Horizontal adduction				
Horizontal abduction				
Internal rotation				
External rotation				
ELBOW AND FOREARM				
Flexion				
Supination				
Pronation				
WRIST				
Flexion				
Extension				
Radial deviation				
Ulnar deviation				
FINGERS				
Metacarpophalangeal (MP)				
Flexion				
Extension				
Proximal interphalangeal (PIP)				
Flexion				
Extension				
Distal interphalangeal (DIP)				
Flexion				
Extension				
THUMB				
MP Flexion				
IP Flexion				
Abduction				
Adduction				

FOLLOW-UP

✔ Complete the Application of Competencies at the end of this chapter.

Exercise 83

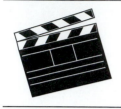

"I cried because I had no shoes until I met a man who had no feet."

PERSIAN SAYING

ACTIVITIES OF DAILY LIVING

OBJECTIVES

✔ Detail adaptive techniques and or devices used to facilitate a client's independence in activities of daily living (ADLs)

✔ Describe how the occupational therapy performance areas relate to a specific ADL task

✔ Provide instruction in the completion of a client's ADL tasks, including standard precautions and safety techniques

DESCRIPTION

This exercise will facilitate your understanding of your role as an occupational therapy (OT) practitioner when working with clients in a physical rehabilitation setting who are gaining independence in their activities of daily living (ADLs). Referrals for clients needing therapeutic intervention for ADLs are frequent in a physical rehabilitation setting. Basic ADLs or self-maintenance tasks are some of the most important skills a client wants and needs to learn in the process of restoring function. Being able to feed and dress oneself is a task taken for granted until the ability to do so is thwarted by injury, illness, or disease. Relearning the basic ADLs often signals an individual's return to function.

PREPARATION

Suggested Readings

AOTA (latest edition)
Christiansen (2000)
Neidstadt and Crepeau (1998)
Pedretti (1996)
Trombly (1995)

Study Questions

1. Define basic ADLs and list terms that are frequently substituted for the same.

2. Describe what is meant by instrumental activities of daily living (IADLs).

3. Identify the performance area as indicated by the uniform terminology document (AOTA, latest edition) that classifies each of the following tasks.

TASK	PERFORMANCE AREA
Transfers	
Grooming	
Telephoning	
Vacuuming	
Shopping	
Preparing meals	
Operating light switches	
Handling medication	
Ability to call 911	

4. Describe the role of the OT practitioner in treating clients with deficits in the performance of ADLs.

5. List and describe factors that must be considered in evaluating and treating a client for deficits in ADL.

6. List possible causes of performance problems that may be observed during ADL tasks.

7. Give a description of each of the terms used to describe performance levels:
   a. Independent

   b. Supervised

   c. Minimal assistance

   d. Moderate assistance

   e. Maximal assistance

   f. Dependent

8. Describe several methods that an occupational therapy practitioner may use to teach improved functioning in ADLs.

9. List a technique or adaptive device that may be used to assist a client with the following performance area deficits in ADLs. The first one is completed for you.

PERFORMANCE AREA	TECHNIQUE OR DEVICE FOR LIMITED ROM AND/OR STRENGTH	TECHNIQUE OR DEVICE FOR PROBLEMS OF INCOORDINATION
Dressing	A reacher may assist in putting on pants.	Velcro may be used to replace buttons.
Feeding and eating		
Grooming		
Oral hygiene		
Functional communication		
Functional mobility		

10. When teaching a person with hemiplegia to dress:

   a. Which arm or leg should be put in the garment first?

   b. Which should be taken out first?

11. Using the latest edition of uniform terminology (AOTA), complete the following abbreviated occupational analysis on an activity of daily living task in which you participate such as taking a shower. To assist you in filling out the analysis, begin by identifying the steps involved in the task. The tactile section for this task has been done for you.

	ABBREVIATED OCCUPATIONAL ANALYSIS				HOW IS THE COMPONENT/ CONCEPT USED IN THIS TASK?	HOW CAN THIS BE ADAPTED?
	DEGREE TO WHICH IT IS USED					
	NONE	MIN.	MOD.	MAX.		
COMPONENTS						
Tactile				X	To feel hair is rinsed of shampoo feel waterspray, feel dirt on skin	Mirror to check for residual soap and dirt, take tub baths, position body under showerhead.

	ABBREVIATED OCCUPATIONAL ANALYSIS				HOW IS THE COMPONENT/ CONTEXT USED IN THIS TASK?	HOW CAN THIS BE ADAPTED?
	DEGREE TO WHICH IT IS USED					
	NONE	MIN.	MOD.	MAX.		
COMPONENTS						

					OCCUPATIONAL ANALYSIS	
	DEGREE TO WHICH IT IS USED				HOW IS THE COMPONENT/ CONTEXT UTILIZED?	HOW CAN THIS BE ADAPTED?
	NONE	MIN.	MOD.	MAX.		
COMPONENTS						

12. Identify assessments appropriate for identifying ADL functioning.

13. Summarize your impression on the personal meaning of self-care. Use Christiansen (2000) as a reference.

Note: In preparation for the following activities, bring the following items to be used in class: pants, skirt, front opening skirt, bra, socks, shoes that tie.

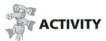 **ACTIVITY**

Materials

Bed, hospital bed, chair, bathroom, bedside commode, washcloth, towel, basin for water, bar of soap, raised commode, razors, deodorant, toothbrush, toothpaste, hairbrush or comb, clothes (pants, pullover shirt, front-opening shirt, bra, socks, shoes that tie); Case Studies 37, 38, 39 and 40 located at the end of this chapter.

Instructions

1. As a class, discuss and record conditions that interfere with successful completion of self-care activities. Include in your discussion ways in which this condition may interfere with functioning as well as precautions and safety techniques that need to be used with a person having this condition. Finally, discuss treatment techniques that may be implemented to increase independence. Fill in the following chart as your discussion progresses. The first item is completed for you.

CONDITION	HOW IT INTERFERES	PRECAUTIONS/SAFETY	TECHNIQUE
Impulsivity	The client may fall while trying to get up on his or her own.	Don't leave the client unattended.	Verbal and physical cueing and repetition of safety techniques.

2. Watch your instructor demonstrate adaptive techniques in dressing for individuals with the diagnosis in the following chart. Practice and then teach a partner, who will role-play a person with the diagnosis listed, how to perform these skills. Write comments on the chart about your performance as you solicit feedback from your peers and instructor.

DRESSING SKILL	CEREBRAL VASCULAR ACCIDENT	PARAPLEGIA	QUADRIPLEGIA	OTHER
Front-opening shirt				
Slipover shirt				
Pants				
Socks				
Shoes				
Bra				

3. Watch your instructor demonstrate adaptive techniques in bathing, toileting, and grooming for the diagnoses in the following chart. Practice and then teach a partner, who will role-play a person with the diagnosis listed, how to perform these skills. Write comments in the chart about your performance as you solicit feedback from your peers and instructor.

BATHING				
	GENERALIZED WEAKNESS	CEREBRAL VASCULAR ACCIDENT	PARAPLEGIA	QUADRIPLEGIA
In bed				
Sitting on side of bed				
In chair at bedside				

In chair at sink				
In the tub				
In shower				

TOILETING				
	GENERALIZED WEAKNESS	CEREBRAL VASCULAR ACCIDENT	PARAPLEGIA	QUADRIPLEGIA
Beside commode				
Raised commode				
Regular commode				

GROOMING				
	GENERALIZED WEAKNESS	CEREBRAL VASCULAR ACCIDENT	PARAPLEGIA	QUADRIPLEGIA
Shaving face				
Shaving legs				
Applying deodorant				
Brushing teeth				
Applying make-up				
Combing hair				

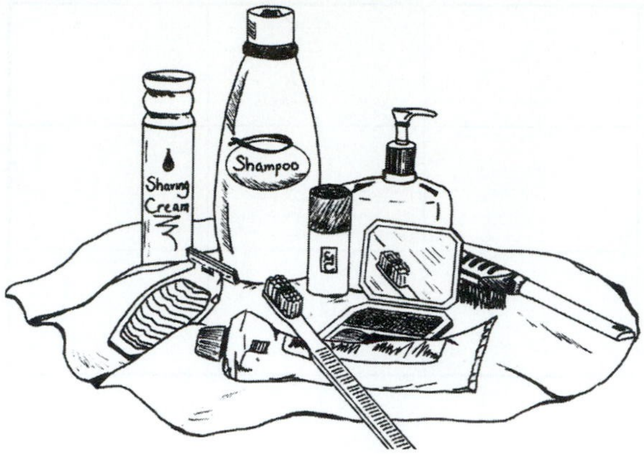

Fig. 5-12

4. Work with a partner on several assigned case studies. Describe how you would begin ADL treatment and how you plan to grade your treatment as the client begins making improvements. An example is given for you.

	PLAN TO GRADE TREATMENT		
DESCRIBE INITIAL SETUP	1	2	3
Patient bathing at the sink in a chair	Patient bathing on a tub seat in bath tub	Client bathing in shower with adaptive equipment	Patient bathing independently in shower

Case No.: _____

	PLAN TO GRADE TREATMENT		
DESCRIBE INITIAL SETUP	1	2	3

Case No.: _____

	PLAN TO GRADE TREATMENT		
DESCRIBE INITIAL SETUP	1	2	3

Case No.: _____

DESCRIBE INITIAL SETUP	PLAN TO GRADE TREATMENT		
	1	2	3

FOLLOW-UP

✔ Complete the Application of Competencies at the end of this chapter.

WHEELCHAIRS

OBJECTIVES

✔ Discuss criteria that are considered in recommending a specific wheelchair for a client
✔ Detail the correct wheelchair measurement procedure needed to complete a wheelchair prescription
✔ Instruct a client in the use of a wheelchair, including component use, safety, and mobility

DESCRIPTION

A wheelchair provides mobility for clients of many different abilities. For some clients it will be a temporary means of mobility; for others it will be a permanent one. In either case it is imperative that as an occupational therapy practitioner you are knowledgeable about all that needs to be taken into consideration in ordering a wheelchair. Your client's goals, needs, lifestyle, and financial means will become factors in the selection process. When recommending a wheelchair, you will likely be a part of a team. With the growing number of types of wheelchairs and wheelchair accessories available, the additional expertise of your fellow team members, such as a rehabilitation supplier, durable medical supplier, and physical therapist will be invaluable. Instructing your client in the proper use, care, and safety procedures in using a wheelchair will help to ensure that the wheelchair offers the maximal services possible to the client.

PREPARATION

Suggesting Readings

Angelo (1997)
Mayall and Desharnais (1990)
Pedretti (1996)
Sacred Heart General Hospital Oregon Rehabilitation Center (1987)
Trefler, Hobson, Taylor, Monochan, & Shaw (1993)
Trombly (1995)

Exercise 84

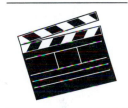

"Of course we make mistakes; it's how we learn."

DAN MILLMAN

Study Questions

1. For what conditions might a client need a wheelchair?

2. What do you need to know about the client's level of functioning before recommending a wheelchair?

3. What do you need to know about the client and his or her lifestyle before recommending a wheelchair?

4. Describe the role of the following team members who may work together in recommending and obtaining a wheelchair for a client.

   a. Rehabilitation technology supplier

   b. Durable medical supplier

   c. Physical therapist

   d. Other

5. Fill in the information about the following wheelchair measurement:

	SEAT WIDTH	SEAT DEPTH	SEAT HEIGHT	BACK HEIGHT	ARM HEIGHT
Objectives					
Measurement procedure					
Wheelchair clearance					
Check for fit					
Other considerations					

6. Describe the methods to assess a client's fit for a wheelchair.

7. View the wheelchair instructional video series "New Moves" (Sacred Heart General Hospital Oregon Rehabilitation Center, 1987) and describe the technique used in performing the following mobility skills:

   Propel on level surfaces

   Turn wheelchair

   Maneuver on ramps

   Maneuver up/down curbs

8. Describe the advantages and disadvantages of the following wheelchairs:
   a. Manual versus electric

   b. Manual recline versus power recline

   c. Folding versus rigid manual

   d. Lightweight versus standard weight

   e. Top of the line versus bottom of the line

9. What safety issues need to be conveyed to the client regarding wheelchair use?

10. Describe the advantages and disadvantages of renting versus purchasing a wheelchair.

11. Describe the funding guidelines set forth by the following agencies in purchasing or renting a wheelchair:

    a. Medicaid

    b. Medicare

    c. Private insurance

12. What questions need to be asked before recommending a specific wheelchair?

13. What assessments need to be completed to recommend the proper wheelchair for a client?

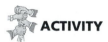 **ACTIVITY**

Materials

Wheelchairs, tape measures, wheelchair prescription form.

Instructions

1. Locate, remove and replace, where applicable, the following parts of a wheelchair. Place a check mark in each box as you are finished.

WHEELCHAIR PARTS	LOCATE	REMOVE	REPLACE
Arm rests			
Leg rests			
Brakes			
Tipping levers			
Heel loops			
Hand grips			
Front casters			
Large wheels			
Crossbrace			
Other			
Other			
Other			

2. Assess your partner in a wheelchair noting proper fit or lack thereof:
   a. Seat width

   b. Seat depth

   c. Leg length

   d. Seat height

   e. Arm height

   f. Back height

3. Measure your partner and record the information on a wheelchair prescription form. Document your partner's measurement as well as the actual size of the wheelchair part(s) you'll need. Fill out the wheelchair options section also.

4a. Instruct your partner in the use of the wheelchair. Use the following chart as a guide to ensure that your instructions are thorough and complete. Repeat your instructions without using the chart and have your partner check off the components as you review them. Practice your wheelchair instruction techniques outside of structured class time. Use the columns below to document your practice on the different dates.

INSTRUCTION IN THE USE OF A WHEELCHAIR	DATE	DATE	DATE	DATE
CLIENT WAS INSTRUCTED IN THE USE OF THE FOLLOWING:				
Folding/unfolding the wheelchair				
Locking/unlocking wheels				
Folding/unfolding the foot plates				
Releasing, swinging away leg rests				
Elevating leg rest				
Removing, replacing the detachable arms				
Adjusting foot rest length				
CLIENT WAS INSTRUCTED IN SAFETY POINTS:				
Maintenance check on wheelchair				
Fit considerations due to weight change				
Pressure sores				
Leaning forward				
Inclines				
Use of seat belt				
Use of brakes				

CLIENT WAS INSTRUCTED IN WHEELCHAIR MOBILITY:				
Propelling self on level surface				
Maneuvering over incline surfaces				
Maneuvering up/down curbs				
Instructing caregiver in negotiating steps				
Going in/out of elevators				
Managing doors from a wheelchair				
Other				
INSTRUCTIONS WERE GIVEN IN A CLEAR, LOGICAL SEQUENCE				
Patient demonstrated that instructions were understood				

4b. Record below feedback you received on your instruction of wheelchair use to your partner.

FOLLOW-UP

✔ Complete the Application of Competencies at the end of this chapter.

Exercise 85

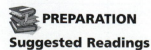

"God gave us memories so that we might enjoy roses in December."

JAMES BARRIE

COGNITIVE IMPAIRMENTS

OBJECTIVES

✔ Select assessment tools that are useful in identifying cognitive impairments
✔ Describe intervention approaches that are used for individuals with cognitive impairments
✔ Determine specific treatment strategies to increase a client's functional performance

Description

This exercise will help you to understand some of the needs of the client with cognitive impairments. Many of the clients with whom you will be working will have some kind of cognitive impairment. It is imperative that you be equipped to work with such individuals. There are numerous intervention approaches that can be used to minimize a client's functional limitations that at the same time assist in facilitating the client's task and role performance. Cognitive impairments are varied and complex. You will need to sharpen your observation skills as well as adjust the task, environment, and strategy for your client, as he or she will present you with challenging cognitive concerns.

PREPARATION
Suggested Readings

Pedretti (1996)
Trombly (1995)
Zoltan (1996)

Study Questions

1. Define cognition.

2. Define executive functions.

3. Describe what may cause a cognitive impairment in a person. List several diagnoses in which this may occur.

4. Describe the importance of approaching each person at an age-appropriate level.

5. Describe the following treatment approaches:
   a. Adaptive

   b. Remedial

   c. Process

   d. Multicontext treatment

   e. Applied behavioral analysis

   f. Sensory integration

   g. Eclectic

   h. Functional

   i. Dynamic interactional

   j. Affolter

   k. Neurodevelopmental

6. Describe the following components of performance, how they can be assessed, and an activity that could be used in treatment of impairment for each component.

DESCRIPTION	ASSESSMENT	TREATMENT
Attention		
Memory		
Initiation		
Awareness/insight		
Planning and organization		
Problem solving		
Mental flexibility		
Generalization and transfer		
Acalculia		

7. List the eight levels identified by the Ranchos Los Amigos Scale of Cognitive Functioning (Ranchos Los Amigos Medical Center, 1980, as cited in Pedretti, 1996).

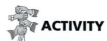 **ACTIVITY**

Materials

Index cards with cognitive terms, calculator, paper, pencil, math worksheets, simple cooking activity, money, phone book, phone, computer program entitled *Captain's Log: Cognitive Training System* (Sanford, Browne, and Turner, 1985–95); Case Studies 41 and 42 located at the end of this chapter.

Instructions

GAME

1. Divide into several teams, with no more than four on each team, to play a game of cognitive charades. Use the typical rules of charades. Take turns acting out the key terms below that were previously written on index cards and placed face down on the table. Use the space below to circle the terms you know as well as to keep score.

KEY TERMS

Cognition	Initiation
Executive functions	Awareness
Attention	Planning and organization
Orientation	Impulsivity
Memory	Problem solving
Mental flexibility	Generalization and transfer
Acalculia	

2. Participate in cognitive activities available in your lab or clinic using the materials listed. List the activity and its therapeutic purpose.

ACTIVITY	PURPOSE

3. With a partner, work on the assigned case studies. For each case, identify assessments that may need to be performed. For the cognitive deficits identified, describe what treatment activities you will use, the rationale for your choice, and how you will set up the activities. Finally, include safety precautions that should be implemented. Once you have completed the planning, share your ideas with your class in a role-play situation.

Case No.: _____

Assessments:

COGNITIVE IMPAIRMENTS	TREATMENT	RATIONALE	SETUP

Safety precautions:

Case No.: _____

Assessments:

COGNITIVE IMPAIRMENTS	TREATMENT	RATIONALE	SETUP

Safety precautions:

FOLLOW-UP

✔ Complete the Application of Competencies at the end of this chapter.

Exercise 86

"The important thing is not to stop questioning."

ALBERT EINSTEIN

PERCEPTUAL IMPAIRMENTS

OBJECTIVES

✔ Select assessment tools that are useful in identifying perceptual impairments
✔ Describe intervention approaches that are used for individuals with perceptual impairments
✔ Determine strategies to increase a client's functional perceptual performance

DESCRIPTION

This exercise will acquaint you with the many types of perceptual impairments that may occur in a client receiving occupational therapy services. Often, perceptual impairments are linked to cognitive impairments, and it is difficult to determine which has the greater impact on the other. Perceptual and cognitive difficulties often overlap and are interrelated to one another. As you work with the neurologically impaired individual, you will quickly see the power and importance of the brain and the intricacies of its functioning. As you work with your client toward increased skill and performance, you will be amazed at the plasticity of the brain through the life span.

PREPARATION

Suggested Readings

Pedretti (1996)
Trombly (1995)
Zoltan (1996)

Study Questions

1. What is perception?

2. Describe the cause of perceptual impairments as well as some of the more common diagnoses with which these deficits may be linked.

3. Describe the following approaches that may be used in the treatment of perception difficulties.
   a. Remedial

   b. Sensory integrative

   c. Affolter

   d. Neurodevelopmental

   e. Transfer of training

   f. Adaptive

   g. Functional

   h. Occupational performance

   i. Dynamic interactional

4. Describe the following perceptual impairments, how they can be assessed, and one activity that can be used in treatment of each deficit.

DEFICIT	ASSESSMENT	TREATMENT
Astereognosis		
Somatognosia		
Ideation ideamotor apraxia		
Ideamotor apraxia		
Constructional apraxia		
Dressing apraxia		
Tactile perception		
Figure-ground perception		
Homonymous hemiopsia		
Unilateral neglect		

ACTIVITY

Materials

Index cards with a perceptual deficit written on each one, chalkboard, markerboard, or flip charts; shirt, pants, toothbrush, hairbrush, paper, pencil, vibrator, washcloth, electric razor, weighted cuff; masking tape, kitchen utensils, wheelchair, figure-ground worksheet; Case Studies 39 and 45 located at the end of this chapter.

Instructions

GAME

1. As a class, divide into two or more teams. Play a game similar to Pictionary™, using the perceptual terms listed below. Follow the rules for playing Pictionary™ by taking turns drawing the term (written on an index card placed face down on the table) on a chalkboard or flip chart page. See whether your team can guess what you are drawing. Score by noting how many correct responses your team is able to make. A time limit for each answer and for the entire game needs to be decided before beginning.

   TERMS

Body scheme	Sensory integration	Astereognosis
Praxis	Affolter	Somatognosia
Graphesthesia	Neurodevelopmental	Dressing apraxia
Tactile	Transfer of training	Tactile perception
Inattention	Adaptive	Figure-ground
Apraxia	Functional approach	Oral apraxia
Occupational performance	Plasticity	Unilateral neglect
Homonymous hemianopsia	Dynamic interaction approach	Constructional apraxia

   Score: _____

2. Observe your instructor demonstrating perceptual training techniques using the materials listed, for example, training someone with a perceptual deficit to put on a shirt or having the client complete a figure-ground activity. Participate in these same activities.

3. With a partner or in a small group, use the assigned case studies to complete the following chart. Read the case study and determine the perceptual deficits of the client. Select a treatment approach, activities you will use with this approach, and how you will set up the activities. List the safety precautions you will need to take. Share and demonstrate your treatment ideas in a role-play situation to the class.

Case No.: _____

PERCEPTUAL IMPAIRMENT	TREATMENT APPROACH	TREATMENT ACTIVITIES	SETUP

Safety precautions:

Case No.: _____

PERCEPTUAL IMPAIRMENT	TREATMENT APPROACH	TREATMENT ACTIVITIES	SETUP

Safety precautions:

FOLLOW-UP

✔   Complete the Application of Competencies at the end of this chapter.

NEURODEVELOPMENTAL TREATMENT

Exercise 87

OBJECTIVES

✔   Define and describe neurodevelopmental treatment (NDT) techniques that are used for adults with hemiplegia
✔   Perform handling and treatment techniques
✔   Select appropriate activities incorporating a NDT approach

DESCRIPTION

Neurodevelopmental treatment (NDT) was originated by Berta and Karl Bobath, a physical therapist and physician, respectively, as well as a wife/husband team. Their work began in England in the 1940s and has increasingly been incorporated in the United States since that time. It is a treatment approach that is appropriate for individuals with cerebral palsy or hemiplegia. This exercise will focus on the adult client with hemiplegia and will acquaint you with the basic principles and techniques that are used. To become proficient in the use of such techniques, further study is necessary. Current certification in either neurodevelopmental theory and treatment for adults or neurodevelopmental theory and treatment for infants and children from the National NDT Association is available.

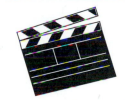

"We should have much peace if we would not bury ourselves with the sayings and doings of others."

THOMAS LAMPIS

 PREPARATION

Suggested Readings

Pedretti (1996)
Trombly (1995)

Study Questions

1. Describe how the following techniques may be incorporated into treatment of the adult with hemiplegia:

    a. Weight bearing

   b. Trunk rotation

   c. Scapular protraction

   d. Anterior pelvic tilt position

   e. Slow, controlled movements

   f. Proper positioning

2. Describe the importance of using everyday activities in treatment.

3. What should the occupational therapy practitioner constantly assess when providing treatment?

4. Describe the typical problems of hemiplegia:
   a. Flaccidity

   b. Mixed tone

   c. Spasticity

   d. Unilateral neglect

5. Differentiate between an inhibition technique and a facilitation technique and list several of each.

INHIBITION	FACILITATION

6. Describe the NDT evaluation process.

ACTIVITY

Materials

Case study 48 located at the end of this chapter.

Instructions

1. As a class, discuss, review, and list the basic principles of NDT.

2. Discuss and list the normal development of a functional upright position.
   a.

   b.

   c.

   d.

   e.

3. Observe a classmate with normal movement patterns and watch your instructor demonstrating abnormal movement patterns. Describe how each performs the following movements and/or maintains the following postures.

MOVEMENT OR POSTURE	NORMAL	IMPAIRED
Rolling		
Supine to sit		
Sitting		
Sit to stand		
Standing		

4. Watch your instructor demonstrate how to physically handle a person with a neurological impairment. Assess your partner to determine whether the following factors are present for upper extremity functioning.

FACTOR	DEMONSTRATION	PARTNER
Trunk stability/mobility (anterior pelvic tilt)		
Scapular stability/mobility		
Balance of muscle tone		

5. Watch your instructor perform the following treatment techniques in handling. Record notes from your observation in the space provided. Practice these treatment techniques on each other. Have your instructor observe your performance and give you feedback. Record instructor's feedback in the space provided.

NDT TECHNIQUE	NOTES	INSTRUCTOR FEEDBACK
TRUNK MOBILIZATION		
Supine		
Side-lying		
SCAPULAR MOBILIZATION		
Sidelying/sitting		
Supine		
ROLLING		
To noninvolved side		
To involved side		
SUPINE TO SITTING		
Roll to side		

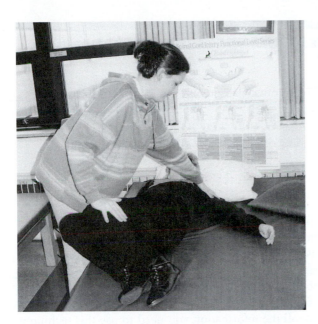

Fig. 5-13 Applying NDT trunk mobilization technique.
Photo courtesy of Gina Knab.

6. Work with a partner or small group to plan a treatment session for the individual described, in the assigned case study, using NDT principles. Outline below the activities you selected, the rationale for doing so, the setup you will need, and the approximate time needed to complete the activity.

    a. Occupation Selected: _____   Time: _____

       Rationale: _____

       Setup: _____

    b. Occupation Selected: _____   Time: _____

       Rationale: _____

       Setup: _____

    c. Occupation Selected: _____   Time: _____

       Rationale: _____

       Setup: _____

7. Share ideas with your classmates. Ask yourself, "Do they meet the requirements of NDT?" List the ideas you wish to remember.

FOLLOW-UP

✔ Complete the Application of Competencies at the end of this chapter.

Exercise 88

"When we long for life without difficulties, remind us that oaks grow strong in contrary winds and diamonds are made under pressure."

PETER MARSHALL

PROPRIOCEPTIVE NEUROMUSCULAR FACILITATION

OBJECTIVES

✔ Identify the proprioceptive neuromuscular facilitation (PNF) treatment principles, procedures, and techniques

✔ Demonstrate diagonal patterns used in intervention

✔ Plan treatment activities incorporating PNF techniques

DESCRIPTION

Proprioceptive neuromuscular facilitation (PNF) is a technique used in a physical rehabilitation setting. It originated from the work of Herman Kabat, Margaret Knott, and Dorothy Voss in the 1950s. It is intended to facilitate functional return for those with paralysis. The techniques are based on normal movement and motor development. Functional activities are emphasized and many movements as well as diagonal patterns are incorporated. At times this technique may be used exclusively; at other times PNF may be used in conjunction with other therapeutic techniques. Additional training will be beneficial in providing you with all the information you need to use this technique in the most advantageous manner.

 PREPARATION

Suggested Readings

Pedretti (1996)
Trombly (1995)

Study Questions

1. List the eleven PNF treatment principles:

   a.

   b.

   c.

   d.

   e.

   f.

g.

h.

i.

j.

k.

2. Describe the sensory and motor systems that may be used in PNF treatment:
   a. Auditory (verbal comments)

   b. Vision (visual aids)

   c. Motor (repetitive practice)

   d. Tactile (manual contact)

3. Perform the following movements and then list the diagonal that it represents:
   a. Hand to mouth

   b. Buttoning clothing parts on the opposite body side

   c. Combing hair on the same body side as the hand

   d. Pushing a car door open from inside the car

  e. Putting on an earring

  f. Putting on a cap or hat with both hands

4. Describe how the following procedures are used in PNF treatment:
   a. Manual contact

   b. Stretch

   c. Traction

   d. Approximation

   e. Maximal resistance

5. Describe how the following techniques are used with the procedures in Study Question 4.
   a. Repeated contraction

   b. Rhythmical initiation

   c. Slow reversal

   d. Rhythmical stabilization

   e. Contract-relax

   f. Hold-relax

g. Slow reversal-hold-relax

h. Rhythmic rotation

6. What developmental postures are helpful for treatment?

7. Describe the PNF evaluation process.

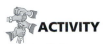

ACTIVITY

Materials

Case study 48 located at the end of this chapter.

Instructions

1. Watch a demonstration of your instructor exhibiting the diagonal patterns (D) listed below. Practice with a partner and verbally state what you would tell a client performing these motions. Record your verbal directions in the following chart. After the demonstration, have your partner check off whether you completed the motion and the verbal directions correctly. Have your partner do one of the movements while you state which diagonal and flexion or extension pattern is being used. Take turns checking each other's accuracy.

	VERBAL DIRECTIONS	MOTION	VERBAL	PARTNER'S DIAGONAL AND FLEXION/EXTENSION PATTERN
D₁				
Extension				
Flexion				
D₂				
Extension				
Flexion				
Bilateral Lifting				
Down				
Up				
Bilateral Chop				
Down				
Up				

2. Using the assigned case study with your partner, determine the main physical and functional deficits present in that individual. Plan three occupations incorporating PNF techniques and principles that would be appropriate to facilitate return to function for the client. Include your rationale for the activities chosen, the setup you will need, the diagonal pattern facilitated, and the approximate amount of time the activity will take to complete.

    a. Occupation 1: _____ Time: _____

        Rationale: _____

        Setup: _____

        Diagonal: _____

    b. Occupation 2: _____ Time: _____

        Rationale: _____

        Setup: _____

        Diagonal: _____

    c. Occupation 3: _____ Time: _____

        Rationale: _____

        Setup: _____

        Diagonal: _____

3. Share your ideas with your class.

FOLLOW-UP

✔ Complete the Application of Competencies at the end of this chapter.

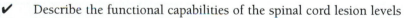

Exercise 89

"If I have a patient who is afraid, I can grasp his hand reassuringly and he will feel better. This happens even under anesthesia."

DEPAK CHOPRA

SPINAL CORD INJURY

OBJECTIVES

✔ Describe the functional capabilities of the spinal cord lesion levels
✔ Identify appropriate treatment techniques that can be used with the client who has a spinal cord injury
✔ Plan and demonstrate a treatment session for a client with a specified level of spinal cord injury

DESCRIPTION

This exercise will acquaint you with spinal cord injuries. Spinal cord injuries can be seen across the life span but are commonly seen in the adolescent and young adult, often resulting from an automobile accident or some other trauma. A spinal cord injury can result in a complete or incomplete lesion, which leads to paralysis, termed either tetraplegia or paraplegia. Along with the resulting physical trauma, emotional and psychological trauma are also incurred. Adjusting to a spinal cord injury will be an ongoing process throughout the individual's life. As an occupational therapy practitioner you will need to be aware of your client's many and varied needs. You will provide not only services to the newly injured client but to the client who has lived with an injury for decades.

PREPARATION

Suggested Readings

AOTA (1998)
Daniel and Strickland (1992)
Pedretti (1996)
Pierson (1999)
Trombly (1995)

Study Questions

1. Define quadriplegia, tetraplegia, and paraplegia.

2. Differentiate between a complete and an incomplete lesion.

3. Describe precautions that must be adhered to in treating a person with quadriplegia/tetraplegia.

4. In each of the following areas, list at least one treatment technique that may be implemented in working with a person with quadriplegia and paraplegia.

AREA	TREATMENT TECHNIQUES	
	TETRAPLEGIA	PARAPLEGIA
Maintain ROM		
Increase muscle strength		
Improve coordination/ dexterity		
Manage spasticity		
Improve awareness of sensory deficits		
Improve endurance		
Improve mobility		
Facilitate client and family teaching		
Promote independence in activities of daily living		
Pursue vocational/ avocational activities interests		
Facilitate emotional adjustment		
Maximize home safety and accessibility		

Pursue community independence		
Investigate driving potential		
Facilitate social and interpersonal adjustment		

5. Fill in the following chart, indicating the primary muscle groups involved, the primary movement patterns available for use, and the expected functional outcome for each spinal cord level of lesion listed.

SPINAL CORD LEVEL OF LESION	PRIMARY MUSCLE GROUPS	PRIMARY MOVEMENT	EXPECTED FUNCTIONAL OUTCOME
C1–C3			
C3–C4			
C5			
C6			
C7–C8			
C8–T1			
T4–9			
T10–L2			
L3–L4			
L5–S3			

6. Summarize three significant areas of emotional adjustment an individual must deal with after a spinal cord injury.

a.

b.

c.

7. Describe when you think it might be appropriate and necessary to refer a client with a spinal cord injury for treatment by another discipline (e.g., physical therapy, counseling).

8. Identify the frame of reference(s) most likely to be used in working with a client who has a spinal cord injury.

9. List and briefly describe the purpose of six assessments that would be appropriate to administer to the client with a spinal cord injury.

    a.

    b.

    c.

    d.

    e.

    f.

10. Read AOTA's position paper entitled "Broadening the Construct of Independence" (AOTA, 1998) and describe how it is possible for a person with quadriplegia to be independent.

11. Describe several general accommodations that may be necessary to make, according to the Americans with Disabilities Act, for someone who has a spinal cord injury.

    Note: In preparation for the following activity, bring items of clothing large enough to put on over student's own clothing.

 ACTIVITY

Materials

Wheelchairs, sliding boards, transfer belts, clothes that are large enough to be put on over student's own clothes, cooking equipment, reachers, long-handled sponges, bath mitt, universal cuff, bath benches, raised commode, dycem, mat tables, kitchen, and bathroom.

Fig. 5-14 An individual with a spinal cord injury talks to students about his disability.

Photo courtesy of Nick Puhlman, Christie Tuttle, Traci Holt, and Charlene Kennedy.

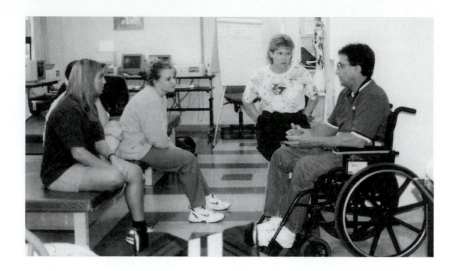

Instructions

1a. Invite one or two guest speakers who have had a spinal cord injury to talk to your class about their injury and current functional level. Ask questions to obtain information on their performance in the following areas:

PERFORMANCE AREA	GUEST 1 LEVEL OF INJURY	GUEST 2 LEVEL OF INJURY
Dressing		
Bathing/showering		
Toilet hygiene		
Grooming		
Feeding and eating		
Socialization		
Functional communication		
Community mobility		
Sexual expression		
Home management		
Other		

1b. Query your guests further and describe their emotional adjustment to their spinal cord injury.

2a. Have your guests role-play being a newly injured client. Teach them to do a sliding board transfer. Take turns until all students have had a chance to teach a sliding board transfer. After each transfer, give feedback to classmates on their performance. Record the feedback that you receive.

Introduction to the transfer

Demonstration

Body mechanics

Bedside manner (use of self)

2b. Summarize your feelings and the learning that occurred during this activity. Summarize your strengths and areas of concern in completing sliding board transfers.

3a. Divide into small groups. With an assigned level of spinal cord lesion, practice and then role-play with a peer, teaching him or her the various activities of daily living and home management tasks listed below. Continue practicing until all group members are proficient in performing and teaching the task. Use adaptive equipment as needed. List the adaptive equipment needed. Check each box as you complete the skill.

Level of injury: _____

ADL AND HOME MANAGEMENT TASKS	PRACTICE PERFORMING TASK AS A CLIENT	TEACHING TASK TO CLIENT	ADAPTIVE EQUIPMENT NEEDED
Sliding board transfers			
Donning/doffing			
Shirt			
Pants			
Bra			
Socks			
Shoes			
Toilet hygiene			
Bathing/showering			
Wheelchair mobility			
Grooming			
Kitchen/homemaking tasks			

3b. When each person in your group is proficient at performing each task and teaching the task for that particular level of spinal cord injury, take turns demonstrating the activities to your entire class.

3c. With your small group, plan a treatment session in the clinic with your client. Describe the session, including the activities you will use, the setup needed, the estimated time the activities will require, and the rationale for your choice of activities. Present your ideas to the class.

OCCUPATION	SETUP	TIME	RATIONALE

3d. Use the space below to record ideas from classmates that you would like to remember.

INJURY LEVEL	TREATMENT IDEAS

FOLLOW-UP

✔ Complete the Application of Competencies at the end of this chapter.
✔ Complete Performance Skill 5A on Disability Simulation.

HOME MANAGEMENT

OBJECTIVES

✔ Identify tasks associated with home management
✔ Prepare a meal with an assumed deficit in independent functioning
✔ Select adaptive techniques and equipment to facilitate independence in home management

DESCRIPTION

This exercise will begin to prepare you to work with the client who lacks independence in the area of home management. Home management is an important aspect of work and productive activities. In some settings, home management tasks are a part of activities of daily living (ADLs), as they are considered self-maintenance tasks. In such instances home management tasks would be called instrumental ADLs or advanced ADLs, connoting their role of allowing an individual to live independently. With either designation it is important for you to understand all the components involved and problem-solve with your clients about the most efficient adaptive techniques and equipment that they might benefit from using.

"If each of us sweeps in front of our own steps, the whole world will be clean."

GOETHE

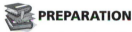

PREPARATION

Suggesting Readings

AOTA (latest edition)
AOTA (1998)
Christiansen (2000)
Klinger (1997)
Pedretti (1996)
Trombly (1995)

Study Questions

1. You may use the *Reference Manual of the Official Documents of AOTA* (latest edition) to assist you. List all of the activities involved in the subcategories of each home management task area taken from Uniform Terminolgy for Occupational Therapy, 3rd ed. (AOTA, 1998). Once you have listed each activity, find one adaptive technique that could be used to perform this activity and at least one piece of adaptive equipment that may assist in performance. If you are unable to find a technique or piece of equipment for a particular activity think of one on your own. Put a star by these. The first one is completed for you.

TASK: CLOTHING CARE		
ACTIVITIES	ADAPTIVE TECHNIQUE	ADAPTIVE EQUIPMENT
Obtaining and using supplies	Use a wheeled cart	Use a reacher
Sorting	Having separate baskets for each clothing type	Use a reacher if necessary to pick up items from the floor
Laundering—hand	Roll clothes in a towel instead of wringing	Have someone assist as needed
Laundering—machine	Wash small loads during week	Stacked laundry center
Folding	Avoid bending by organizing area	Use hangers if this is easier*
Ironing	Select non-ironing clothes	Adjustable ironing board so you can sit
Storing	Store on low shelves*	Hang clothes on hangers*
Mending	Send mending out for repair*	Use a needle threader*

a. Task: cleaning

ACTIVITIES	ADAPTIVE TECHNIQUE	ADAPTIVE EQUIPMENT

b. Task: meal preparation and clean-up

ACTIVITIES	ADAPTIVE TECHNIQUE	ADAPTIVE EQUIPMENT

c. Task: shopping

ACTIVITIES	ADAPTIVE TECHNIQUE	ADAPTIVE EQUIPMENT

d. Task: money management

ACTIVITIES	ADAPTIVE TECHNIQUE	ADAPTIVE EQUIPMENT

e. Task: household maintenance		
ACTIVITIES	ADAPTIVE TECHNIQUE	ADAPTIVE EQUIPMENT

f. Task: safety procedures		
ACTIVITIES	ADAPTIVE TECHNIQUE	ADAPTIVE EQUIPMENT

2. For each of the following deficits, write several home management suggestions that may be used to increase independence. Add to the example given below.

DEFICIT	HOME MANAGEMENT SUGGESTIONS
Decreased range of motion/strength	Example: use a wheeled cart in the kitchen to transport cooking supplies
Incoordination	
Use of only one hand	
Using a wheelchair for mobility with good upper extremity (UE) function	
Using a wheelchair for mobility with UE weakness	

ACTIVITY

Materials

Stove, oven, refrigerator, microwave, blender, mixer, can opener, bowls, pans, measuring spoons and cups, cooking utensils, baking dishes, towels, washcloths, eating utensils and plates, drinking glasses, grater, blindfolds, wheelchairs, walker, all ingredients necessary to make the food items planned by the students; Case Study 44 located at the end of this chapter.

Instructions

1a. As a class, prepare a meal while assuming that you are an individual with a deficit that would interfere with your independence in your home management abilities. First, plan the meal by making sure each of the skills listed below is used at least once during the meal preparation. Use the following chart for your planning. List the food item to be prepared and the person who is responsible for bringing the ingredients of that particular item to lab on the day the meal will be prepared. Put a check mark in each box below the food item being prepared to identify the skills needed to prepare that item.

	MAIN DISH	DRINK	DESSERT	SIDE DISH	SIDE DISH	SIDE DISH
Food/Person responsible						
Grating						
Opening package						
Opening jar						
Cutting						
Baking with oven						
Cooking with stovetop						
Opening can						
Peeling						
Mixing						
Reading directions						

1b. Pair with a partner and take turns assuming the role of a client with a disability (as indicated in the following chart) and the therapist working with that client. Get together adaptive equipment that your client may need for the meal preparation. Decide as a class who will be responsible for making the menu items. Halfway through the preparation, switch roles so that everyone will have the opportunity to be the client and the therapist.

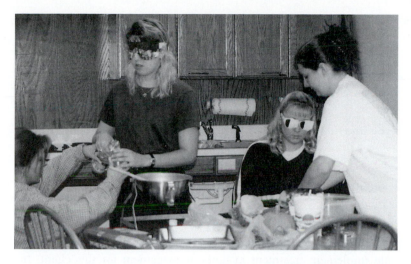

Fig. 5-15   Cooking a meal while simulating blindness and hemianopsia.

Photo courtesy of Jessica Johantges, Gina Knab, Kim Meyer, and Christie Tuttle.

STUDENT ROLES	STUDENT	MENU ITEM	ADAPTIVE EQUIPMENT
Client with right-sided hemiplegia			
Therapist			
Client who is blind			
Therapist			
Client in a wheelchair with right-sided hemiplegia			
Therapist			
Client with rheumatoid arthritis and a total hip replacement			
Therapist			
Other client			
Therapist			

1c.   Eat the meal your class has prepared. Afterward, clean up using only your non-dominant hand. As a group, select some minor consequence to anyone who is caught using two hands and/or his or her dominant hand; for example, any student who is caught will have to sing a song in class. Following your meal planning, preparation, and cleanup, write your impressions of these activities from the point of view of a client with a disability. Use the following questions as a guide. Discuss impressions with your class.

   a.   What was the most difficult component or task?

b. What technique/s did you find helpful?

c. What was the most frustrating?

d. What did you like that your therapist did?

e. What did you not like that your therapist did?

2. With a partner, using Case Study 44 located at the end of this chapter, describe how you would implement treatment in home management for this client. Include the activities you might use and the setup needed for those activities.

TREATMENT ACTIVITIES	SETUP

FOLLOW-UP

✔ Complete the Application of Competencies at the end of this chapter.
✔ For your participation in the meal preparation complete an Analysis of Self located in Appendix B.

Exercise 91

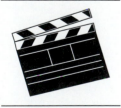

"Do the one thing you fear and the death of fear is certain."

RALPH WALDO EMERSON

ASSISTIVE TECHNOLOGIES

OBJECTIVES

✔ Define assistive technology related terms
✔ Determine the therapeutic implications of assistive technology
✔ Locate local supply and funding sources for assistive technology

DESCRIPTION

This exercise will familiarize you with assistive technologies. Assistive technology can be defined as any device, service, strategy, or practice that improves the functional capabilities of individuals with disabilities. Because of recent advances in the scientific field, assistive technologies have become much more commonplace and accessible. As an occupational therapy practitioner you may help in assessing a client's need for a particular technology as well as training the client and/or caregiver in its use. You may also find yourself in the role of consultant as you pass on information to other professionals and caregivers about your client's needs. It will be an exciting challenge to keep yourself abreast of the latest assistive technologies available.

PREPARATION

Suggested Readings

Alliance for Technology Access (1994)
AOTA (latest edition)
Cook and Hussey (1995)
Cromwell (1986)
Neidstadt and Crepeau (1998)
Trombly (1995)

Study Questions

1. Define the following technology related terms and give an example of each:

   a. Impairment

   b. Disability

   c. Handicap

   d. Assistive technology

   e. Rehabilitative technology

   f. Low technology

   g. High technology

   h. Soft technology

   i. Hard technology

   j. Appliances

k.   Tool

l.   Prosthetic device

m. Minimal technology

n.   Maximal technology

o.   General-purpose technology

p.   Specific-purpose technology

q.   Commercial technology

r.   Custom technology

2.   Define the following computer-related terms:
a.   Hardware

b.   Software

c.   Application

d.   Program

e.   Input

f.   Processing

g. Output

h. Operating system

i. ROM

j. RAM

k. Floppy disks

l. ECU

3. List examples of conventional and assistive technologies associated with their mode of input, processing, and output.

CONVENTIONAL TECHNOLOGY	ASSISTIVE TECHNOLOGY
Input	
Processing	
Output	

4. Describe how the following laws affect a person's use of assistive technology.
   a. Individuals with Disabilities Education Act (IDEA)

   b. Americans with Disabilities Act (ADA) of 1990

   c. Technology-Related Assistance for Individuals with Disabilities Act of 1988

   d. 1986 Amendments to the Rehabilitation Act of 1973

5. What does the acronym RESNA represent and what is their purpose?

6. List potential resource organizations related to assistive technology. Include their addresses and phone numbers.

ORGANIZATION	ADDRESS	TELEPHONE

7. Summarize the service delivery process in assistive technology.

8. Describe how computers can be used in occupational therapy as a treatment technique.

9. For each of the following difficulties, find at least one approach or technology that may be used to increase the independence of an individual with that difficulty. Assume that the individual needs to access a computer.

   a. Use of one hand

   b. Low vision

   c. No vision

   d. Difficulty isolating fingers

   e. No use of hands

   f. Very short attention span

10. Briefly summarize AOTA's position on assistive technology.

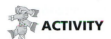
ACTIVITY

Materials

Computers, assistive technology that is available for use, such as alternative keyboards, touch screens, mouthsticks, joystick, talking word processors, trackball, arm and wrist supports, electronic pointing devices, environmental control units, computer software to promote cognition, memory, visual spatial perception, Internet access; telephone and a set of telephone books for each group; AOTA (latest edition), Americans with Disabilities Act of 1990; Case Studies 37, 40, 44, 45, and 47 located at the end of this chapter.

Instructions

1. Participate in various computer software programs designed to promote cognition, memory, and/or visual spatial perception. Analyze the programs according to the performance components that would be needed for a client to use the program.

   a. Program:

      Components:

   b. Program:

      Components:

   c. Program:

      Components:

   d. Program:

      Components:

   e. Program:

      Components:

2. Work with a partner and access various assistive technologies (as listed under the materials section). Determine their therapeutic implications.

ASSISTIVE TECHNOLOGY	THERAPEUTIC IMPLICATIONS

3. Working with a partner or small group, select a computer software program and/or any other assistive technology that could be used in treatment for the client in one of the two case studies assigned. List your selections below. Include the rationale for your choice. Share your case study with your classmates. Record their ideas below also.

Case No.: _____

COMPUTER PROGRAM	ASSISTIVE TECHNOLOGY	RATIONALE

Case No.: _____

COMPUTER PROGRAM	ASSISTIVE TECHNOLOGY	RATIONALE

🎲 GAME

4a. Divide into teams of no more than three or four. Play a scavenger hunt game in which the first team that finds all the requested information is the winner. Each team will be given a different case study. After your group has studied the case, fill out the following chart, giving one example of a piece of equipment for each of the following areas that may be beneficial for the person in your case study. Include where you found this information, where it could be purchased locally, to whom you spoke, and the price to purchase the item. Obtain the information from your readings, local resources, Internet, and so on. When you have completed the information or when your allotted time limit is up, come back to the room and claim your prize. Share your information with your classmates and take notes on the information they have obtained.

Case No.: _____

AREA	EQUIPMENT	SOURCE	WHERE PURCHASED	SALESPERSON	PRICE
Low tech					
High tech					
Soft tech					
Hard tech					
Appliance					
Tool					
Prosthetic					
Minimal tech					
Maximal tech					

4b. Locate a possible funding source that may cover all or some of the equipment listed above. Indicate the person to whom you spoke and the available assistance that source might have to offer.

SOURCE	PERSON TO WHOM YOU SPOKE	ASSISTANCE AVAILABLE

4c. Locate an Internet site that is available to this person so that he or she might speak with others who have a similar diagnosis.

4d. Locate a support group in your area that is available for this person to attend.

SUPPORT GROUP	TIME AND PLACE OF MEETING

4e. Describe a job this person may be able to do and necessary accommodations he or she may need to fulfill the job responsibilities. Cite a section in the Americans with Disabilities Act of 1990 that supports having this accommodation.

JOB	ACCOMMODATION	CITATION

4f. Share your information with your classmates. Record the information below that you would like to remember.

FOLLOW-UP

✔ Complete the Application of Competencies at the end of this chapter.

✔ Complete Performance Skill 5B on Fabrication Adaptive Device.

Exercise 92

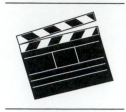

"A pupil from whom nothing is ever demanded which he cannot do, never does all he can."

JOHN STUART MILL

THERAPEUTIC ADAPTATIONS

OBJECTIVES

✔ Describe the adaptive equipment that might be used for deficits in the performance areas
✔ Identify low-cost, readily available adaptive equipment
✔ Identify the source, cost, and availability of commercially made adaptive equipment devices

DESCRIPTION

Therapeutic adaptations are frequently needed by clients in a physical rehabilitation setting. Adaptations can facilitate a client's independent functioning and interaction with the environment. Many excellent and frequently used adaptive devices are available commercially. Alternatively, in some cases, a client may have a more economical and readily available device or technique already in his or her home. When you need adaptive equipment and technique, be sure to problem-solve with the client. Certain expenses cannot be avoided; however, a little creativity and problem solving can help to avoid some of the costs. Additionally, remember that some adaptive devices can be rented rather than purchased. This may or may not cut down on the cost but is an important consideration to keep in mind.

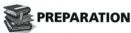 **PREPARATION**

Suggested Readings

> Arthritis Foundation (1988)
> Christiansen (2000)
> Neidstadt and Crepeau (1998)
> Pedretti (1996)

Study Questions

1. When might it be necessary to adapt an activity?

2. What are some general adaptive options for clients with the following deficits?
   a. Range of motion

   b. Strength

   c. Coordination

   d. Hand function

   e. Endurance

   f. Use of one hand

3. What factors must be considered in determining whether or not a piece of adaptive equipment may be necessary for a particular client?

4. Describe the collaboration that must occur between the client and the therapist.

5. Describe the collaboration that must occur between the client's family or caregiver and the therapist.

6. For each of the performance areas (AOTA, 1998) name two pieces of adaptive equipment that may be used to promote an increase in a client's functional level.

   a. Grooming

   b. Oral hygiene

   c. Bathing/showering

   d. Toilet hygiene

   e. Personal device care

   f. Dressing

   g. Feeding and eating

   h. Medication routine

i. Health maintenance

j. Socialization

k. Functional communication

l. Functional mobility

m. Community mobility

n. Emergency response

o. Sexual expression

p. Clothing care

q. Meal preparation and cleanup

r. Shopping

s. Money management

t. Household maintenance

u. Safety procedures

v. Care of others

w. Educational activities

x. Vocational activities

y. Play or leisure activities

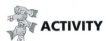 **ACTIVITY**

Materials

Adaptive equipment samples representing as many performance areas as possible; catalogues exhibiting adaptive equipment; yellow pages of the phone book.

Instructions

1a. With a partner or small group, look through the catalogues provided and find as many pieces of adaptive equipment from your study questions as possible. Fill in the first four columns in the following chart, documenting the availability of that particular item. Explore your lab or facility, and if that piece of adaptive equipment is available there, place a check mark in the appropriate column if it is. Finally, determine at least one diagnostic condition a client may have that would require or benefit from the use of this piece of adaptive equipment.

ADAPTIVE EQUIPMENT	CATALOGUE NAME	PAGE NO.	PRICE	CHECK IF AVAILABLE	DIAGNOSIS

Fig. 5-16 Display of basic adaptive equipment.

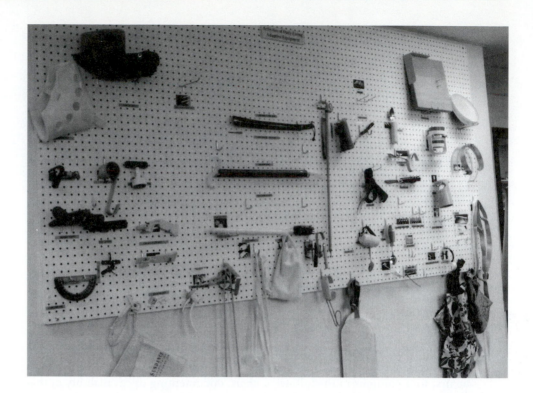

1b. List additional equipment you find in your lab or facility that was not included on any of the lists completed by your classmates. Find these pieces of equipment in a catalogue and fill in the information in the following chart.

ADAPTIVE EQUIPMENT	CATALOGUE NAME	PAGE NO.	PRICE	CHECK IF AVAILABLE	DIAGNOSIS

2a. Brainstorm and problem-solve with your partner or small group to determine what adaptive technique (or materials a person would normally have in his or her home) can be used instead of a commercially purchased piece of equipment to adapt the following occupations. An example is given for you. Share your ideas with your classmates when completed.

OCCUPATION	ADAPTIVE TECHNIQUE
Holding a bowl while stirring	Place a damp washcloth under the bowl
Opening a jar	
Reaching dishes in overhead cabinet	
Holding paper while writing	
Gripping a fork	
Standing in the shower	
Using the telephone	
Remembering to take medicine	

2b. Identify at least one other occupation (not mentioned in Activity 2a) and list an adapted technique for the same. Share this idea with your class and record your classmates' ideas below.

OCCUPATION	ADAPTIVE TECHNIQUE

3. Divide into pairs or small groups. Using your local telephone book or yellow pages, identify local vendors of medical equipment. Use a sign-up method to indicate which ones your group will call. Call the vendors and inquire about their rental policy and costs to rent and own the following items. Share your findings with your class.

ITEM	VENDOR'S NAME	POLICY	COST TO RENT	COST TO OWN
Bathtub bench	1.			
	2.			
	3.			
Commode	1.			
	2.			
	3.			
Hospital bed	1.			
	2.			
	3.			
Wheelchair	1.			
	2.			
	3.			
Wheelchair ramp	1.			
	2.			
	3.			
Electric power scooter	1.			
	2.			
	3.			
Hoyer lift	1.			
	2.			
	3.			
Stair lift	1.			
	2.			
	3.			

FOLLOW-UP

✔ Complete the Application of Competencies at the end of this chapter.
✔ Complete Performance Skill 5D on Activity Adaptation.

Exercise 93

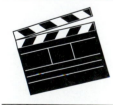

"Confidence is half the victory."

Hebrew proverb

MEDICAL EQUIPMENT IN CLIENT CARE

OBJECTIVES

✔ Identify medical equipment that is used to monitor and maintain a client's physiological status
✔ Describe safety precautions to be considered when working with medical equipment
✔ Select treatment activities appropriate for a client with compromised medical status

DESCRIPTION

This exercise will acquaint you with specialized medical equipment that is used to monitor and maintain a client's physiological status. You may encounter this equipment in either an outpatient or an inpatient setting. Generally, the more compromised the client's health is, the more lines, monitors, and tubes you will need to be knowledgeable about. Clients in such condition are still very much in need of your services, and often more so as inactivity leads to further decline in their health status. As you engage clients in the evaluation and intervention process, you will need to grade the activities in relationship to their physiological status.

PREPARATION

Suggested Readings

Early (1998)
Pedretti (1996)
Pierson (1999)

Study Questions

1. Define the following:

   a. Nasal cannula

   b. Dialysis

   c. Fistula

   d. Endotracheal tube

   e. Infusion pump

   f. Electrocardiogram

   g. Intravenous therapy

   h. Nasal gastric tube

   i. Shunt

   j. Ventilator

   k. Arterial line

     l. Gastric tube

     m. Foley catheter

     n. External catheter

     o. Suprapubis catheter

     p. Ostomy device

2. List several diagnoses of clients whom you may be treating in a special care environment.

3. Describe what you may do before treating a client in an intensive care environment.

4. If you are treating a client with lines, monitors, or tubes in the clinic, identify the information that you need to work with such medical equipment:

   a. Care of the lines, monitors, or tubes

   b. Positioning and transferring the client with lines, monitors, or tubes

   c. Precautions regarding lines, monitors, and tubes

ACTIVITY

Materials

Access to hospital intensive care unit, Case Study 46 located at the end of this chapter.

Instructions

1a. As a class, visit a hospital intensive care unit. Have a medical professional describe equipment used, its purpose, and any precautions to which you would need to adhere. Record this information in the following chart.

EQUIPMENT	PURPOSE	PRECAUTIONS

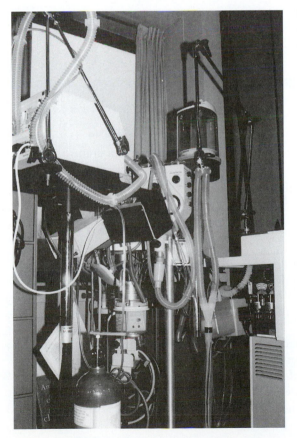

Fig. 5-17 Working in ICU can be quite overwhelming until all of the equipment procedures are learned.

1b. Record and discuss your impressions from this visit.

2a. Work with a partner on the case study assigned to determine appropriate therapeutic activities for intervention, their rationale, how you would set up the activities, and any precautions and/or assistance you may need in performing your treatment procedures.

Case No: _____

ACTIVITY	RATIONALE	SETUP	PRECAUTIONS

2b. Discuss your intervention ideas with your classmates.

FOLLOW-UP

✔ Complete the Application of Competencies at the end of this chapter.

Exercise 94

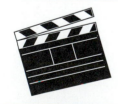

"Do today what you want to postpone until tomorrow."

LEBANESE PROVERB

HOME HEALTH

OBJECTIVES

✔ Identify important client safety issues that are encountered in a home health setting
✔ Discuss treatment techniques that are used in a home health setting
✔ Outline home health activities for therapeutic intervention

Description

This exercise will acquaint you with the practice area of home health. This is an expanding area of practice as it facilitates independent functioning within a client's familiar and natural environment. In a home health setting, a variety of clients will be seen, and each client will have his or her own individual needs. Various legislative initiatives are supporting the continuation of such services as positive outcomes are documented. Basing medical care in the client's home aligns well with the philosophy of occupational therapy in providing occupation in a climate that is meaningful to the client. A word of caution, though; when working in this climate, you will need to be a self-starter, as your schedule and system of support in the work environment will probably not be as available and obvious as in other settings.

PREPARATION

Suggested Readings

Lewis (1989)
Commission on Practice in Home Health Task Force (1995)

Study Questions

1. According to Medicare guidelines, how does a person qualify for home health services?

2. List therapeutic interventions that are used in the home.

3. Explain why teaching is important in delivering home care services.

4. Explain why a therapist working in home health care needs to adapt to clients' different lifestyles.

5. Describe the relationship between the occupational therapist and the occupational therapy assistant (OTA) in home health care.

6. What team members are likely to provide services in a home health setting and what are their responsibilities?

7. Has there been a recent increase in need for occupational therapy services in the home?

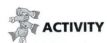 ACTIVITY

Materials

Case Studies 47 and 48 located at the end of this chapter.

Instructions

1. Work with a partner or small group and use the two case studies assigned by your instructor to answer the following questions.

Case No.: _____

   a. What safety considerations will you need to evaluate in the home?

b. What are the client's adaptive equipment needs?

c. List the intervention concerns that you will want to discuss and assess with the caregiver.

d. Write one long-term goal and two short-term goals and for this client.

e. How will you begin your intervention services? List possible activities, the needed setup, and the approximate time needed for your first session.

ACTIVITY	SETUP	TIME

f. What additional activities might you use in future treatment sessions?

g. Assume that you have met the initial short-term goals written for this client. Write two new short-term goals.

h. Describe the kind of supervision needed if the treatment for this client were provided by an OTA.

i. Discuss as a class and record below treatment ideas you would like to remember.

Case No.: _____

a. What safety considerations will you need to evaluate in the home?

b. What are the client's adaptive equipment needs?

c. List the intervention concerns that you will want to discuss and assess with the caregiver.

d. Write one long-term goal and two short-term goals for this client.

e. How will you begin your intervention services? List possible activities, the needed setup, and the approximate time needed for your first session.

ACTIVITY	SETUP	TIME

f. What additional activities might you use in future treatment sessions?

g. Assume that you have met the initial short-term goals written for this client. Write two new short-term goals.

h. Describe the kind of supervision needed if the treatment for this client were provided by an OTA.

i. Discuss as a class and record below treatment ideas you would like to remember.

FOLLOW-UP

✔ Complete the Application of Competencies at the end of this chapter.

WORK HARDENING

Exercise 95

OBJECTIVES

✔ Identify the diagnoses of clients seen in a work hardening setting
✔ Identify components of a work hardening program
✔ Determine a three-week schedule of activities for a client in a work hardening program

DESCRIPTION

This exercise will introduce you to the practice area of work hardening. Work hardening programs are most often provided in a hospital-based program or in an industrial setting. With current federal legislation more workers injured on the job are able to return to work. The Americans with Disabilities Act of 1990 allows that responsible ac-

"Adversity causes some men to break; others to break records."

WILLIAM A. WARD

commodations be made to expedite the return to work. When in a work hardening setting, you will be part of a team working together to return the injured worker to the labor market as efficiently and safely as possible. Advocating and consulting to prevent job-related injuries might also be part of the services you provide.

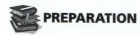 **PREPARATION**

Suggested Readings

AOTA (latest edition)
Internet
Jacobs (1991)
Neidstadt and Crepeau (1998)
Pedretti (1996)
Occupational Safety & Health Administration (OSHA) web site:
http://www.osha.gov

Study Questions

1. Define the following terms:
   a. Work practice

   b. Work hardening

   c. Work conditioning

2. Describe the history of work practice in occupational therapy.

3. Describe the objectives of a work hardening program.

4. List the type of clients who are treated in work-related practice and the kinds of occupational therapy programs that are available.

CLIENTS	PROGRAMS

5. Who are the team members that are generally involved in a work hardening program?

6. Briefly summarize guidelines for a work hardening program in the following areas:
    a. Entrance criteria:

    b. Services included:

    c. Exit criteria:

7. What is the length of a typical work hardening program?

8. What work hardening assessments are available for use?

9. Describe how an occupational therapy (OT) practitioner might use a job simulation as part of the evaluation process and/or as an intervention modality.

10. Describe a job site analysis and its contribution to a work hardening program.

11. Discuss the role of prevention education.

12. Summarize AOTA's position on work-related and industrial rehabilitation practice.

13. Visit OSHA's Web site. Summarize the current ergonomic standards.

14. Locate and describe three Internet sites related to industrial rehabilitation.

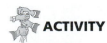 **ACTIVITY**

Materials

Access to a work hardening facility or a slide or video presentation from such a facility; Case Studies 43, 49, and 53, located at the end of this chapter.

Fig. 5-18 A work hardening tour.

Photo courtesy of Ralph Dehner.

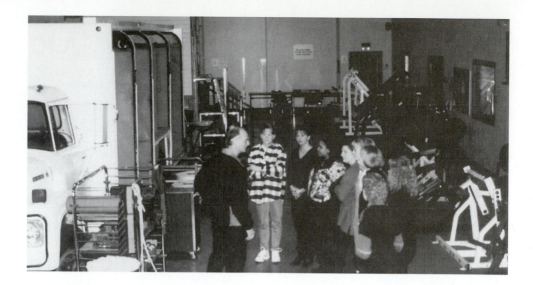

Instructions

1. As a class, visit a local occupational therapy center that focuses on work hardening. Obtain the information identified below. If you are unable to visit a center, gather information from sources available to you, such as slides, a video, or guest speakers.

    a. List the type of injuries and conditions treated.

    b. Name the equipment used.

    c. Describe the types of programs that are available to clients. Include the amount of time spent in therapy and duration of time in the program.

    d. Describe the OT practitioner's responsibilities on the job sites of the clients.

    e. Give your general impressions of the facility and this practice setting.

2a. Working with a partner or small group, plan a three-week program for the client in Case Study 49 located at the end of this chapter. Grade the client's schedule so that he or she will ultimately be involved in activities eight hours a day in your clinic. Include in your schedule the time your client will need to spend with related team members, such as a psychologist, physical therapist, exercise physiologist, and/or vocational counselor. Write two short-term goals and a schedule of appropriate activities.

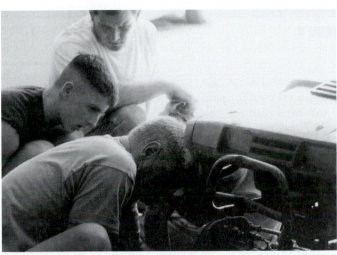 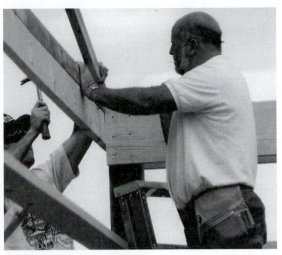

Fig. 5-19a,b In work hardening settings, occupational therapy must prepare clients to meet the demands of a real-life job. *Photo 19a courtesy of Bill Kief, Rob Kief, and Craig Sacksteder. Photo 19b courtesy of Gary Detmer and Dennis Nixon.*

Case No.: _____

    Goals:

    1.

    2.

    Week 1 schedule of activities

    Week 2 schedule of activities

    Week 3 schedule of activities

2b. Share your weekly schedule with your classmates. Note below ideas from your peers that were different from yours.

FOLLOW-UP

✔   Complete the Application of Competencies at the end of this chapter.
✔   Complete Performance Skill 5F on Non-traditional Interventions.

Exercise 96

"Difficulties teach a man."

TURKISH PROVERB

PAIN MANAGEMENT

OBJECTIVES

✔ Differentiate between chronic and acute pain
✔ Describe intervention methods used for pain management
✔ Plan a one-week schedule for a pain management group

DESCRIPTION

This exercise will help you to understand the occupational therapy practitioner's role in pain management. You will encounter the need for pain management in many areas of practice. Both acute and chronic pain can impair an individual's functioning level. As an occupational therapy practitioner you will often be working with individuals with chronic pain. With some conditions and under some circumstances, pain can be alleviated. At other times pain can only be tolerated, and coping strategies must be taught to the client. In therapy you will most often use a variety of approaches to assist in managing pain. In dealing with pain, the behavioral aspects cannot be overlooked, as the interaction of the client with his or her environmental supports needs to be considered.

 PREPARATION

Suggested Readings

Catalano (1987)
Jacobs (1991)
Neidstadt and Crepeau (1998)
Trombly (1995)

Study Questions

1. Describe what is meant by chronic pain.

2. Describe some of the causes of chronic pain.

3. Describe some of the psychosocial characteristics of clients who have chronic pain.

4. List what are considered pain behaviors.

5. In addition to occupational therapy, what other professionals might be on the pain management team providing services to clients?

6. Describe treatment methods used in occupational therapy for pain management.

7. Describe how a client's interaction with his or her environment might prolong chronic pain.

8. List methods of assessing pain intensity.

9. List additional assessment measures that are appropriate for using with the client presenting with acute and or chronic pain.

10. Describe the relationship between pain and stress management.

11. List strategies that may be helpful in decreasing resistant behaviors in your client.

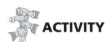 **ACTIVITY**

Materials

None.

Instructions

1a. In a small group, plan a weekly schedule for an outpatient pain management group. The group will be in your clinic eight hours each day, Monday through Saturday. Create four brief case studies of clients who will be in your group. Determine the needs of these clients and activities to address those needs. List at least three goals of your group and plan a weekly schedule for these clients. Include in your schedule the time your client will spend with other team members, such as a psychologist, physical therapy, and or rehabilitation counselor.

CASE DESCRIPTIONS	
1.	2.
3.	4.

NEEDS OF THE CLIENTS	ACTIVITIES TO ADDRESS NEEDS

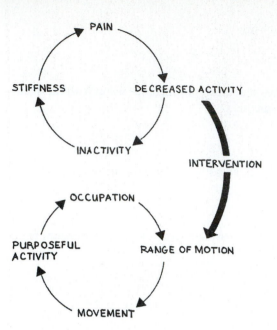

Fig. 5-20 Occupational therapy will help to interrupt the pain cycle and assist the person in returning to functional activities.

GROUP GOALS:

1.

2.

3.

WEEKLY SCHEDULE						
TIME	MONDAY	TUESDAY	WEDNESDAY	THURSDAY	FRIDAY	SATURDAY

1b. Share and discuss ideas with your class. Record below ideas generated by your peers that you had not thought about.

FOLLOW-UP

✔   Complete the Application of Competencies at the end of this chapter.

SPLINTING

Exercise 97

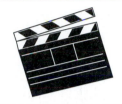

OBJECTIVES

✔   Identify anatomical landmarks of the hand
✔   Describe the biomechanical principles of splinting
✔   Create a splint to facilitate the normal resting position of the hand

DESCRIPTION

This exercise will give you an opportunity to create a hand splint. Splints are made to restore or facilitate function of the hand. Each hand is uniquely different, and an occupational therapy practitioner fabricating splints needs to be knowledgeable about the many types of splints that can be made and splinting materials that can be used. Instructing a client in the use of the splint, the wearing schedule, and associated precautions will all be part of your role. The hand is a very important tool of function. Facilitating that function will enable your clients to interact and communicate with their environment.

"The human hand may be viewed as the brain's most important instrument with which to explore and master the world. It is the only body part that can substitute for other senses."

CARROLL ENGLISH

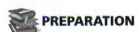 **PREPARATION**

Suggested Readings

Coppard and Lohman (1996)
Neidstadt and Crepeau (1998)
Pedretti (1996)
Rehabilitation Division, Smith and Nephew (1998)

Study Questions

1. Describe the role of occupational therapy in splinting.

2. Complete the crossword puzzle, identifying splinting-related terms.

3. Describe several purposes of splinting.

4. Summarize the biomechanical principles of splinting.

5. List precautions associated with splinting.

DOWN

1. Ability to return to a shape
2. Temporary and part of treatment
3. Sticks to itself
4. Movable parts

ACROSS

1. Resistance to stretching
2. Used to replace lost function
3. Immovable part
4. Conforms easily

6. Watch the CD-ROM *Splinting Made Easy: Just Add Water* (Rehabilitation Division, Smith and Nephew, 1998). Answer the following questions:

   a. What materials are being used?

   b. What is important to remember about the creases and arches of the hand?

   c. What is important to remember in finishing a splint?

7. Describe the antideformity (functional) position of the hand for splinting.

 ACTIVITY

Materials

Variety of thermoplastic, electric fry pans, scissors, paper towels, towels, spatulas, hook and loop closure material, padding, sample splints.

Instructions

1. Locate the following anatomical landmarks on several classmate's hands. Place the name of the person who has the arch or crease you identified in the designated space on the table on page 527. Check your answers with one of the suggested reading resources.

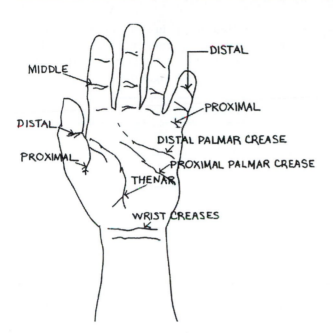

MIDDLE

DISTAL

DISTAL

PROXIMAL

PROXIMAL

DISTAL PALMAR CREASE

PROXIMAL PALMAR CREASE

THENAR

WRIST CREASES

Fig. 5-21 In splinting, it is important to know the creases and arches of the hand.

ARCHES	NAMES OF CLASSMATES		
Distal transverse arch			
Proximal transverse arch			
Longitudinal arch			
CREASES			
Distal digital crease			
Middle digital crease			
Proximal digital crease			
Distal palmar crease			
Proximal palmar crease			
Thenar crease			
Wrist crease dorsal/volar			

2. Manipulate the following splints in your lab. Write a brief description of the splint and the hand condition it may be used to treat.

SPLINT	DESCRIPTION	CONDITION
Volar wrist cock-up		
Dorsal wrist cock-up		
Resting hand		
Thumb spica		
Finger spreader		
Hard cone design		
Arthritis-mitt splint		
Soft splints		
Other:		
Other:		

3. Experiment with various splinting materials available in your lab. Heat, manipulate, and cut them to become familiar with their properties. In the following chart, list the various splinting materials, the temperature used to heat them, their characteristics, and the qualities you observed as the heating process took place.

MATERIAL	TEMPERATURE	CHARACTERISTICS	QUALITIES

4a. Fabricate the three splints indicated below for your partner. Have your instructor check for quality. Record comments on the characteristics of your splint as indicated below.

	WRIST COCK-UP	THUMB SPICA	RESTING HAND
Proper fit			
Absence of pressure areas			
Appealing cosmesis			
Proper position			

4b. Give your partner instructions for the care of his or her splint, a recommended wearing schedule, and precautions for wearing. Write directions below that are given to you by your partner.

CARE	WEARING SCHEDULE	PRECAUTIONS

4c. Wear the splint that has been made for you as directed by your partner. Record your partner's impressions below. Make certain to give this feedback to your partner during the next class period.

1. Comfort:

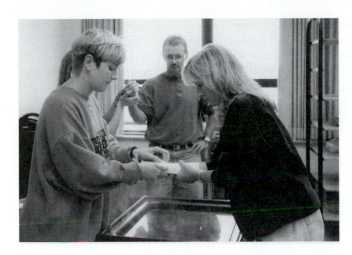

Fig. 5-22 Learning the art of splinting.
Photo courtesy of Tim Dirr, Laurie Brady, and Michelle Kenkel.

2. Effect on function:

3. Overall impression/comments:

4d. Record below your partner's feedback on your splint fabrication.
1. Comfort:

2. Effect on function:

3. Overall impression/comments:

FOLLOW-UP

✔ Complete the Application of Competencies at the end of this chapter.
✔ For your splint fabrication skills complete an Analysis of Self located in Appendix B.

UPPER EXTREMITY AMPUTATIONS AND PROSTHETICS

Exercise 98

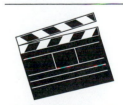

OBJECTIVES

✔ Identify the amputation levels of the upper extremity
✔ Describe various upper extremity prosthetic devices
✔ Detail the care of and training in use of a prosthetic device

DESCRIPTION

This exercise will help you to understand your role in working with a client who has an upper extremity amputation. Most often clients with an upper extremity amputation are fitted with a prosthetic device. It will be your role to help determine whether a de-

"Questioning is the door of knowledge."

IRISH PROVERB

vice is necessary, what device, the correct size, and type, as well as educating the client in its care and use. In this role you will be part of a team providing support and services to the individual with an upper extremity amputation. All team members will need to work together closely to ensure a match between the user's needs and abilities and the potential of the prosthetic device. Additionally, a client's psychological and emotional adjustment to his or her changed body image and function will be important considerations in your intervention.

PREPARATION

Suggested Readings

Pedretti (1996)
Trombly (1995)

Study Questions

1. Identify conditions or circumstances that may result in an upper extremity amputation.

2. Indicate the levels of upper extremity amputation, the loss of function, and the suggested functional prosthetic components required to operate a prosthetic device.
   a. Level of amputation

   b. Loss of function

   c. Suggested functional prosthetic components

3. Briefly describe types of occupational therapy intervention techniques that are used in the treatment of upper extremity amputation.

INTERVENTION TECHNIQUE	DESCRIPTION

4. Describe related medical problems and precautions you will need to follow in working with a client with an upper extremity amputation.

5. Describe potential psychological adjustments that a person may experience after an amputation and what can be done to facilitate recovery.

6. Name and describe the two most common types of terminal devices.

    a.

    b.

7. Describe the client training you may want to consider using in the following areas:

    a. Prehension training

    b. Independent living skills

    c. Leisure interests

    d. Driving training

    e. Work-related activities

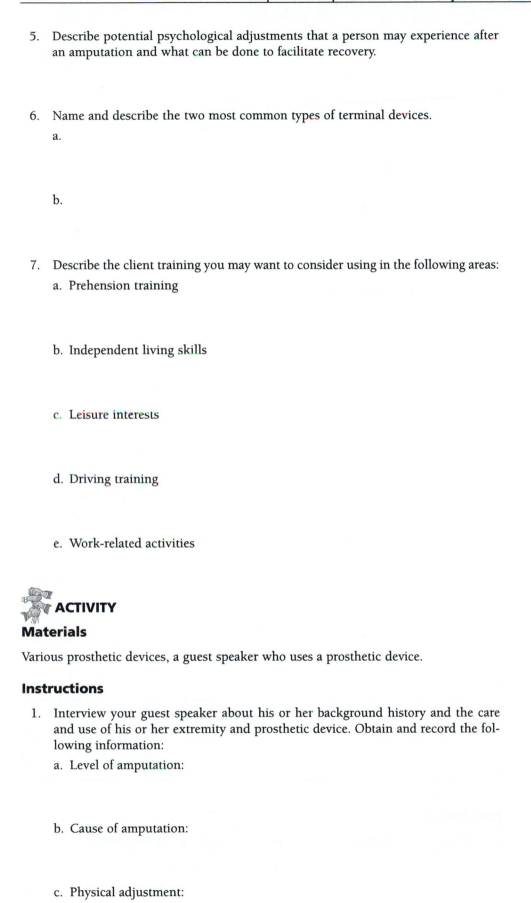 **ACTIVITY**

Materials

Various prosthetic devices, a guest speaker who uses a prosthetic device.

Instructions

1. Interview your guest speaker about his or her background history and the care and use of his or her extremity and prosthetic device. Obtain and record the following information:

    a. Level of amputation:

    b. Cause of amputation:

    c. Physical adjustment:

    d. Participation in rehab services:

    e. Application/removal procedure for prosthesis:

    f. Control of prosthetic device:

    g. Performance of ADL skills:

    h. Psychological adjustment:

    i. Any other comments:

2. Experiment with the various prosthetic devices available during class. Record the type and description below.

PROSTHETIC DEVICE	DESCRIPTION

FOLLOW-UP

✔   Complete the Application of Competencies at the end of this chapter.

HAND THERAPY AND PHYSICAL AGENT MODALITIES

Exercise 99

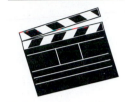

OBJECTIVES

✔ Summarize occupational therapy's national and state position on the use of physical agent modalities (PAMs) in occupational therapy

✔ Identify the treatment implications of commonly used PAMs in a hand therapy setting

✔ Select appropriate functional treatment activities to be used before, during, or after the use of PAMs

DESCRIPTION

This exercise will introduce you to the use of physical agent modalities (PAMs) used in a hand therapy setting. PAMs are used in hand therapy settings, though not exclusively so. PAMs represent an array of modalities that produce a soft tissue response in a client through using light, water, temperature, sound, or electricity. They are used either before, during, or after the client engages in functional activities and are considered an adjunct modality. To be competent in the use of PAMs, further education and experience will be necessary, as the use of PAMs is not considered an entry-level skill. Additionally, some state licensure laws restrict the use of PAMs, so you will need to review your state licensure laws for indication of their use in your state.

"Hands: Who does not know the value of a gentle touch? A fine made chair? A delicious pie? Hands are the tools of productivity and sensitivity."

SANDRA LEWIS

PREPARATION

Suggested Readings

AOTA (latest edition)
Pedretti (1996)
Trombly (1995)
State licensure laws

Study Questions

1. List the most common diagnoses clients may have who are treated in hand therapy.

2. List one technique used for each of the following conditions:

   a. Reflex sympathetic dystrophy

   b. Hypertrophic scar

   c. Flexor tendon injuries

   d. Edema

   e. Nerve repair

3. Describe the following PAMs and list a corresponding treatment implication as well as a contraindication to treatment.

PHYSICAL AGENT	DESCRIBE	TREATMENT IMPLICATION	CONTRAINDICATION
Paraffin			
Hot packs			
Cryotherapy			
Whirlpool			
Electrical stimulation			
Fluidotherapy			
Transcutaneous electrical nerve stimulation			

4. Describe the role of the occupational therapy practitioner in the use of PAMs.

5. Briefly summarize AOTA's position on the use of physical agent modalities in occupational therapy.

6. Briefly summarize your state licensure laws regarding the use of PAMs.

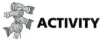 **ACTIVITY**

Materials

Access to a hand therapy clinic where physical agent modalities are used; Case Studies 50 and 51 located at the end of this chapter.

Instructions

1a. As a class, visit a hand therapy clinic. Observe and interact with the modalities used at this facility. Record each modality, how it is used in treatment, and your reaction to its use on you.

MODALITY	TREATMENT PURPOSE	YOUR REACTION

1b. Obtain information from the hand therapist on injuries, conditions, and functional limitations of people who are most commonly seen in occupational therapy, their referral source, and the intervention that may be indicated. Record this information below.

INJURIES/ CONDITIONS	FUNCTIONAL LIMITATIONS	REFERRAL SOURCE	INTERVENTION PROGRAM

2. Using the modalities available to you, describe how they could be used with Case Studies 50 and 51, found at the end of this chapter. Describe the modality and then demonstrate functional activities you would implement before, during, or after use of the modality to the class.

BRIEF CASE DESCRIPTION	MODALITY AND DESCRIPTION	ACTIVITIES

FOLLOW-UP

✔   Complete the Application of Competencies at the end of this chapter.

Exercise 100

"For most occupational therapy practitioners, cones would not be considered an occupational form nor would stacking be part of occupational performance unless that patient worked at Diary Queen or spent time on his or her job sorting those large orange cones used to indicate road construction."

AIMEE LEUBBEN

INTERVENTION PLANNING

OBJECTIVES

✔ Describe the intervention continuum
✔ Select intervention activities based on client's wants, needs, and role expectations
✔ Explain what is meant by a client-centered approach

DESCRIPTION

This exercise will introduce you to the concept of the intervention continuum. Activities for intervention need to be based on the client's wants, needs, and occupational role performance expectations. Interventions that are occupation-based will have the most transferability to a client's current life experiences. Getting a client to this level is the goal of intervention and purposeful activities, enabling activities, as well as adjunctive methods can help a client reach that goal. Therapeutic exercise is an adjunctive modality that is often used in a physical rehabilitation setting and its role and place along the continuum needs to be thoroughly understood. Focusing on your client's goals as you work up the intervention continuum facilitates effective intervention. Occupation-based interventions using a client-centered approach help produce the most rewarding and meaningful results.

PREPARATION

Suggested Readings

AOTA (1998)
Law (1998)
Pedretti (1996)
Trombly (1995)

STUDY QUESTIONS

1. Describe what is meant by the treatment continuum. Detail and give examples of activities you may see in each of the following along the continuum.

   a. Adjunctive methods:

   b. Enabling activities:

   c. Purposeful activities:

   d. Occupational performance/roles:

2. Define therapeutic exercise as it is used as an adjunctive modality.

3. State several purposes for using therapeutic exercise as a treatment technique.

4. Describe the populations for whom the use of therapeutic exercise is most appropriate and for whom it is contraindicated.

5. List examples of exercises used to work on the target areas below.
   a. Cardiovascular fitness

   b. Range of motion

   c. Coordination

   d. Strength

   e. Range of motion (gravity eliminated)

   f. Muscle strength with no motion

6. Draw lines to match each of the following terms with its closest description:

   - Eccentric contraction
   - Isotonic resistive exercise

   - Isometric contraction
   - Isotonic active exercise

   - Active-assistive exercise
   - Passive exercise
   - Isotonic or concentric contraction
   - Active stretch
   - Isometric exercise without resistance
   - Passive stretch

   - Isometric exercise with resistance

   - Moves through range with no resistance
   - Moves through partial range then assisted to completion
   - As muscle lengthens, tension is the same
   - Holding a weight in the hand while the wrist is stabilized
   - Muscle contraction with no joint motion
   - No muscle contraction
   - Applied pressure at the end range
   - Joint movement with muscle shortening
   - Joint movement against a load
   - Actively contracting muscles without movement
   - Force of agonist increases the antagonist

7. What principles should be considered in selecting activities or occupations to be therapeutic?

8. What characteristics must activities have to be used for physical restoration?

9. Describe methods an occupational therapy practitioner may use to individualize activity selection.

10. Describe the relationship between exercise and purposeful activity.

11. Describe techniques to apply the "The Psychosocial Core of Occupational Therapy" (AOTA, 1998) with clients in a physical disability setting.

12. Describe what is meant by a client-centered approach to intervention.

13. List several strategies that you may use to incorporate the client-centered approach into your treatment.

14. Describe how the treatment approach and goaling process affect a client's motivation.

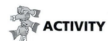 **ACTIVITY**

Materials

Index cards, Case Studies 48, 50, and 52 located at the end of this chapter.

Instructions

1. For each of the performance components selected below state one adjunctive method, one enabling activity, one purposeful activity, and one occupational performance based activity that could be used in treatment of each component. Share ideas with your class and taking notes on those you want to remember. The first one is completed for you.

COMPONENT	ADJUNCTIVE METHOD	ENABLING ACTIVITY	PURPOSEFUL ACTIVITY	OCCUPATIONAL PERFORMANCE ACTIVITY
Fine motor coordination	Passive range of motion and retrograde massage	Manipulate theraputty into small balls	Play a game of checkers with small pegs	Write thank you notes to friends who have sent you flowers
Range of motion				
Strength				
Memory				

Postural control				
Problem solving				
Gross motor coordination				
Praxis				
Sequencing				
Oral/motor control				

2. With your partner or small group, use the case study assigned by your instructor to plan a treatment session incorporating a variety of activities from the different stages of the treatment or intervention continuum. First, have your partner role-play the client in the case taking on a chosen identity and culture. Interview your client to determine what he/she wants, what he/she needs, and what he/she is expected to do in his/her occupational roles. Next, work with the client discussing the goals he/she would like to achieve. Rank order the importance of the goals. Discontinue the role play and together work on planning intervention for that client. Based on the interview information, select three goals with accompanying activities. Use the designated spaces below to describe the simulated client and plan intervention. With each goal, describe your activity selection in the intervention continuum stage where it most closely aligns. Activities are not needed in stages one and two, but they must be included in stages three and four. Share your completed plan with the class.

Case study description

a. Client's wants, needs, and expected occupational performance/roles:

b. Three goals valued by client and conjointly agreed to:

c. Selected occupations for each goal:

Goal No. 1:

ADJUNCTIVE METHODS	ENABLING ACTIVITIES	PURPOSEFUL ACTIVITIES	OCCUPATIONAL/ROLE PERFORMANCE

Goal No. 2:

ADJUNCTIVE METHODS	ENABLING ACTIVITIES	PURPOSEFUL ACTIVITIES	OCCUPATIONAL/ROLE PERFORMANCE

Goal No. 3

ADJUNCTIVE METHODS	ENABLING ACTIVITIES	PURPOSEFUL ACTIVITIES	OCCUPATIONAL/ROLE PERFORMANCE

d. What safety precautions would you need to follow with this client?

e. Describe how you would include family members/caregivers in treatment.

f. Describe how group treatment could be used with this client.

g. Describe how you will determine when this client is ready for discharge.

h. Describe what related services this client may need including outside referrals.

i. Describe the role of the OTA and the OT in this client's progression through treatment.

GAME

3. With your class play the game "Who Wants to Be an OT Practitioner" based on the popular television show "Who Wants to Be a Millionaire?" To prepare for the game, generate one question based on the study questions and activities in this exercise. Put the question on an index card and include the answer on the other side. (Several sample questions have been provided for you to jumpstart your thinking). Divide into two groups. Select one student from each group to answer the questions. Give each student an opportunity to answer four questions previously generated from the other group in your class. To answer the questions, each student may select one assist for three out of the four questions; one of the four questions needs to be completed without an assist. Assists include: asking the entire group for help; asking to have two wrong answers taken away delimiting the answer to two choices; and consulting one resource book of his/her choice for 60 seconds. Declare the winning team by which student answers the most questions correctly. If both students correctly answer the same number of questions, have the game go to a final round. Participate with your entire group during the final round having the entire group rather than an individual representative answer the questions. Declare the winner by which group first gives a correct answer. Final round questions may be selected from instructor-generated questions.

Study Questions

1. Put the following activities in order according to what stage (1 = adjunctive modalities; 2 = enabling activities; 3 = purposeful activities; 4 = occupational performance) they occur in the treatment continuum.

   a. Stacking cones
   b. Passive range of motion
   c. Reaching for supplies to make your favorite lunch
   d. Putting away groceries in the clinic kitchen

2. Which of the following would be an occupational performance activity?

   a. Dowel rod exercises to improve strength to do home management
   b. Transfer training from mat to chair
   c. Folding hospital towels
   d. Doing personal laundry

3. In the movie "Karate Kid" Mr Miagie gives Daniel activities to do to prepare him to learn karate. In fact he refuses to teach him karate until he completes these ac-

tivities. Select which aspect of the intervention continuum the preparation activities would be considered.

a. Adjunctive methods
b. Enabling activities
c. Purposeful activity
d. Occupational performance

FOLLOW-UP

✔   Complete the Application of Competencies at the end of this chapter.
✔   Complete Performance Skill 5C on Adding to Your Files.
✔   Complete Performance 5E on Intervention Planning.

Application of Competencies   After completing each exercise, record one concept you learned and how you anticipate that learning will influence your interaction and intervention with clients.

Exercise 76 Observation Skills
Application:

Exercise 77 Standardized Assessments
Application:

Exercise 78 Muscle Testing
Application:

Exercise 79 Vital Signs
Application:

Exercise 80 Sensory Assessment and Reeducation
Application:

Exercise 81 Transfers and Positioning
Application:

Exercise 82 Range of Motion
Application:

Exercise 83 Activities of Daily Living
Application:

Exercise 84 Wheelchairs
Application:

Exercise 85 Cognitive Impairments
Application:

Exercise 86 Perceptual Impairments
Application:

Exercise 87 Neurodevelopmental Treatment
Application:

Exercise 88 Proprioceptive Neuromuscular Facilitation
Application:

Exercise 89 Spinal Cord Injury
Application:

Exercise 90 Home Management
Application:

Exercise 91 Assistive Technologies
Application:

Exercise 92 Therapeutic Adaptations
Application:

Exercise 93 Medical Equipment in Client Care
Application:

Exercise 94 Home Health
Application:

Exercise 95 Work Hardening
Application:

Exercise 96 Pain Management
Application:

Exercise 97 Splinting
Application:

Exercise 98 Upper Extremity Amputations and Prosthetics
Application:

Exercise 99 Hand Therapy and Physical Agent Modalities
Application:

Exercise 100 Intervention Planning
Application:

Performance Skill 5A

DISABILITY SIMULATION

Assume a disability for six to eight hours on arising. Assemble needed equipment and supplies the night before. Experience what a typical day may be like for someone with a disability. Listed below are several suggestions of activities in which you may engage, but be creative and don't limit yourself to this list. You may need to take a friend to provide assistance. The more you do, the more you will learn!

Disability assumed _____

☐ Perform all ADLs

☐ Access public transportation

☐ Access private transportation

☐ Go shopping

☐ Go out to dinner

☐ Cross an intersection

☐ Use a public restroom

☐ Go to the bank

☐ Other: _____

☐ Other: _____

☐ Other: _____

Check all the activities that you experienced. Write a paper describing your experiences, barriers, and limitations.

Performance Skill 5B

FABRICATION OF ADAPTIVE DEVICE

Select a case study from a client with whom you worked on fieldwork or a case study given to you by your instructor. Make a piece of adaptive equipment for this client or case study. Create your own device or make modifications to a piece of equipment that is already used in occupational therapy. Record your creation here.

Case description or number: _____

_____

_____

Device created: _____

Materials used: _____

Cost: _____   Commercial cost: _____

Goals met by device: _____

_____

_____

_____

ADDING TO YOUR FILES

Search and add to your activity file for adults. Type a paper for each activity with the information in the chart and assemble these with a table of contents. Include in your file at least one activity that will work on the targeted areas listed below. Note on each occupation the ages for which it is intended. Be sure to have activities for a wide variety of ages. Include activities that have diverse cultural and contextual qualities. Use at least three references that you have not used previously. List the occupations and activities you have gathered. Check each box as you complete the requirements. When the chart is completed, you will have at least eighteen new activities.

Check as you complete each section

TARGETED AREA	OCCUPATION	RATIONALE	PERFORMANCE CONTEXT	SUPPLIES/ MATERIALS	STEPS TO PERFORM	ADAPTATIONS	PRECAUTIONS	REFERENCES
UE strength								
Hand strength								
Fine motor								
ROM								
Endurance								
Functional standing balance								
UE bilateral								
Functional transfers								
Dynamic sitting balance								
Trunk rotation								
Memory								
Figure ground								
Tactile discrimination								
Weight bearing on UE								
Reaching to the floor from sitting								
Reaching to the floor from standing								
Keyboard skills								
Eye-hand coordination								

Performance Skill 5D

ACTIVITY ADAPTATION

Select and adapt an activity for three different disabilities. The activity can either be a leisure time or work activity. Make a different physical change for each disability chosen. Use this sheet to record your results. An example is completed for you.

ACTIVITY ADAPTED: FISHING		
DISABILITY	CHANGE(S) MADE	MATERIALS AND COST
Left CVA	Fishing pole adapted with a holder that is attached around the client's waist	Webbing: $6.00 Velcro: $3.00 Leather: $10.00 Foam: $1.00

Activity Adapted: _____

DISABILITY	CHANGE(S) MADE	MATERIALS AND COST

Performance Skill 5E

INTERVENTION PLANNING

Given a case study, plan two one-hour intervention sessions using the treatment planning guide below. Vary your treatment, spending time in at least two settings in the clinic (homemaking, ADL, general treatment setting). Use the space below to begin planning, then formally type up the plan. Identify your client's problem areas and strengths. On the basis of that information, write three to five short-term goals, determine the frame of reference you will use, select occupations to meet the goals, describe the setup you will need, and explain your rationale for your activity choices.

Case description or number: _____

Problems identified:

_____

_____

_____

_____

Strengths:

_____

_____

_____

Goals:

_____

_____

_____

_____

GOAL	FRAME OF REFERENCE	OCCUPATIONS	SETUP	RATIONALE

NONTRADITIONAL INTERVENTIONS

Performance Skill 5F

With a partner, find information on one nontraditional intervention used in occupational therapy. Interview at least one OT practitioner who uses this therapeutic technique to gain information about it. Plan to present the information to your classmates. Make your presentation interesting and include resources for the class to use at a later date. Some of the nontraditional interventions on which you may want to gather information include aquatics, tai chi, craniosacral, pet therapy, hippotherapy, and forensic. This list is far from inclusive; feel free to investigate other interventions. Use the following space to prepare your presentation and record the information from the presentation of your peers. After your peers' presentations, critique their performance on the form provided. Look at the scoring criteria ahead of time so that you know the criteria from which you will be critiqued.

Topic chosen: _____

Description:

Resources:

Therapeutic implications:

Topic: _____

Description:

Resources:

Therapeutic implications:

Topic: _____

Description:

Resources:

Therapeutic implications:

Nontraditional Interventions Peer Evaluation Form

Topic: _____

Group members presenting:

Group appeared organized and prepared.

Group shared equally in the presentation.

Information presented in a clear and logical format.

Presentation completed in a professional manner.

Resources provided to students.

Group related this topic to actual practice setting.

ACUTE CARE

Type:
Intensive Care

Age:
27 years old

Sex:
Male

Culture/Religion:

Insurance Information:

Diagnosis:
MVA: Multiple trauma

Social History:
Eric is a young adult living with his parents and two younger sisters in a rural community about thirty miles from the hospital. His family is very supportive, visiting him at the hospital every day. Eric fell asleep while driving his friend home from a party; his friend suffered fatal injuries.

Medical History:
Eric is currently in intensive care and has assisted breathing on a ventilator. He is semi-comatose. When alert, he will follow with his eyes. Verbal responses cannot be assessed owing to ventilator status. On command, he can move his right foot. Eric has a possible brachial plexus injury to his right UE, a T_{12} compression fracture, flail right arm, right humeral head fracture, and a lacerated liver. He lost the third, fourth, and fifth fingers on his left hand. He has skin grafts on this area. He also has a large open area on his occipital area, which has been grafted. His OT orders are for general rehabilitation, scar massage, ROM, and splinting. He has weight-bearing and ROM restrictions in the right UE and right LE. He tolerates sitting on the edge of the bed with maximal assistance of two for five minutes before tiring. He appears to have extensive sensory deficits in both UEs at this time.

ADULT REHABILITATION

Type:
Inpatient

Age:
26 years old

Sex:
Male

Culture/Religion:

Insurance Information:

Diagnosis:
Spinal cord injury, C4–7

Social History:

David is single and lives in his own apartment. He played the guitar and enjoys all kinds of music. David is very social and enjoys going to nightclubs with his friends.

David's parents live out of town and would probably not be willing to assist. They have three other teenage children at home. They live in a four-bedroom, bilevel home, and both parents work full-time.

Medical History:

David fell off a ladder at a construction site where he was working. He has a halo applied and is agitated and noncompliant. He has C5–6 UE movement and some spasticity. He can move both elbows to 40° flexion, and he has no grasp.

David has phila collar from the brace shop, teds, and abdominal binder; sits on a ROHO; and has resting hand splints. He requires maximum assistance of two for sliding board transfers. He is currently dependent in all self-care.

CASE STUDY 38

ADULT REHABILITATION

Type:
Inpatient

Age:
56 years old

Sex:
Male

Culture/Religion:

Insurance Information:

Diagnosis:
Perforated viscous; S/P repair one month ago, M.S., COPD

Social History:
James lives alone in a one-bedroom apartment. He has 18 steps to his floor. He is divorced and has seven children, but none keep in touch. He is on disability and has no other interests besides watching television.

Medical History:
James is oriented and intact perceptually. He c/o double vision. His endurance is fair, and he walks with a cane. He transfers and demonstrates independent mobility in his room. James describes increased difficulty bathing, walking, climbing stairs, and standing to cook.

At this time James is independent in feeding and UE dressing. He requires assistance with LEs. James has full active ROM in both UEs; strength is fair bilaterally. He has impaired stereognosis in his fingers, but all other sensation is intact.

James reports being very apprehensive about going home.

CASE STUDY 39

ACUTE CARE

Type:
Acute Care

Age:
36 years old

Sex:
Male

Culture/Religion:

Insurance Information:

Diagnosis:
Mitral endocarditis, embolic CVA

Social History:
Mike has a history of drug abuse, shared needles, and multiple sex partners. He smokes two packs of cigarettes a day. He lives alone in an efficiency apartment and does odd jobs for a living.

Medical History:
Mike has undergone a valve replacement. This is his third admission for endocarditis. Mike has expressive aphasia, is dysarthric, and has been choking on liquids. He is scheduled to have a Hickman catheter placed and will need six weeks of therapy at a skilled nursing facility to monitor this.

Mike has been uncooperative, becoming angry and refusing to participate in many tasks.

His left UE is WNL. His right UE is beginning to move in flexion synergy patterns. It appears to have little voluntary control and is generally held close to body with the elbow bent at 90°, the wrist in slight flexion and the hand fisted. Mike is independent in chair to bed transfers, but is at times unsteady. He moves quickly and is at times impulsive.

Mike is set up at the sink to perform his ADLs. He is independent in washing his face, chest, and top of legs. He requires cueing and directions to wash his arms, legs, and back. Dressing is performed with moderate assistance to demonstrate. Mike is frustrated frequently, and therapy sessions are often terminated early because of this.

ADULT REHABILITATION

CASE STUDY 40

Type:
Inpatient

Age:
58 years old

Sex:
Male

Culture/Religion:

Insurance Information:

Diagnosis:
General debility with deconditioning, S/P right CVA with left hemiparesis, admitted with femoral neck fracture, S/P bipolar arthroplasty left hip, major depressive disorder

Social History:
Jesse lives with his wife, who is currently not working. He is noncompliant with his care and is becoming extremely difficult for his wife to care for. He formerly worked as a short-order cook. There are plans to be made about alternative placement at this time.

Medical History:

Jesse has end-stage renal disease and receives hemodialysis on MWF. He had a spleenectomy, hypertension, hypothyroidism, and history of DVT. He has been on disability for fifteen years.

Jesse is able to do his feeding and grooming independently. He requires minimum assistance with dressing UEs and maximum assistance with LEs. He bathes with minimum assistance and transfers with maximum assistance.

His muscle strength in UEs is G to G− on right, F to F− on left. He has 60 pounds grip on right and 27 pounds on left. His AROM in left UE is 65 degrees shoulder flexion and 75 degrees abduction. He is oriented x3 and able to follow two-step directions.

CASE STUDY 41

ADULT REHABILITATION

Type:
Inpatient

Age:
42 years old

Sex:
Male

Culture/Religion:

Insurance Information:

Diagnosis:
Multiple trauma motorcycle accident—head-on collision without helmet, CHI/TBI, Ranchos Los Amigos Scale 5

Social History:
Before the accident Carlos lived alone on a farm that has a one-story house with two steps. He works the crops on the farm for his living. Several close friends are involved in his recovery.

Medical History:
Carlos is ten days post-accident, transferred from the general hospital. He has multiple rib fractures and right distal clavicular fracture, left retinal hemorrhage, right sphenoid fracture, and right zygomatic arch fracture.

Carlos has right ROM WNL in both UEs but complains of pain in left shoulder. His grip strength is 35 in the right hand and 36 on the left.

He is oriented x1, agitated, combatant, and easily distracted. At this time he is unable to follow one-step commands. He is an extreme safety risk and should have a seat belt in bed and chair.

He currently requires maximal assistance with ADLs, minimum assistance to supine to sit, and SBA sitting at bedside.

He ambulates quickly when given the chance but is very unsafe in his manner.

ACUTE CARE

Type:
Acute Care

Age:
56 years old

Sex:
Female

Culture/Religion:

Insurance Information:

Diagnosis:
23% burns to face, arms, and legs; schizophrenia; mild mental retardation

Social History:
Linda lives with her husband and 20-year-old son. She is not employed outside the home. She spends her time at home caring for the house, listening to music, and painting.

Medical History:
Linda set herself on fire at her home. She had been refusing to take her Clozaril for the past several weeks. She was diagnosed with schizophrenia when she was 25 years old. She is currently in the intensive care unit, where she is to be seen for rehabilitation, including ROM and splinting. Linda responds appropriately to yes and no questions but does not follow commands. She yells while being ranged, saying that this is not doing any good and that it should be stopped. She has increased bleeding in her left hand while being ranged. Her elbows are tight due to H.O. PROM is WNL at this time, except for elbow flexion which is 120°. MMT is 3/5 grossly, and she has edema in both hands. She wears safe position splints at all times.

Linda requires maximum assistance of two to move in bed, come to sit, and transfer to a chair.

WORK HARDENING

Type:
Outpatient

Age:
45 years old

Sex:
Male

Culture/Religion:

Insurance Information:

Diagnosis:
Lumbar sprain

Social History:
Tyrone lives with his wife and five children. His wife works at a department store. He is a groundskeeper for the city ballpark.

Medical History:
Tyrone injured his back at work, lifting heavy supplies. He began experiencing difficulty with pain and spasms approximately five months ago; his condition has been getting worse. He is no longer able to work and is afraid of reinjury. On evaluation he has decreased hip abductors and hip extensors. He is very deconditioned and has weight problems.

Tyrone demonstrates inconsistent use of proper body mechanics and moves very stiffly.

CASE STUDY 44

ADULT REHABILITATION

Type:
Outpatient

Age:
32 years old

Sex:
Female

Culture/Religion:

Insurance Information:

Diagnosis:
Rheumatoid arthritis

Social History:
Stephanie is a full-time teacher and is married to a firefighter. They have three small children and all live in a two-story home with a full basement. She is in an acute flare-up of her R.A.

Stephanie's leisure mostly consists of caring for her children. However, she used to enjoy bowling and dancing.

Stephanie has been finding all work extremely difficult and has taken a leave of absence from her job.

Medical History:
Stephanie has been referred by her doctor for evaluation, treatment, and education regarding her arthritis. She has orders for two visits a week.

Stephanie reports having difficulty with fine motor activities, such as buttons, snaps, and handwriting. She has pain in all extremities but complains of most severe pain in her neck, shoulders, and fingers. She has full ROM except for shoulder flexion, which is 110° bilaterally. She is currently walking with a cane in the morning and late evening.

CASE STUDY 45

ACUTE CARE

Type:
Acute Care

Age:
36 years old

Sex:
Female

Culture/Religion:

Insurance Information:

Diagnosis:
MS

Social History:
Juanita lives alone in a one-bedroom apartment; her husband died in a car accident one year ago. She moved out of their house shortly after his death. Juanita worked as a nurse in a pediatrics office. She has been collecting disability for two years now. She enjoys old movies, cooking, and baking. These activities have been increasingly difficult for her to do.

Medical History:
Juanita is admitted with inability to urinate and is unable to catheterize herself for relief. She is also extremely weak, requiring moderate assistance with all mobility and minimum assistance with all self-care.

She has been using a wheelchair for most of her mobility but was able to do a standing transfer independently to all surfaces.

Juanita complains of double vision and lack of stereognosis in her hands. It is becoming more difficult for her to catheterize herself, and her bladder does not empty on its own.

CASE STUDY 46

INTENSIVE CARE

Type:
SICU

Age:
56 years old

Sex:
Male

Culture/Religion:

Insurance Information:

Diagnosis:
Necroticizing pancreatitis, possible CVA, diabetes, HTN

Social History:
Phil came to the hospital from a homeless shelter. He has reportedly been on the streets for several years. It is unknown whether he has any living relatives. No other history has been obtained.

Medical History:
Phil has been in the hospital for forty days. He has been having surgery every other day for debridement. He was admitted with acute abdominal pain. He does not follow commands or open his eyes in response to his name. Orders have been written to keep the patient from deteriorating any further physically.

On arrival in the patient's room, the following equipment was observed:
1. Ventilator
2. Hickman catheter with seven IVs attached
3. Two blood pressure cuffs, one on each arm
4. NG feeding tube
5. NG suction tube
6. Leads from the heart to the heart monitor
7. Two abdominal drainage tubes
8. Catheter
9. Pulse monitor on index finger
10. Electric pump stockings on both legs

PT and OT will co-treat Phil. The initial setup to get him to the side of the bed took 20 minutes and assist from nursing to manage all the leads. He required maximum assistance of two to come to and maintain sitting on edge of bed. While sitting, he did show an increased level of alertness. He responded to simple commands with his right hands and appeared to mouth some words in response to questions. No active movement was noted in his left UE.

CASE STUDY 47

HOME HEALTH

Type:
Home Health

Age:
85 years old

Sex:
Female

Culture/Religion:

Insurance Information:

Diagnosis:
S/P fractured hip and pelvis PMH; NIDDM CABGx3 in 1984, S/P amputation of right great toe, artificial right eye

Living Situation:
Maude lives alone on tenth-floor apartment with elevator. Patient has been receiving rehabilitation in nursing facility for two months.

Prior Level of Functioning:
Maude walked with a cane before she fell.

Strengths:
Maude is alert, oriented, and cooperative. Strength and coordination are WFL. Transfers from lift chair to wheelchair. Standing, sitting balance good.

Problem List:
Maude is sedentary, using a wheelchair for ambulation. She requires moderate assistance with LE bathing and dressing. She requires assistance for meal preparation and laundry.

HOME HEALTH

Type:
Home Health

Age:
67 years old

Sex:
Male

Culture/Religion:

Insurance Information:

Diagnosis:
Right CVA

Social History:
Daniel lives by himself in a small house on ten acres of land; his wife died two years ago. Daniel has no children. He has three brothers, all of whom live out of town. He is retired and spends most of his time with his animals; he has two cats and two dogs, which he has had for years. He enjoys playing cards, which he doesn't get to do often.

Medical History:
Daniel has a history of HTN; he smokes one pack of cigarettes per day. His infarct is in the basal ganglia and thalamic region. His cognitive abilities appear within normal limits. He is currently NPO owing to swallowing difficulties.

On evaluation Daniel presents with intact sensation, proprioception, and stereognosis. He is able to actively flex his left shoulder to 45 degrees and bend his elbow WNL; he has only slight wrist and hand movement.

At this time he requires total assistance in all areas of self-care and is taking maximal assistance of one to move in bed and transfer. He is two weeks post-stroke.

WORK HARDENING

Type:
Outpatient

Age:
48 years old

Sex:
Female

Culture/Religion:

Insurance Information:

Diagnosis:
Disc herniation at L1–S1

Social History:
Valerie is a single mother of six children, ages 6 to 16. They live in a small home. She works at a fast-food restaurant, full-time days. Valerie's husband was shot and killed in a fight. He was very abusive to her and the children, and he was often in trouble with the law.

Medical History:

Valerie injured her back at work while reaching for something on a high shelf. She had a lumbar laminectomy one month ago with no relief and is unable to return to work.

She has diabetes, high blood pressure, TKR, and post surgery: disc removed. Valerie is in constant aching pain with shooting pain in her lower right side.

Valerie complains of being very frustrated, barely able to take care of her children. She appears depressed and withdrawn.

Valerie demonstrates many pain behaviors and moves in a rigid, guarded fashion.

CASE STUDY 50

HAND THERAPY

Type:
Outpatient

Age:
35 years old

Sex:
Female

Culture/Religion:

Insurance Information:

Diagnosis:
Right colles fracture

Social History:
Alice is a homemaker who lives with her husband and two children, ages 6 and 10. She sews for a hobby and has a part-time job. She does alterations, working out of her home.

Medical History:
Alice is three months post fracture with continued decrease functional use of her right hand including pain. She reports pain to be 8/10 with use and 5/10 with rest. She reports burning pain with touch to ulnar border. She has increased hair growth, especially on the ulnar border.

Alice has marked edema in her right hand. She has decreased functional use, decreased wrist flexion/extension, decreased supination, and decreased strength.

She has been referred by her doctor to evaluate and treat.

CASE STUDY 51

HAND THERAPY

Type:
Outpatient

Age:
38 years old

Sex:
Female

Culture/Religion:

Insurance Information:

Diagnosis:
Left wrist pain

Social History:
Heather lives with her girlfriend in a homosexual relationship in their own home. Heather works in a warehouse, doing manual labor, mostly lifting and grabbing. She likes to sew and make crafts.

Medical History:
Heather reports falling on the concrete getting into her car and catching herself with her left hand. She is unable to use her left UE owing to pain. She has not worked in two weeks.

Heather has 35 degrees flexion and 45 degrees wrist extension. Radial and ulnar deviation are both 15 degrees. She has decreased ROM in the thumb along with edema, decreased strength, and function. She has been ordered to come to outpatient therapy three times a week.

WORK HARDENING

Type:
Outpatient

Age:
45 years old

Sex:
Female

Culture/Religion:

Insurance Information:

Diagnosis:
Lumbosacral sprain

Social History:
Wilma is divorced and has custody of her two teenage daughters, both of whom are having behavior problems. In her leisure she used to like to go to the racetrack, watch TV, and garden. Currently, she has no leisure interests in which she feels capable of participating.

Wilma works in a department store in the stock department.

Medical History:
Wilma sprained her back while dropping a box that she was getting off a shelf. Wilma has high blood pressure. On evaluation she presents with decreased trunk mobility and minimal decreased strength lower and upper extremities. She has poor abdominal and back strength, deconditioning, weight problems, decreased endurance, and poor lifting techniques. Wilma exhibits excessive pain behaviors and seems to lack knowledge of pain management techniques and work capabilities.

WORK HARDENING

Type:
Outpatient

Age:
55 years old

Sex:
Male

Culture/Religion:

Insurance Information:

Diagnosis:
Lumbar displacement hernia—hernia operation

Social History:
Steve lives with his wife and three teenage children. The children are all boys and help around the house as needed. Steve is a sheet metal worker in a large factory. He enjoys fishing, golfing, and coaching his boys' sports.

Medical History:
Steve hurt his back at work five months ago. He has been receiving P.T. for two months, but he does not seem to be getting any better. Steve complains of on-and-off sharp, stabbing pain in his back for most of the day. He has received three epidural steroid injections.

Since his injury, Steve has been very sedentary. He reports that the only way he is comfortable is lying down or standing up. He spends most of the day on the couch or walking around the block. He reports being very discouraged with his progress and wishes he could sue someone to make himself feel better.

REFERENCES

Alliance for Technology Access. 1994. *Complete Resources for People with Disabilities: A Guide to Exploring Today's Assistive Technology.* Alameda, CA: Hunter House.

American Guidance Service. 1969. *Pennsylvania Bi-Manual Test.* Circle Pines, MN: Author.

American Occupational Therapy Association. 1998. *Reference Manual of the Official Documents of the American Occupational Therapy Association.* Bethesda, MD: Author.

American Occupational Therapy Association. latest edition. *Reference Manual of the Official Documents of the American Occupational Therapy Association.* Bethesda, MD: Author.

Americans with Disabilities Act of 1996. (PL101-336), 42 U.S.C., 12101, Federal Register, vol. 56:144, 35543–35691.

Angelo, J. 1997. *Assistive Technology for Rehabilitation Therapists.* Philadelphia: F. A. Davis.

Arthritis Foundation. 1988. *Guide to Independent Living for People with Arthritis.* Atlanta, GA: Author.

Catalano, E. M. 1987. *The Chronic Pain Control Workbook: A Step-by-Step Guide for Coping with and Overcoming Your Pain.* Oakland, CA: New Harbinger Publications.

Christiansen, C. ed. 2000. *Ways of Living: Self-Care Strategies for Special Needs.* 2d ed. Rockville, MD: American Occupational Therapy Association.

Colarusso, R. P., D. D. Hammill, and L. Merceir. 1995. *Motor-Free Visual Perception Test.* Rev. Novato, CA: Academic Therapy Publications.

Commission on Practice Home Health Task Force. 1995. *Guidelines for Occupational Therapy Practice in Home Health.* Bethesda, MD: Author.

Cook, A. M., and S. M. Hussey. 1995. *Assistive Technologies: Principles and Practice.* Boston: Mosby.

Coppard, B. M., and H. L. Lohman. 1996. *Introduction to Splinting: A Critical-Thinking and Problem-Solving Approach.* St. Louis, MO: Mosby.

Cromwell, F. S. 1986. *Computer Applications in Occupational Therapy.* New York: Haworth Press.

Daniel, M. S., and L. R. Strickland. 1992. *Occupational Therapy Protocol Management in Adult Physical Dysfunction.* Gaithersburg, MD: Aspen Publishers.

Daniels, L., and C. Worthington. 1986. *Muscle Testing: Techniques of Manual Examination.* 5th ed. Philadelphia: W. B. Saunders.

Early, M. B. 1998. *Physical Dysfunction Practice Skills for the Occupational Therapy Assistant.* St. Louis: Mosby.

Jacobs, K. 1991. *Work-Related Programs and Assessments.* 2d ed. Boston: Little, Brown.

Jebsen, R. H., N. Taylor, R. B. Trieschmann, M. J. Trotter, and L. A. Howard. 1996. "An Objective and Standardized Test of Hand Function." *Archives of Physical Medicine and Rehabilitation* (June): 311–319.

Kendall, F. P., E. K. McCreary, and P. G. Provance. 1993. *Muscles: Testing and Function.* 4th ed. Baltimore, MD: Williams & Wilkins.

Klinger, J. L. 1997. *Meal Preparation and Training: The Health Care Professional's Guide.* Thorofare, NJ: Slack.

Law, M. ed. 1998. *Client-centered occupational therapy.* Thorofare, NJ: Slack.

Lewis, S. C. 1989. *Elder Care in Occupational Therapy.* Thorofare, NJ: Slack.

Mathiowetz, V., K. Weber, N. Kashman, and G. Volland. 1985. Nine Hole Peg Test of Fine Motor Coordination. Bolingbrook, IL: Sammons Preston.

Mayall, J. K., and G. Desharnais. 1990. *Positioning in a Wheelchair: A Guide for Professional Care Givers of the Disabled Adult.* Thorofare, NJ: Slack.

Neidstadt, M. E., and E. B. Crepeau. eds. 1998. *Willard and Spackman's Occupational Therapy.* 9th ed. Philadelphia: Lippincott.

Occupational Safety and Health Administration: web site: http:/www.osha.gov.

Pedretti, L. W. 1996. *Occupational Therapy: Practice Skills for Physical Dysfunction.* 4th ed. St. Louis, MO: Mosby.

Pierson, F. M. 1999. *Principles and Techniques of Patient Care.* Philadelphia: W. B. Saunders.

Ramsammy, H., and P. Brand. *Hand Volumeter.* Idyllwild, CA: Volumeters Unlimited.

Rothstein, J. M., S. H. Roy, and S. L. Wolf. 1998. *The Rehabilitation Specialist's Handbook.* Philadelphia: F. A. Davis.

Rehabilitation Division, Smith and Nephew. 1998. *Splinting Made Easy: Just Add Water.* Germantown, WI: Author.

Sacred Heart General Hospital Oregon Rehabilitation Center. 1987. *New Moves: Wheelchair Skills Video Series.* Programs 1 to 4. Eugene, OR: Author.

Sanford, J. A., R. J. Browne, and A. Turner. 1985–95. *Captain's Log: Cognitive Training System.* Richmond, VA: Braintrain.

Tiffin, J. 1960. *Purdue Pegboard.* Lafayette, IN: Lafayette Instrument.

Trefler, E., D. A. Hobson, S. J. Taylor, L.C. Monahan, and C. G. Shaw. 1993. *Seating and Mobility for Persons with Physical Disabilities.* San Antonio, TX: Therapy Skill Builders.

Trombly, C. A. 1995. *Occupational Therapy for Physical Dysfunction.* 4th ed. Baltimore, MD: Williams & Wilkins.

University of Minnesota Employment Stabilization Research Institute. 1993. *Minnesota Rate of Manipulation Test.* Circle Pines, MN: American Guidance Service.

Zoltan, B. 1996. *Vision, Perception, and Cognition: A Manual for the Evaluation and Treatment of the Neurologically Impaired Adult.* 3d ed. Thorofare, NJ: Slack.

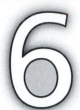

Competencies in Geriatric Practice

Exercise 101

"If you wish to know the road ahead, inquire of those who have traveled it."

CHINESE PROVERB

GETTING IN TOUCH

OBJECTIVES

✔ Identify myths related to the aging process
✔ Analyze personal perceptions about aging and elderly people
✔ Summarize how perceptions affect one's interaction with elderly individuals

DESCRIPTION

Our society is quickly aging, and as it does, the practice area of geriatrics draws more and more occupational therapy practitioners. To work with the geriatric population, you will need much insight and understanding. Abounding myths color our perception of the aging process and people who are elderly. As an occupational therapy practitioner, you need to analyze your own perceptions and sort through those myths to fully understand the persons who are elderly with whom you will be working. Theories on aging will help you with this analysis. When we get in touch with the individuals who are developmentally in the last stages of life, the vibrancy and wisdom that they bring to us can easily be seen.

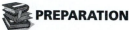**PREPARATION**

Suggested Readings

AOTA (latest edition)
Larson, Stevens-Ratchford, Pedretti, and Crabtree (1996)
Lewis (1989)

Study Questions

1. Before you complete the readings, answer the following questions as they relate to people who are elderly. After answering the questions, go to the references and compare your answers. How accurate were your perceptions?

   a. What percentage of people over age 65 are women?

   b. Are minority people who are elderly more at risk for health concerns than non-minority elderly people?

   c. Is it normal for all people who are elderly to lose cognitive abilities as they age?

   d. Is it true that it is much more difficult to learn when you are over 65?

   e. Will most people who are elderly live in a nursing home in the later stages of life?

2. Describe the people who are elderly you know and your view of the aging process through them.

3. The number of older people in the United States continues to climb. Why does this group of people consume one third of all health care costs?

4. Describe society's attitude toward aging.

5. Describe how the following laws and public initiatives help to protect the rights of the elderly:

   a. Social Security Act

   b. Supplemental Security Income

   c. Older Americans Act

   d. National Institute on Aging

   e. Medicare

   f. Medicaid

6. Outline the following theories as they relate to aging and describe how they may influence your practice as an occupational therapy practitioner:

   a. Activity

   b. Disengagement

   c. Erikson's stages of personality development

   d. Peck's developmental stages

   e. Kohlberg's theory of moral development

7. Describe AOTA's (latest edition) position on occupational therapy and long-term care.

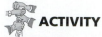 **ACTIVITY**

Materials

Game entitled *Into Aging* (Dempsey-Lyle and Hoffman, n.d.), poem entitled "Preserve Me from the Occupational Therapist, Lord" (MacLay, 1977), essay entitled "My World Now" (Seaver, 1994).

Instructions

1a. Participate in the game *Into Aging* (Dempsey-Lyle and Hoffman, n.d.). What areas of living did the following tables represent and how were they designed?

TABLE	AREA OF LIVING	DESCRIPTION
One		
Two		
Three		

1b. Discuss and record on the following chart the feelings you experienced while playing the game, what made you feel that way, the myth regarding that behavior, and the truth that dispels the myth. A sample is completed for you.

FEELING	BEHAVIOR THAT PRODUCED FEELING	MYTH REGARDING THAT BEHAVIOR	TRUTH TO DISPEL THAT MYTH
Angry	Leader told me that she needed to keep my money so I won't lose it.	Elderly people are all forgetful and unable to manage money on their own.	Most elderly people are able to remain independent in such matters.

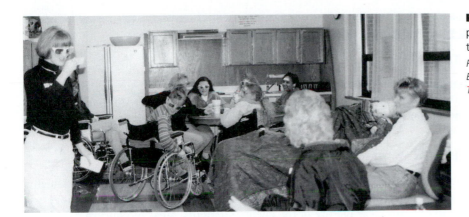

Fig. 6–1 Experiencing life as a person who is elderly when playing the game Into Aging.

Photo courtesy of Leanne Pitcher, Pam Boone, Jessica Johantges, Gina Knab, Tiffany Walker, and Traci Holt.

1c. Discuss and record your summary and overall impressions of the game. Include your thoughts on how this experience can help you to deal more effectively with the elderly.

2a. Listen to the poem "Preserve Me from the Occupational Therapist, Lord" (MacLay, 1977) read aloud. Describe your feelings after listening to the poem.

2b. What assumptions does the occupational therapy practitioner make about the client?

2c. Describe one or more alternative approaches that could be used with this client. Role-play these with your class.

2d. How will you use this information in your work with the elderly?

2e. With what theory about aging does your alternative approach most closely align?

3. Listen to the short essay "My World Now" (Seaver, 1994) read aloud. Record your impressions below as well as the influence this essay may have on your interactions and intervention with the elderly person.

    a. Impressions

    b. Influence on intervention

FOLLOW-UP

✔ Complete the Application of Competencies at the end of this chapter.

Exercise 102

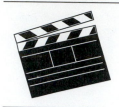

"Hear twice before you speak once."

ENGLISH PROVERB

EVALUATION IN GERIATRICS

OBJECTIVES

✔ Identify assessments that are used in a geriatric setting
✔ Compile questions to complete an occupational performance interview
✔ Administer screening tools that are used with clients who are elderly

DESCRIPTION

As in the other treatment settings, there are many occupational therapy assessments that are available for use with the geriatric population. Using multiple assessments is necessary to obtain a clear picture of the client's strengths, areas of concern, and functional performance. In evaluating geriatric clients, it is important to keep an open mind and be deliberate in the conclusions reached. Individuals who are elderly are often able to adapt to their changing health status and take cues from their environment to maintain their functioning level in ways that are creative and often unusual. These sometimes out-of-the-ordinary methods can allow them to remain in their natural environments longer and preserve their dignity. You will need to be an astute observer to note an individual's myriad ways of coping. Be careful in interpreting the assessments you administer and look beyond the scores obtained to the client's functional performance.

 PREPARATION

Suggested Readings

Asher (1996)
Emlet, Crabtree, Condon, and Treml (1996)
Lewis (1989)
Watts, Brollier, Bauer, and Schmidt (1989)

Study Questions

1. Describe the methods and specific assessments used in the occupational therapy and/or other medical professionals in evaluating elderly clients in the following areas:

   a. In-home assessment

   b. Home safety and accessibility assessment

   c. Activities of daily living assessment

   d. Basic mobility assessment

   e. Physical examination and body systems assessment

    f. Medication management assessment

    g. Nutritional assessment

    h. Assessment of elder abuse

    i. Assessment of mood and thought disorders

    j. Assessing memory and other cognitive functions

    k. Assessing the caregiver

2. What accommodations might you need to make to ensure that the person who is elderly clearly understands your assessment or interview?

3. Identify the components of the three internal subsystems of the human occupation system as identified by Kielhofner.
    a. Volitional

    b. Habituation

    c. Performance

4. Describe the "Occupational Performance History Interview" by Kielhofner, Henry, and Whalens as cited in Asher (1996) and how it is used in assessment.

5. Plan for a one-hour interview of a volunteer person who is elderly. Use the semi-structured interview schedule of the "Assessment of Occupational Functioning" (Watts, Brollier, Bauer, and Schmidt, 1989) to guide your interview. Ask questions that address each subsystem of the human occupation frame of reference. Use the space below to prepare your questions.
    a. Volition

b. Habituation

c. Performance

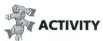 **ACTIVITY**

Materials

Questions each student has prepared, community volunteers, Set Test (Issacs and Kinnie, 1973), Mini Mental State (Folstein, Folstein, and Mettugn, 1975), Paracheck Geriatric Rating Scale (Paracheck, 1986).

Instructions

1a. As a class, prepare for your interview by first discussing and recording how you will introduce yourself to the resident.

1b. What could go wrong during your interview? Problem-solve. See the example to help you anticipate how the interview may proceed.

PROBLEM	SOLUTION
A person is unable to hear you.	Have a paper and pencil ready to write down questions.

1c. Interview a community volunteer, using the questions you have prepared. Administer the Set Test (Issacs and Kinnie, 1973) and the Mini Mental State (Folstein, Folstein, and Mettugn, 1975) to this person, also. Additionally, have the person describe for you what he or she does in a typical week and record that information below.

SUN.	MON.	TUES.	WED.	THURS.	FRI.	SAT.

1d. Record the Set Test (Issacs and Kinnie, 1973) and Mini Mental State (Folstein, Folstein, and Mettugn, 1975) scores below:

Set Test _____   Mini Mental State _____

1e. Score the person you interviewed on the Parachek Geriatric Rating Scale (Paracheck, 1986) and list the score obtained. _____

1f. From information gathered in your interview, list the activities the resident performs in the following categories.

SELF-CARE	WORK	PLAY/LEISURE

1g. Describe what you learned about this person's culture.

1h. Identify activities that might be available to this person that could be included in his or her schedule to help balance the time spent in the areas of ADL, work, and play/leisure.

1i. Describe the observed strengths and areas of concern of this person.

STRENGTHS	AREAS OF CONCERN

1j. Summarize your observations from the interview.

1k. Critique your own performance. Note the modifications you plan to make the next time you administer this interview and these screening tools.

1l. Share the above information with your classmates. Record the points you want to remember from your classmates' presentations.

FOLLOW-UP

✔ Complete the Application of Competencies at the end of this chapter.
✔ Complete a Therapeutic Use of Self Analysis found in Appendix B on your performance of standardized testing.

Exercise 103

SAFETY AND FALL PREVENTION

OBJECTIVES

✔ List barriers to home safety
✔ Discuss the importance of an emergency plan in providing home safety
✔ Plan an inservice on fall prevention

DESCRIPTION

Safety in the elderly population is a critical issue. Making sure a person who is elderly is safe in his or her home environment will help to prevent injuries and unnecessary medical expenses. As an occupational therapy practitioner you will be in a key position to assess the client's indoor and outdoor environments as well as their functional skills. Maintaining safety is often an issue of thorough thinking and planning ahead. Fall prevention is an important and significant component of home safety. Falls frequently alter an elderly client's level of independence and cause financial strain due to incurred medical expenses. Prevention of falls will be critical. Anticipating emergencies and making a plan for the same will also help in providing support to the client who is elderly in remaining healthy and independently functioning as long as possible.

 PREPARATION

Suggested Readings

Emlet, Crabtree, Condon, and Treml (1996)
Larson, Stevens-Ratchford, Pedretti, and Crabtree (1996)
Boston University Roybal Center for Late Life Enhancement:
    http://www.bu.edu/roybal

Study Questions

1. List barriers to home safety.

2. Detail the importance and the components of an emergency plan that is appropriate to use with the elderly.

3. Summarize the demographics and causes of falls in the elderly.

4. List the intrinsic and extrinsic causes of falls:
   a. Intrinsic

   b. Extrinsic

5. Describe the primary, secondary, and tertiary methods of fall prevention:
   a. Primary

    b. Secondary

    c. Tertiary

6. What do the initials in the acronym SPLAT represent?

    a. S

    b. P

    c. L

    d. A

    e. T

7. Summarize the information from the Boston University Roybal Center for Late Life Enhancement web page.

8. Describe treatment ideas that can be used in occupational therapy for fall prevention.

9. Identify several specific home safety assessments that would be helpful to use in facilitating safety and preventing falls in the elderly population.

10. List key questions that need to be asked as part of the safety assessment to obtain information about a client's indoor environment.

11. What levels of outdoor accessibility does an individual need?

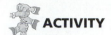 **ACTIVITY**

Materials

Posterboard, markers, flip charts, yellow pages of the local phone book, Case Study 54 located at the end of this chapter.

Instructions

1a. Divide into small groups. Select a setting from those listed below and plan an in-service on fall prevention for a group in that setting. Use a flip chart to make a draft of a handout you might like to distribute. Use posterboard to make a visual display to accompany your presentation. Use the space below to prepare your presentation. Present your inservice to the class. Rate and give feedback to each group on their presentation (use the form in Activity 1b.)

GROUP SETTINGS

a. Staff at a nursing home

b. Independent living residents in a retirement community

c. Assisted living residents in a retirement community

d. Caregivers' support group

e. Well elderly at a community senior citizens center

OUTLINE FOR PRESENTATION	
Group setting:	
FORMAT	STUDENT RESPONSIBLE

1b. Use the following chart to record feedback on your peers' presentations. Do this by placing the letter for that group setting next to the number that best represents the quality of the presentation. For example, if you were scoring the group that presented to the staff at a nursing home you would place an "a" on number 10 if you thought that they did an excellent job of displaying professional behavior during their presentation. Add additional comments as appropriate for each group.

EVALUATION OF GROUP PRESENTATIONS	1	2	3	4	5	6	7	8	9	10
Professional behavior										
Organized and prepared										
Teamwork evident										
Handouts were clear and organized										
Poster display was helpful and informative										
Content was easily understood for the elderly population										
Information was comprehensive										
Met time limits										

Comments on each group:

a.

b.

c.

d.

e.

1c. Rejoin your small group when all the presentations have been completed and feedback has been given. Discuss the feedback and your impressions. Record the changes you would like to make in your presentation before giving it to an actual community facility.

2. Using Case Study 54, work with a partner and detail an emergency plan for this client. Include an exit plan and a support system complete with necessary phone numbers and/or medical alert systems. Discuss your plan with your classmates.

   a. Exit plan:

   b. Support system:

EXIT PLAN

- you are here

←←←← escape routes

Fig. 6–2   Sample emergency plan.

FOLLOW-UP

✔   Complete the Application of Competencies at the end of this chapter.
✔   Complete Performance Skill 6D on Health and Wellness Presentation.

Exercise 104

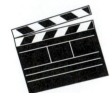

"Don't laugh at him who is old; the same will assuredly happen to us."

CHINESE PROVERB

ADAPTING OCCUPATIONS AND ENVIRONMENT

OBJECTIVES

✔   Identify techniques and adaptations that benefit the elderly
✔   Detail necessary adaptations for specific activities and environments
✔   Select occupational and environmental adaptations for a given situation

DESCRIPTION

Adaptations for an occupation and for the environment will help to provide support for individuals who are elderly. Providing support, ranging from minimal to maximal, to an individual can enable the person to remain healthy and free from injury. As an occupational therapy practitioner you will play a key role in analyzing the needs of the elderly and problem solving with them and their family and/or caregivers on the best way to provide support for them. Many simple environmental and occupational adaptations can be made that will make a significant difference in the level of performance for a client who is elderly. A client's level of care and living arrangements will, in part, determine the adaptations that are needed. Your creativity and ingenuity will be important as you adapt activities and the environment for persons who are elderly.

PREPARATION

Suggested Readings

Christiansen (2000)
Lewis (1989)
Pierson (1999)

Study Questions

1.   List systems and organs of the body that experience change as a result of the aging process.

2. List precautions that need to be taken to prevent injuries and/or illness in working with clients who are elderly.

3. List techniques and adaptations that may be used for a person who is elderly and experiencing deficits in the following abilities:

   a. Vision

   b. Hearing

   c. Mobility

   d. Balance

   e. Memory

4. Describe what is meant by the term *negotiability* and the equipment and human and environmental factors that affect it.

5. Identify at least seven types of living arrangements that are available to the elderly.

6. List levels of care that a person who is elderly may need.

7. Describe the role of the client, family, and caregivers in problem solving about needed adaptations to an activity or the environment.

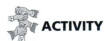 **ACTIVITY**

Materials

Videotape entitled "Adapting the Home for the Physically Challenged" (A/V Health Services, n.d.) videocassette recorder, Case Study 55 located at the end of this chapter.

Instructions

1. View the video entitled *Adapting the Home for the Physically Challenged* (A/V Health Services, n.d.) on adaptations and/or discuss ways to adapt a person's home. Use the following form to record information obtained from viewing the video and/or discussing adaptation of a person's home.

AREA	WAYS TO ADAPT
Ramp construction	
Entrance/doorways	
Kitchen	
Bedroom	
Bathroom	
Laundry/housekeeping	
Living room	

2a. List adaption techniques for several activities that older people living in a community setting typically participate in, such as baking, bingo, cards, and sing-alongs. As a group, decide which occupations you want to include. With a partner, fill in the chart with ways in which the occupations can be adapted to fit the condition listed in the first column.

CONDITIONS	OCCUPATIONS				
Tremors					
Poor fine motor coordination					
Low vision					
Poor hearing					
Confusion					
Use of only one hand					
Aggressiveness					
Psychosis					
Poor balance					
Weak grasp					

No use of lower extremities				
Decreased range of motion				
Poor endurance				
Active rheumatoid arthritis				
Osteoarthritis				
Oral motor deficits				
Inability to verbalize				
Degenerative weakness				
Short attention span				

2b. Discuss and record how the living environment of a client may influence the above adaptations.

3. Using Case Study 55, determine what type of adaptations the client may need, as well as the level of care you foresee the client will need in the future. Write this below and share your thoughts with the class.

FOLLOW-UP

✔   Complete the Application of Competencies at the end of this chapter.
✔   Complete Performance Skill 6F on Home Assessment.

JOINT PROTECTION, ENERGY CONSERVATION, AND WORK SIMPLIFICATION

Exercise 105

OBJECTIVES

✔   List the principles of joint protection, energy conservation, and work simplification
✔   Plan an educational presentation on protecting joints, conserving energy, and simplifying work
✔   Identify case-specific joint protection, energy conservation, and work simplification techniques

"Good sense comes only with old age."
IRISH PROVERB

DESCRIPTION

As an occupational therapy practitioner you will be working with clients who will need educational information and training in joint protection, energy conservation, and work simplification or efficiency. Clients with decreased strength and endurance as well as those with chronic pain and/or cardiac and pulmonary difficulties will need such training. Your clients will need to incorporate these techniques into their typical daily routines in all components of their self-care, work, and play or leisure activities. You will play an important role in helping them to determine how to do this. The benefits to your client in using these techniques will be realized in their reduced pain as well as greater independence and functional performance.

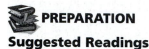 **PREPARATION**

Suggested Readings

Lewis (1989)
Melvin (1989)
Neidstadt and Crepeau (1998)

STUDY QUESTIONS

1. Briefly define and describe principles of each of the following treatment techniques as well as their use in intervention.

TECHNIQUE	DEFINITION	PRINCIPLES	USE
Joint Protection			
Energy conservation			
Work simplification/ efficiency			

2a. Describe how you can apply the three techniques to some activity of daily living task that you performed today. A brief example is shown in the task of making breakfast.

TASK	JOINT PROTECTION	ENERGY CONSERVATION	WORK SIMPLIFICATION
Making breakfast	Use a lighter-weight pan to make my omelet	Microwave water for tea in the cup from which I will be drinking	Eat a cold breakfast

2b. Describe why the three treatment techniques must be used with clients who have rheumatoid arthritis.

3. Identify other diagnostic conditions in which joint protection, energy conservation, and work simplification must be used.

4. How can the use of assistive devices be implemented in the three treatment techniques. Give examples.

   a. Joint protection

   b. Energy conservation

   c. Work simplification

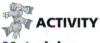 **ACTIVITY**

Materials

Posterboard, markers.

Instructions

1. With a partner or small group, prepare an infomercial to sell membership in your joint protection, energy conservation, and work simplification group. Use the posterboard to display your infomercial. Be creative, be persuasive, be educational, and have fun. Use the space below to plan your presentation.

2. Write the following scenarios on the top of blank 8 1/2 × 11 inch piece of paper (one scenario per page). Distribute the papers to classmates. On the paper you receive, write a treatment suggestion that incorporates a work simplification, energy conservation, and/or joint protection technique. Sign your name to your idea. Pass the paper to a classmate and receive a paper from another classmate. Add an idea not previously given. If you are unable to think of a suggestion, write "pass" and your name. Continue to pass the forms until all ideas have been exhausted. Redistribute the papers and take turns reading the scenarios and the ideas given. Use the space below to record ideas you would like to remember.

   a. A client with a total hip replacement wants to visit friends, but she doesn't know how she will be able to use the restroom.

   b. A client is afraid to travel in a wheelchair.

c. A client has difficulty locking and unlocking doors.

d. A client complains of joint pain during and after sexual intercourse.

e. A client complains of body aches when working at the desk for two hours at a time. Her boss is threatening to fire her.

f. It is very difficult for a client to get up and move about after sitting for long periods of time.

g. A client has a very large kitchen with many workstations and large storage areas. She becomes exhausted very quickly when working.

h. Because of declining function a client is not fixing meals and therefore is not eating properly.

i. Grocery shopping is almost impossible because the client would have to carry groceries up two flights of stairs.

j. A client loves gardening, but it is becoming very difficult to do the necessary bending over.

k. The client's washer and dryer are down the stairs at the apartment building. He is unable to carry laundry baskets and walk up or down the stairs at the same time.

l. Using the vacuum cleaner is an impossible task for this client because of low endurance.

FOLLOW-UP

✔   Complete the Application of Competencies at the end of this chapter.

JOINT REPLACEMENT

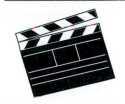

OBJECTIVES

✔ Describe the incidence of and intervention for joint replacement procedures
✔ Identify adaptive equipment that is useful for a client with a joint replacement
✔ Explain the procedures and precautions for a client's postoperative engagement in activities of daily living and home management

DESCRIPTION

"Reverence your elder, for the man excelling in age excels in wisdom."

AFRICAN PROVERB

Individuals with surgical replacements of their hip or knee joints are seen quite commonly in the population of elderly people. Such a client with an orthopedic condition will be seen briefly for occupational therapy intervention. The intervention you provide will be postsurgical and of a practical nature, helping the client to relearn basic essential activities of daily living and home management. Some of the tasks, activities, and precautions you will teach your clients may come as a surprise to them, as they may not have realized that they would need training in those areas. Using simple techniques and adaptations, you can help the client to recover more quickly and gain independence faster. If the client can also be seen preoperatively for some of the retraining you will provide, the postoperative procedures and training will be further expedited.

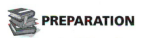 **PREPARATION**

Suggested Readings

Melvin (1989)
Platt, Begun, and Murphy (1992a, 1992b)

Study Questions

1. Describe the indications for, occurrence of, functional goals for, and precautions needed after surgery for both a knee and hip replacement.

	TOTAL KNEE	TOTAL HIP
Indications		
Occurrence		
Goals		
Precautions		

2. Describe the occupational therapy intervention process that will be used with the client who has undergone a total knee replacement (TKR) and a total hip replacement (THR).

   a. Total knee replacement

   b. Total hip replacement

3. Describe the postoperative training procedure and precautions after a THR in the following daily activities:

   a. Sitting

   b. Use of a walker

   c. Transfers to bath and shower

   d. Bed positioning

   e. Bed transfer

   f. Car transfer

   g. Dressing

   h. Toilet transfer

   i. Homemaking

4. What are common pieces of equipment that a client may need:

   a. After a THR?

   b. After a TKR?

ACTIVITY

Materials

Walker, bathroom, wheelchair, knee immobilizer, bed, hospital bed, bedside commode, raised commode, reachers, dressing sticks, sock aid, long-handled sponge, long-handled shoehorn, elastic shoe laces, kitchen stool, tub benches, hand-held shower extension, rolling kitchen cart; Case Studies 56, 57, 58 located at the end of this chapter.

Instructions

1. Watch your instructor demonstrate a typical treatment session that might occur with a client who has undergone a THR. Take notes below as each area is covered.

    a. Precautions

    b. Dressing

    c. Home management

    d. Chair positioning

    e. Using a walker

    f. Bed transfer

    g. Bed positioning

    h. Car transfer

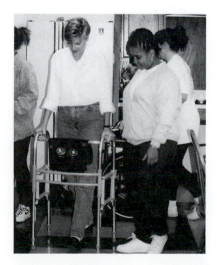

Fig. 6–3 Following hip replacement precautions.
Photo courtesy of Tiffany Walker and Pam Boone.

    i. Shower transfer

    j. Tub transfer

    k. Toilet transfer

2a. Participate in a role-play with a partner who is assuming the role of the client from the case study assigned. Instruct your partner in how to follow the recommended precautions and perform the following skills. Record the feedback you received on your instructional accuracy and techniques from your peers and/or instructor.

    a. Precautions

    b. Dressing

    c. Homemaking

    d. Chair positioning

    e. Using a walker

    f. Bed positioning

    g. Tub transfer

    h. Toilet transfer

    i. Bed transfer

    j. Car transfer

     k.   Pants

     l.   Socks

     m. Undergarments

     n.   Hose

     o.   Shoes

2b. Discuss your case study with your classmates. Record the variations in treatment sessions and case studies.

FOLLOW-UP

✔   Complete the Application of Competencies at the end of this chapter.

REMOTIVATION AND REALITY ORIENTATION

Exercise 107

OBJECTIVES

✔   Differentiate between remotivation and reality orientation
✔   Plan a reality orientation group
✔   Identify activities to use in remotivation groups

DESCRIPTION

In working with clients who have impairments in cognition, judgment, and memory, remotivation and reality orientation will be two useful tools that you will need to learn how to use. Remotivation is appropriately used in group sessions. Reality orientation is also used in group situations, and its techniques can be used effectively 24 hours a day. Orienting clients to reality can take place in a formal session or in informal encounters. The impact of dementia can be lessened by the activities and interaction guidelines given by remotivation and reality orientation therapies. Families and caregivers will also appreciate the helpful hints you will be able to pass on to them as they interact with their loved one.

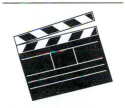

"Respect the elders.
They are our fathers."

Yoruba proverb

PREPARATION

Suggested Readings

> Emlet, Crabtree, Condon, and Treml (1996)
> Lewis (1989)
> Miller, Peckham, and Peckham (1995)

Study Questions

1. Define remotivation therapy.

2. Describe the type of client who would benefit from remotivation therapy and the number of clients who may be involved in a group.

3. List several goals of remotivation therapy.

4. Describe the five steps of a remotivation group and describe what might happen in each step.

   a.

   b.

   c.

   d.

   e.

5. Define reality orientation therapy.

6. For what type of client is reality orientation therapy best suited?

7. What is the 24-hour method of reality orientation?

8. Describe the atmosphere and methods the leader needs to use in a reality orientation group.

9. What reality therapy and remotivation techniques can you pass on to your clients' families and caregivers?

10. Identify at least two assessments that are appropriate for determining a client's current orientation status.

Note: In preparation for the following activities, gather and bring to class various items that may be used in a remotivation group. Raid the attic to find items that are interesting or attractive and that may be good conversation starters, such as jewelry, hats, photos, clothes, and heirlooms. List here the items you found.

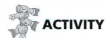 **ACTIVITY**

Materials

Items collected from home to demonstrate a remotivation group.

Instructions

1a. Divide into small groups and design a reality orientation group treatment plan for a long-term care facility. Use the Group Treatment Plan Protocol below, as adapted from Cole (1998). When you have completed the plan, share your ideas with the class.

GROUP TREATMENT PLAN PROTOCOL
Group title:
Frame of reference:
Purpose:
Group membership and size:
Group goals:
Rationale:
Outcome criteria:
Leadership style:
Method:
Time and place of meeting:
Supplies and cost:
Adaptations/variations/modifications:
References:

Adapted with permission from: Cole, M.B. 1998. Group Dynamics in Occupational Therapy: The Theoretical Basis and Practice Application of Group Treatment. 2d ed. Thorofare, NJ: Slack.

1b. Plan how you will carry out two specific group sessions. Use the following outline, as taken from Cole (1998).

FIRST GROUP SESSION
Group title:
Session title:
Format:
Supplies:
Description:

SECOND GROUP SESSION
Group title:
Session title:
Format:
Supplies:
Description:

Used with permission from: Cole, M. B. 1998. Group Dynamics in Occupational Therapy: The Theoretical Basis and Practice Application of Group Treatment. 2d ed. Thorofare, NJ: Slack.

2. Participate in a remotivation group with your instructor as leader. Afterward, discuss and record what was done in each of the five steps, as taken from Miller, Peckham, and Peckham (1995).

   a. Climate of acceptance

   b. Bridge to reality

   c. Exploring the world we live in

    d. Exploring the work of the world

    e. Climate of appreciation

3a. Divide into small groups and share the items you brought that could be used in a remotivation group. Decide on a theme for your group and plan what to do in each step, as outlined by Miller, Peckham, and Peckham (1995). Use the materials you brought and/or any other necessary items as appropriate.

    a. Climate of acceptance

    b. Bridge to reality

    c. Exploring the world we live in

    d. Exploring the work of the world

    e. Climate of appreciation

3b. Share your group ideas with the class. Record interesting ideas that you want to remember from each step.

FOLLOW-UP

✔ Complete the Application of Competencies at the end of this chapter.

DEMENTIA

Exercise 108

OBJECTIVES

✔ Describe the symptoms and causes of dementia
✔ Detail therapeutic responses of reality orientation, attitude therapy, and validation therapy used with clients who have dementia
✔ Select therapeutic intervention techniques for a client with dementia

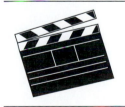

DESCRIPTION

In working with the geriatric population, it will not be uncommon to work with a client who has some type and or level of dementia. You will play a significant role in facilitating communication and interaction with such clients. You will also assist in organizing the environment of a client with dementia to facilitate the individual's orientation and functional performance. As you provide services for a client with dementia, it will

"If you carry your childhood with you, you never become old."

THEODORE ROOSEVELT

be necessary to work closely with that client's family and/or caregivers. They will need your expertise in structuring their loved ones' interactions and environment. The clients with dementia and the unpredictability seen in their cognitive, functional, and behavioral manifestations will benefit from your therapeutic interventions.

PREPARATION

Suggested Readings

> AOTA (latest edition)
> Holden and Woods (1995)
> Larson, Stevens-Ratchford, Pedretti, and Crabtree (1996)
> Lewis (1989)
> Miller, Peckham, and Peckham (1995)

Study Questions

1. Describe what is meant by the term *dementia*.

2. Differentiate between the different types of dementia.

3. Describe the symptoms and causes of dementia.

4. Locate and cite a source that answers the question as to whether dementia is a normal stage in the aging process.

5. Describe strategies that are useful in communicating and interacting with a person who is experiencing dementia.

6. Describe the relationship of sensory deprivation to confusion.

7. Summarize the AOTA's position on services for people with Alzheimer's disease and other dementias.

8. List strategies to assist in dealing with behavior problems encountered in a person with dementia.

BEHAVIOR PROBLEM	STRATEGY

9. List the progressive stages of dementia identified by a formal deterioration scale.

10. Briefly describe validation therapy.

11. In the spaces provided, describe the stages of late life disorientation and the validation technique that may be used to assist a person in this stage.

	DESCRIPTION	VALIDATION TECHNIQUE
Stage 1: Malorientation		
Stage 2: Time confusion		
Stage 3: Repetitive motion		
Stage 4: Vegetation		

12. Briefly describe attitude therapy and the approaches used.
    a. Attitude therapy

    b. Active friendliness

    c. Passive friendliness

    d. Kind firmness

    e. No demand

    f. Matter of fact

13. Describe respite care and its impact on the caregivers of a client with dementia.

14. Summarize methods that will assist in the effectiveness of group work with dementia.

15. List ideas for activity selection for a client with dementia.

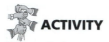 **ACTIVITY**

Materials

Case Study 59 located at the end of this chapter.

Instructions

1. With a partner, formulate a response for each of the following situations of clients with dementia. Put a star by the response you believe may be the most effective. Role-play that response for your class. The first one is completed for you.

SITUATION	REALITY ORIENTATION	ATTITUDE THERAPY	VALIDATION THERAPY
You are approached by an 89-year-old resident about where she can catch the bus home; her parents are going to be worried.	You are 89 years old and live in a nursing home. Your parents have been decreased for many years. Let me show you to your room.	Passive friendliness: I am also very concerned about you. Let me see if your family has been notified, and then I would be happy to help you figure out where to go.	You look worried. But your family all know where you are and are not expecting you home. You are expected in the group down the hall. Let me take you there.
Mrs. Pinsky would like to know who is responsible for that delicious meal. She would like to tell the head chef of the restaurant (dining room) how delicious it was.			
Mr. Tung's wife passed away several months ago. He is asking you again, for the fifth time this morning, where she is. He is not going to your therapy without her.			

When you are working on feeding activities with Mrs. Howard, she tells you she can't eat that food. She can't believe that someone is feeding her worms (spaghetti).			
Mr. Jones has been found rummaging in Mr. Ramirez's room. He said he is looking for his watch and he knows it is in there.			
Mrs. Gates tells you that every night she is asleep a man comes into her room and walks around looking in her drawers.			
Mrs. Washington starts to leave your group and head to the door that leads outside.			
Mr. Pearson refuses to go to therapy because his wallet has been stolen again. He is very angry.			
Mrs. Mathews is finishing her meal, you notice her putting condiment packages into her bra.			
Mrs. Munrich walks up to you frantic and crying because she has lost the children she was babysitting.			

2. After reading Case Study 59, work with a partner to answer the following questions:

   a. Describe the therapeutic approach you will want to use with this client.

   b. List the types of groups and activities that may be helpful.

c. Describe how you would set up this client's morning routine of activities of daily living to maximize independence.

d. What safety precautions would need to be implemented if this client went home?

e. Describe how you would set up and organize this client's room.

f. Detail the supports this client may need.

FOLLOW-UP

✔ Complete the Application of Competencies at the end of this chapter.

Exercise 109

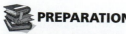

"Youth has a beautiful face and old age a beautiful soul."

SWEDISH PROVERB

SENSORY STIMULATION

OBJECTIVES

✔ Identify the effects of sensory deprivation on elderly individuals
✔ Describe the purpose and goals of a sensory stimulation group
✔ Plan a theme-based sensory stimulation and a Ross five-stage approach group

DESCRIPTION

As an occupational therapy practitioner working with elderly clients, you may find yourself in a long-term care setting. In such a setting, it is common to have residents who can benefit from sensory stimulation. Sensory stimulation is also known by other names, such as sensory training. Sensory stimulation or training, refers to the process of stimulating the senses for an elderly person who may be sensorily deprived. As an individual ages and skills deteriorate, sensory deprivation can occur quickly if and when the person loses the ability to perform his or her typical tasks and roles. Mildred Ross, an occupational therapist known for the work with the geriatric population, has developed an organized, systematic, and effective approach to group work that provides sensory input using a sensory integration theory base. You will need to be familiar with her work.

PREPARATION

Suggested Readings

Holden and Woods (1995)
Lewis (1989)
Miller, Peckham, and Peckham (1995)
Ross (1997)

Study Questions

1. What are the effects of sensory deprivation in people who are elderly?

2. How might you create a sensory-rich environment for a client in a long-term care facility?

3. Describe sensory stimulation as it relates to an activity that is provided in a long-term care setting.

4. What is the major goal of using sensory stimulation with a client?

5. Describe the number and types of clients who benefit from a sensory stimulation group.

6. Describe the use of sensory stimulation in a one-to-one setting.

7. Define and identify activities that may be used by the following senses in a group and/or individual setting:
   a. Tactile

   b. Kinesthesia/proprioception

   c. Auditory

   d. Visual

   e. Gustatory

8. Briefly outline the format that may be used in a sensory stimulation group.

9. Describe Ross's (1997) five-stage approach to group work by answering the following questions:

   a. What type and functioning level of clients might benefit from this approach?

   b. What is the purpose of the group?

   c. What are the neurophysiological assumptions underlying the five-stage approach?

   d. List the five stages and identify three activities that would be appropriate for each stage.

STAGES	ACTIVITIES

10. Bring one object to class that may be used to stimulate each sensory system. List here the items you will bring:

    a. Tactile

    b. Kinesthesia

    c. Olfactory

    d. Auditory

    e. Vision

    f. Gustatory

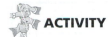 **ACTIVITY**

Materials

Sensory objects brought by the students.

Instructions

1a. Join a small group of students and place all sensory items on the table to share and discuss. Plan a sensory stimulation group using some or all of these materials. Use the space below to plan. Lead a sensory stimulation group, having your classmates role-play clients who may benefit from such a group.

GROUP PLAN
Welcome:
Introduction:
Simple exercise:
Senses stimulated
Tactile:
Kinesthesia/proprioception:
Olfactory:
Visual:
Auditory:
Gustatory:

1b. As other groups are presented, list ideas from their presentation you want to remember. Give feedback to each group when their presentation is completed. Record feedback you received also.

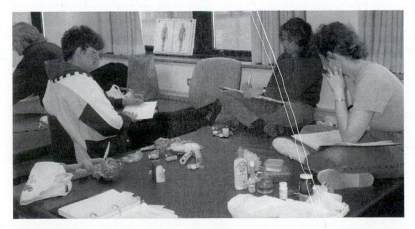

Fig. 6–4 Planning a sensory stimulation group.

Photo courtesy of Linda Ferguson, Nikki Shubenski, and Julie Banks.

Welcome:			
Introduction:			
Simple exercise:			
SENSES STIMULATED	FEEDBACK FOR GROUP 1	FEEDBACK FOR GROUP 2	FEEDBACK FOR GROUP 3
Tactile			
Kinesthesia/ proprioception			
Olfactory			
Visual			
Auditory			
Gustatory			
Feedback Received			

2. With a partner or small group, plan a Ross (1997) five-stage approach group. Once your plan is complete, share your ideas with your classmates. Take note of ideas you want to remember.

I.
II.
III.
IV.
V.
Ideas to remember:

FOLLOW-UP

✔ Complete the Application of Competencies at the end of this chapter.
✔ Complete Performance Skill 6C on Prepare/Present Group.

EATING, FEEDING, AND DYSPHAGIA

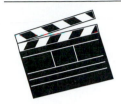

OBJECTIVES

✔ Define and explain the cause of dysphagia
✔ Identify intervention strategies for dysphagia
✔ Develop a treatment plan for a client with self-feeding and/or swallowing disorders

DESCRIPTION

"He who complains much does little."

Swahili proverb

Eating, feeding, and swallowing disorders occur across the life span. However, such disorders appears especially frequently in the elderly population. It is not uncommon to encounter individuals in long-term care facilities with major health issues that affect their feeding and eating. A client with dysphagia compromises a digestive system even further. Adequate nutritional intake is necessary throughout the life span for normal growth and development, but in the later years it becomes increasingly more important in warding off infections and disease. Assessing and treating feeding and eating difficulties, particularly dysphagia, will often be embraced as a team, as the medical ramifications of such conditions are far reaching.

PREPARATION

Suggested Readings

> AOTA (latest edition)
> Early (1998)
> Larson, Stevens-Ratchford, Pedretti, and Crabtree (1996)
> Lewis (1989)
> Reed (1991)

Study Questions

1. Define the term *dysphagia*, explain its causes, and describe the diagnoses of clients who may experience this disorder.

   a. Definition

   b. Causes

   c. Diagnoses

2. Describe what happens in each of the stages involved in the swallowing process:

   a. Anticipatory stage

    b. Oral phrase

    c. Pharyngeal phase

    d. Esophageal phase

3. What are the precautions to which you need to adhere in working with a person with dysphagia?

4. What is the progression of manageability of types of foods from the most easily swallowed to the most difficult to swallow?

5. What problems might a client experience with the task of eating? What strategies may be used to help solve them? What adaptive equipment may be helpful?

PROBLEM	STRATEGY	ADAPTIVE EQUIPMENT

6. List some guidelines that may be helpful in assisting a person with feeding or eating difficulties. Include the necessary environmental conditions.

7. Describe the benefits that may be achieved by having residents in a long-term care facility participate in a dining program.

8. Describe the role of the occupational therapy practitioner in setting up and managing a feeding group.

9. List and describe common problems associated with dysphagia and corresponding treatment suggestions.

PROBLEM	TREATMENT SUGGESTIONS

10. What health care professionals might be on a dysphagia assessment team?

11. Identify several assessments that evaluate dysphagia.

12. Explain the role of videofluoroscopy swallow studies (VFSS) in the assessment process.

13. Summarize the AOTA's position on providing intervention to people with eating dysfunctions (AOTA, latest edition).

14. Differentiate between feeding and eating.
    a. Feeding

    b. Eating

 ACTIVITY

Materials

Videotape entitled *Managing Dysphagia* (Hutchins, 1991); Case Study 60 located at the end of this chapter.

Instructions

1. View the videotape *Managing Dysphagia* (Hutchins, 1991). Describe the purpose and procedures used to perform the VFSS assessment.

2. With a partner, using Case Study 60, devise a brief intervention plan that focuses on the feeding and eating deficits this client is experiencing. Use the space provided below to plan. Share this information with your classmates when complete.

INTERVENTION PLAN
Identified feeding/eating issues:
Long-term goal:
Short-term goal:
Short-term goal:
Short-term goal:
Intervention:
List and describe the collaboration you will have with other team members:

TEAM MEMBER	DESCRIPTION OF COLLABORATION/CONSULTATION

3. With a partner or small group, devise a dining program for elderly residents at a long-term facility who are experiencing difficulty feeding themselves. Use the space below to plan. Share your plan with your classmates when complete.

   a. Population

   b. Environment you will use

   c. Intervention

d. Adaptive equipment needs

e. Collaboration/consultation you will do

FOLLOW-UP

✔ Complete the Application of Competencies at the end of this chapter.

LEISURE TIME

Exercise 111

OBJECTIVES

✔ Describe the role of relaxation and volunteerism in occupying leisure time
✔ Plan a relaxation/guided imagery activity
✔ Identify case-related leisure time activities

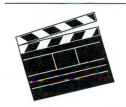

"The trouble with the rat race is even if you win you're still a rat."

LILY TOMLIN

DESCRIPTION

Engaging in leisure time pursuits is important for people who are elderly. The newly retired individual may suddenly find himself or herself with more time than the person is accustomed to filling. Individuals in the later years of life may need to redefine their leisure interests and pursuits because of an accident or injury. In either instance, as an occupational therapy practitioner you will play an important role in facilitating your client's functioning in this important performance area. Individuals may choose to engage in any variety of leisure time pursuits, including but not limited to recreation, relaxation, and volunteerism. Participating in volunteer activities may be considered a part of one's vocational activities. At the same time such activity engagement adds a significant contribution to the lives of others as well as contributing to one's own satisfaction and fulfillment.

PREPARATION

Suggested Readings

AOTA (latest edition)
Asher (1996)
Larson, Stevens-Ratchford, Pedretti, and Crabtree (1996)
Lewis (1996)
Miller, Peckham, and Peckham (1995)

Study Questions

1. What is the definition of leisure?

2. Identify patterns of free time activity that are typical in retirement.

3. Determine what skills you believe are necessary to perform leisure activities successfully.

4. List and describe the skills an occupational therapy practitioner needs to help a client develop leisure activities.

5. Consider the aging process.
   a. List and briefly describe some of the stresses that occur as a result of aging.

   b. Summarize adaptive strategies that may be helpful in coping with the aging process.

6. List and briefly describe at least five types of relaxation techniques that can be used with the elderly.
   a.

   b.

   c.

   d.

   e.

7. Define volunteer participation.

8. List at least ten volunteer and service programs that are available for elderly people to participate in. Put a check mark next to the ones that are available to individuals in the community where you are living.
   a.

   b.

c.

d.

e.

f.

g.

h.

i.

j.

9. Identify several leisure time assessments.

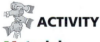 **ACTIVITY**

Materials

Videotape player and monitor, video *Range of Motion (ROM) Dance* (St. Mary's Hospital Medical Center and Board of Regents of the University of Wisconsin System, 1984), tape player, relaxation videotape and/or audiotape (any such tape as found in your local bookstore or library), floor mats, pillows, Case Study 57 located at the end of this chapter.

Instructions

1. Follow the videotape instructions and participate in the *ROM Dance* (St. Mary's Hospital Medical Center and Board of Regents of the University of Wisconsin System, 1984). Describe the therapeutic benefits of this activity. With a partner or small group complete an Abbreviated Occupational Analysis found in Appendix A on the *ROM Dance*.

2. Arrange yourself in a comfortable position. Participate as a class in a relaxation session with an audiotape and/or videotape, following the suggested directions

and guidelines of the tape. Write about this experience, including your reactions, your feelings, and strategies to improve your ability to relax.

3a. Role-play with your partner, taking him or her through another guided imagery and/or progressive relaxation activity. When completed, switch roles. Record the title of your activity, describe the activity, and cite the source of your activity.

Activity title: _____

DESCRIPTION	SOURCE

3b. Describe your performance as the leader of the relaxation activity and as the participant.

4. As a class, brainstorm and record leisure activities that are commonly used in the later years of one's life.

5. Using Case Study 57, work with a partner or small group to focus on leisure interests for this client.

   a. What additional information would you like to have about this client?

   b. Select a least five leisure activities that may be beneficial for this client. Explain the rationale for your choices. Describe how the activity may need to be adapted.

LEISURE ACTIVITY	RATIONALE	ADAPTED

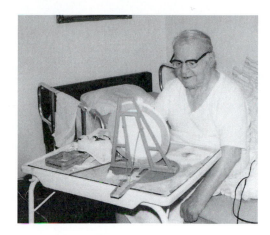

Fig. 6–5 Participation in a leisure time activity of painting can greatly improve the quality of a person's life.
Photo courtesy of Charles Meyer.

c. List three volunteer or service programs in which this individual may be interested in participating.

   a.

   b.

   c.

d. Share your ideas with your classmates.

FOLLOW-UP

✔ Complete the Application of Competencies at the end of this chapter.

INTERVENTION PLANNING   Exercise 112

OBJECTIVES

✔ Identify a variety of intervention strategies
✔ Align intervention activities with diagnostic categories
✔ Develop an intervention plan for a geriatric client

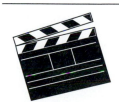

DESCRIPTION

When providing occupational therapy services for the client who is geriatric, you will need to develop a plan for your intervention. This plan will provide a detailed outline of the services you will provide. In developing this plan, it will be important to consult and gather information from the client's family and caregivers as well as the client himself or herself. In selecting the goals and activities for each client, it will be necessary to align these with your client's strengths, interests, and areas of concern. Many treatment modalities and activities are available for the geriatric population, and it will be a challenge for you to select the compatible ones. Keeping informed and abreast of new strategies and techniques will be a continual challenge.

"I used to dread getting older because I thought I would not be able to do all the things I wanted to do, but now that I am older, I find that I don't want to do them."

NANCY ARTHUR

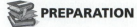 **PREPARATION**

Suggested Readings

Larson, Stevens-Ratchford, Pedretti, and Crabtree (1996)
Lewis (1989)
Neidstadt and Crepeau (1998)

Study Questions

1. Who may be involved in formulating an intervention plan for a client who is geriatric?

2. List and describe the internal and external factors as they relate to intervention planning.

INTERNAL FACTORS	RELATE TO INTERVENTION PLANNING
EXTERNAL FACTORS	RELATED TO INTERVENTION PLANNING

3. Describe how the following questions should be considered when planning intervention:

    a. Who

    b. What

    c. When

    d. Where

    e. How

4. Summarize the characteristics and properties that must be considered when selecting modalities for use with clients in the geriatric setting.

5. Give strategies and/or specific treatment activities that may be used with clients who may have the following diagnoses:
   a. Chronic obstructive pulmonary disease

STRATEGIES	ACTIVITIES

   b. Parkinson's disease

STRATEGIES	ACTIVITIES

   c. Metastatic cancer

STRATEGIES	ACTIVITIES

d. Diabetes

STRATEGIES	ACTIVITIES

e. Cerebral vascular accident (CVA)

STRATEGIES	ACTIVITIES

f. Cardiac conditions

STRATEGIES	ACTIVITIES

6. Describe how the following treatment modalities may be used in intervention:
   a. Aquatic therapy

   b. Pet therapy

c. Horticultural therapy

d. Gentle exercise

e. Cooking

f. Arts and crafts

g. Life review

ACTIVITY

Materials

Case Studies 57, 58, 59, 61, 62, and 63 located at the back of this chapter.

Instructions

1a. Using the assigned case study, with a partner or in a small group, complete the following intervention plan. Be certain to consider the changes in aging along with the disease process.

INTERVENTION PLAN
Client's strengths
Areas of concern to be addressed by occupational therapy
Areas of concern that will be addressed by other team members

CONCERN	TEAM MEMBER

Frame of reference and rationale

Three concerns that you will address in occupational therapy and one short-term goal for each

CONCERN	GOAL

Two or three occupations for each goal, the needed setup, your rationale for the activities, and how you will grade the activity as the client improves

GOAL	OCCUPATION	SETUP	RATIONALE	GRADED

How you have incorporated the client's culture into your planning

Safety precautions you will implement in treatment

1b. Discuss your treatment plan with your class and record any ideas you want to remember from the treatment plans of others.

FOLLOW-UP

✔ Complete the Application of Competencies at the end of this chapter.
✔ Complete Performance Skill 6A Adding to Your Files.
✔ Complete Performance Skill 6E on Intervention Planning.

REMINISCENCE AND LIFE REVIEW

Exercise 113

OBJECTIVES

✔ Describe the therapeutic benefits of reminiscing and life review
✔ Compile a list of reminiscing and life review resources
✔ Plan a reminiscing and life review group for intervention with clients who are elderly

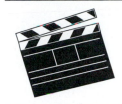

DESCRIPTION

This exercise will help you to understand the role reminiscing, life review, and life stories can play in the elderly population. When working with the elderly, you will need to make sure you do not overlook the important therapeutic benefits of such activities. As an individual enters the final stage of life, closure can be facilitated by reevaluating and interpreting the meaning of one's life. Death and dying can be embraced and accepted more readily when one completes unfinished business and has feelings of fulfillment and efficacy about one's life. As an occupational therapy practitioner you will be in a position to facilitate such occurrences as you lead groups for clients who are elderly.

"The habits of early life will never be forgotten."

TAMIL PROVERB

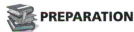 **PREPARATION**

Suggested Readings

> Cole (1998)
> Larson, Stevens-Ratchford, Pedretti, and Crabtree (1996)
> Lewis (1989)

Study Questions

1. Define the terms *reminiscing, life review,* and *life story* and explain what therapeutic purpose each serves.

   a. Reminiscence:

   b. Life review:

   c. Life story:

2. Describe the population that is best served by reminiscing or life review.

3. Describe the format of a reminiscing or life review group.

4. What topics can be included in reminiscing?

5. What goals can be accomplished through the use of reminiscing?

6. Describe several formats or types of reminiscing or life review activities that have therapeutic value.

7. Identify two theorists whose views of aging would be compatible with the therapeutic benefits of a life review.

8. Complete a list of suggested resources that can be used for reminiscing.

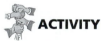 **ACTIVITY**

Materials

The games *A Slice of Life* (Michelson, 1985) and *Pastimes* (Bayles and Tomoeda, 1997).

Instructions

1. Participate in one or both of the above games. Record your observations. Discuss as a class the impact of reminiscing and playing the game(s).
    a. Describe the reactions you observed in individual members.

    b. What was the overall tone of the group? Describe.

    c. Did the tone of the group change? Describe.

    d. How did you feel before, during, and after the game?

    e. Any other comments:

2a. With a small group, begin to plan a reminiscing or life review group (based on Cole's, 1998, group format) to be carried out in class at a later date. Use the space below to begin planning.

Group title:	
Session title:	
Format:	
Supplies:	

DESCRIPTION
Warm-up:
Introduction of activity:
Instructions for activity:
Sharing:

DISCUSSION QUESTIONS
Processing:
Generalizing:
Application:
Summary:

Adapted with permission from: Cole, M. B. 1998. Group Dynamics in Occupational Therapy: The Theoretical Basis and Practice Application of Group Treatment. *2d ed. Thorofare, NJ: Slack*

2b. Decide among the members of your group who will be responsible for bringing the needed supplies for your group. Divide the leadership responsibilities among all group members. For example, one student may lead the warm-up, another may introduce the activity, yet another may lead the discussion, and so on. Write your responsibilities below.

2c. With your small group, lead your reminiscing or life review group for your classmates. Record your classmates' reactions to your group and critique the leadership skills your small group used.

CLASSMATES' REACTIONS	CRITIQUE OF LEADERSHIP SKILLS

FOLLOW-UP

✔ Complete the Application of Competencies at the end of this chapter.
✔ Complete a Therapeutic Use of Self Analysis found in Appendix B on your participation and leadership of reminiscing activities.
✔ Complete Performance Skill 6B on Present a Reminiscing Activity.

Exercise 114

"Though I walk through the valley of the shadow of death, I will fear no evil; for thou are with me."

PSALMS 23:4

TERMINAL ILLNESS

OBJECTIVES

✔ Describe the stages of death and dying
✔ Analyze personal feelings and responses to death and dying
✔ Develop and intervention plan based on prioritized goals of a terminally ill client

DESCRIPTION

In all treatment settings and with all ages of clients you will encounter clients who are terminally ill. In working with the geriatric population, such a situation will probably occur more often. As an occupational therapy practitioner you will have valuable services to provide to the individual who is in or approaching the final stages of life. As you work with such individuals, it will be important to work through your own feelings and responses to death and dying so that you can interact with your client without any negative emotional baggage. It will be important to determine your client's goals and priorities and to avoid allowing your own biases to interfere. Providing the dying client with as much control, quality of life, purpose, and dignity as possible will help him or her to end life with feelings of fulfillment and satisfaction.

PREPARATION

Suggested Readings

AOTA (1998)
AOTA (latest edition)
Davis (1998)
Lewis (1989)

Study Questions

1. Describe the stages of dying identified by Elisabeth Kubler-Ross.

2. Describe cultural and philosophical considerations regarding death.

   a. Cultural

   b. Philosophical

3. Describe several life-sustaining services and several life-terminating services.

4. Describe the role of occupational therapy in the treatment of the terminally ill client.

5. Summarize AOTA's position on hospice care (AOTA, latest edition).

6. Summarize AOTA's position on providing services for people with HIV/AIDS.

7. In what settings do you think an occupational practitioner may provide intervention for terminally ill clients?

8. Describe five stages you may experience as a caregiver in working with a terminally ill client.

9. Highlight the content of "Understanding and Helping People Who Have Cancer" by D. Flomenhoft (as cited in Davis, 1998).

10. To prepare for the experience of working with the dying client, first look at how you might deal with death if it was in your immediate future. Assume that you have just been diagnosed with malignant cancer. You have one year to live, maybe two with chemotherapy. You have had your first dose of chemotherapy, and it made you very sick for five days after the treatment. With this information in mind, answer the following questions:

    a. What goals or tasks would you want to accomplish? Prioritize these tasks and goals.

    b. What are your religious and cultural beliefs about dying and death?

c. Would you want a religious leader or person to assist you? If so, why and how? If not, why not?

d. Would you want to continue chemotherapy to prolong your life even if it made you sick? Why or why not?

e. Which of the following performance areas (as taken from AOTA, 1998) would you be willing to give up first and which ones would you hold onto last? Rank your list with numbers, the highest number being the one you most want to keep. For additional information, ask a family member to complete such a ranking for himself or herself.

PERFORMANCE AREA	NO.	PERFORMANCE AREA	NO.
Grooming		Clothing care	
Oral hygiene		Cleaning	
Bathing/showering		Meal preparation/cleanup	
Toilet hygiene		Shopping	
Personal device care		Money management	
Dressing		Household maintenance	
Feeding and eating		Care of others	
Medication routine		Educational activities (list):	
Socialization			
Functional communication		Vocation (list):	
Community mobility			
Emergency response		Volunteering	
Sexual expression		Play or leisure (list):	

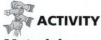

ACTIVITY

Materials

Case Studies 55 and 64 located at the end of this chapter.

Instructions

1. Share your study questions with a partner, a small group, or the class. List the similarities and differences in your answers. Discuss the emotions you experienced while completing the study questions.

SIMILARITIES	DIFFERENCES

2. With the case study assigned, complete the following intervention plan outline with a partner or small group. Share the results with the class when completed.
   a. Determine the frame of reference you will want to use.

   b. Fill in the following information, ranking the order of the goals based on your interpretation of the client's priorities. Select activities to meet these goals and give your rationale for your selection.

NEED/CONCERN/ PRIORITY	GOAL	ACTIVITY	RATIONALE

   c. Describe any adaptive equipment you might construct or recommend.

   d. Describe recommendations to other professionals or agencies you would make.

   e. Describe the influence of your client's culture and religion on your intervention planning.

3. Discuss as a class your ability to work with terminally ill clients. Record here personal growth areas on which you would like to work.

FOLLOW-UP

✔ Complete the Application of Competencies at the end of this chapter.

Exercise 115

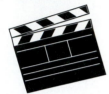

"Lord, I shall be very busy this day. I may forget thee, but do not thou forget me."

SIR JACOB ASTLEY

ACTIVITY PROGRAMMING

OBJECTIVES

✔ Identify the role and qualifications of an activity program coordinator
✔ Determine the beneficial components of programming varied activities in a long-term facility
✔ Establish a weekly activities schedule for a long-term facility

DESCRIPTION

As an occupational therapy practitioner, you will most likely take a job in the field of occupational therapy. On occasion, though, rather than taking a position as a practitioner, you may find yourself accepting the position of an activity program director for a long-term care facility. In such a case you will find that your occupational therapy background has prepared you well. Your understanding of the field of gerontology, the importance of activity, and the significance of balance in one's life will make you an ideal person to accept such a position. Even if that does not occur, you will still need insight into the programming and problem solving that goes into coordinating activities for clients in a long-term care facility. This insight will give you information as a practitioner that can be used in consulting and/or recommending needed activities to the activity program director for the clients with whom you work.

PREPARATION

Suggested Readings

AOTA (latest edition)
Miller, Peckham, and Peckham (1995)
Neidstadt and Crepeau (1998)

Study Questions

1. What is the role of the activity professional in a long-term care facility?

2. What are the purposes of an activities program?

3. List the needs of residents in a long-term care facility and describe how the activities program can improve the residents' quality of life.

4. Locate and cite the source and page number where it is stated that occupational therapy practitioners are able to work as activity program directors or professionals.

5. List information that you will need to obtain for an activity assessment.

6. Describe precautions of which you will need to be aware in planning and implementing activities for residents in a long-term care setting.

7. Give examples of activities that may be included in each of the areas following:

    a. Creative

    b. Cognitive

    c. Expressive

    d. Physical

    e. Social

    f. Spiritual

    g. Work-related

    h. Individual

    i. Community

    j. Grooming

    k. Intergenerational

8. Describe the educational requirements of an occupational therapy practitioner and an activity professional. Delineate the roles and responsibilities of each.

	OT PRACTITIONER	ACTIVITY PROFESSIONAL
Education		
Responsibilities/roles		

ACTIVITY

Materials

Sample activity schedules from local residential care facilities for the elderly.

Instructions

1a. Use the activity schedule given to you and a partner to evaluate the balance in the types of activities available to residents. Use the Characteristics Chart to list the activities and then put check marks in the boxes that apply to the components of that activity. The first one is completed for you. (See page 625.)

1b. Review the characteristics chart and list below the strengths and areas of concern in the balance of the types of activities provided. Note characteristics that may not be addressed by any of the activity groups.

STRENGTHS	AREAS OF CONCERN	CHARACTERISTICS NOT ADDRESSED

1c. List activities and groups that you would recommend adding and others that you would recommend for deletion.

ACTIVITIES/GROUPS TO ADD	ACTIVITIES/GROUPS TO DELETE

CHARACTERISTICS CHART

ACTIVITY	EVENINGS/ WEEKENDS	ACTIVE PARTICIPATION	PASSIVE PARTICIPATION	COGNITIVE	PHYSICAL	PREVENTION	COMMUNITY SOCIALIZATION	PRODUCTIVE CONTACT	SPIRITUAL OUTCOME	AESTHETIC NEEDS	EDUCATIONAL SELF-WORTH	APPRECIATION	NEED	S
Bingo	✓	✓		✓				✓						

1d. Make a new calendar of activities, placing your recommended activities in days and times you have determined to be most beneficial.

SUNDAY	MONDAY	TUESDAY	WEDNESDAY	THURSDAY	FRIDAY	SATURDAY

1e. Divide into small groups, you and your partner being in different groups. In your newly formed group, share your calendar with each other. Merge ideas together to develop a new calendar of activities.

SUNDAY	MONDAY	TUESDAY	WEDNESDAY	THURSDAY	FRIDAY	SATURDAY

FOLLOW-UP

✔ Complete the Application of Competencies at the end of this chapter.

After completing each exercise, record one concept you learned and how you anticipate that learning will influence your interaction and intervention with clients.

Exercise 101 Getting in Touch
Application:

Exercise 102 Evaluation in Geriatrics
Application:

Exercise 103 Safety and Fall Prevention
Application:

Exercise 104 Adapting Occupations and Environment
Application:

Exercise 105 Joint Protection, Energy Conservation, and Work Simplification
Application:

Exercise 106 Joint Replacement
Application:

Exercise 107 Remotivation and Reality Orientation
Application:

Exercise 108 Dementia
Application:

Exercise 109 Sensory Stimulation
Application:

Exercise 110 Eating, Feeding, and Dysphagia
Application:

Exercise 111 Leisure Time
Application:

Exercise 112 Intervention Planning
Application:

Exercise 113 Reminiscence and Life Review
Application:

Exercise 114 Terminal Illness
Application:

Exercise 115 Activity Programming
Application:

ADDING TO YOUR FILES

Add occupations to your activity file for individuals who are elderly. Type a paper on each activity with the information in the chart below and assemble these with a table of contents. Include in your file at least one activity that will work on the targeted areas listed. Note the ages for which each occupation is intended. Include activities that have diverse cultural and contextual qualities. The adaptations can be individual, but many will be applicable to group settings. When the chart is completed, you will have at least twenty new activities. Use at least three references that you have not used previously. A chart follows for you to list the occupations and activities you have gathered. Check each box as you complete the requirements.

TARGETED AREA	OCCUPATION	RATIONALE	PERFORMANCE CONTEXT	SUPPLIES/ MATERIALS	ADAPTATIONS	PRECAUTIONS	REFERENCES
Memory							
Remotivation							
Movement							
Reminiscing							
Reality orientation							
Craft, one-handed							
Sensory stimulation							
Range of motion							
Relaxation							
Socialization							
Griefwork							
Spiritual							
Cooking with joint protection							
House management activity with energy conservation/ work simplification							
Craft with low vision							
Craft with severe arthritic hands							
Leisure with someone in wheelchair							
Leisure with someone unable to get out of bed							
Community outing							
Overall strength endurance							

PRESENT A REMINISCING ACTIVITY

Performance Skill 6B

Divide into small groups to prepare and present a reminiscing activity in a group format. Present this to your classmates or to a group in a nursing home or retirement setting. Use the space below to prepare and divide work among your group members. You may supplement this plan with a more detailed one as discussed by Cole (1998).

Time frame: _____

Number of participants: _____

Age range: _____

Gender: _____

Culture: _____

Identify time or life event(s) to be the theme: _____

ACTIVITIES SELECTED	DESCRIPTION	TIME

Materials needed:

Describe how the duties will be divided among the group members.

STUDENT	DUTY

Performance Skill 6C

PREPARE/PRESENT A GROUP ACTIVITY

Work with several partners to devise and execute a group activity for residents at a specific community facility. Include in your group activity some form of movement, craft, leisure, and/or social activity. Fill in the group plan and session plan outline below, as adapted from Cole (1998). Include adaptations for the stated conditions you may encounter when presenting your group. Additionally, consider the safety precautions that will be needed. Use the worksheet below to assist in planning and use the presentation guidelines at the end to assist in preparation of your presentation. Type the information when completed.

Group Plan

Name of facility where activity will be held:

Name of contact person:

Number of participants to expect:

Functioning level:

Cognitive:

Physical:

Time:

Description of room:

Activity title:

Purpose:

Goals and rationale:

Method:

Outcome criteria:

Session Plan

Session title:

Format:

Supplies and cost:

Description:

    a. Introduction:

    b. Activity:

c. Discussion

Generalization:

Application:

d. Summary:

ADAPTATIONS	
CONDITION	ADAPTATION NECESSARY
Tremors	
One-handed use	
Weakness	
Delusions/hallucinations	
Blindness	

Consider these general safety precautions in your planning process. Keep them in mind and comment on their inclusion in your planning process.

SAFETY CONSIDERATION	COMMENT ON INCLUSION
Any food used should be soft in consistency.	
Edible items should not contain sugar or caffeine.	
Joint protection procedures should be followed.	
Skin protection procedures should be followed.	
Materials used should be checked for toxicity.	
Balance/fall prevention procedures should be followed.	

Presentation of the group should include the following:
Organized format
Thoroughly prepared
Appropriate set up of environment
Adapted format and description as needs arose
Engaged all residents
Used appropriate tone of voice
Implemented safety precautions

Teamwork evident
Time constraints met
Thorough cleanup
Professional behavior demonstrated to residents and staff

Performance Skill 6D

HEALTH AND WELLNESS PRESENTATION

Divide into groups. With your group, plan to present a health and wellness inservice to a group of senior citizens who are independent. Consider doing this at local community centers or facilities that may need such services. Develop a flyer to announce the upcoming event.

Incorporate as many principles of health and wellness as possible in the time allotted. Include examples and resources for adaptive equipment, energy conservation, and joint protection. Be sure to describe occupational therapy and provide information so that a resident might know when to seek a referral from his or her doctor for this service. Also include information on the benefits of participation in occupation. Use the worksheet below to prepare for the presentation and use the questions at the end to check your work.

Time frame:

Facility:

Number of participants:

Age range:

General functioning level:

Culture(s) of audience:

Flyers made and sent to facility:

TOPIC PRESENTED	DESCRIPTION	TIME	STUDENT

List materials you will bring:

Ask yourself these questions when checking your work:

1. Will posters help?
2. Are members of the audience active participants?
3. Is the environment arranged to allow participation, hearing, and seeing?
4. Are duties of the preparation and presentation equally distributed?
5. Is there a smooth transition from one topic to the next?
6. Will you ensure that the presentation will be clearly understood?

INTERVENTION PLANNING

Performance Skill 6E

Given a case study, select three problems of the client to address and select a frame of reference that will direct your intervention. Write the problems in functional terms for clear and concise goal planning. Write one short-term goal for each of the problem statements. State two occupations that you will use during intervention for each problem, describing the setup of the occupation and client. List the reasons you chose this occupation and how it will be graded as the client begins to make improvements. Use the following worksheet to make your plans. Answer the questions at the end to check your work. Type your completed plan.

FUNCTIONALLY STATED PROBLEM 1
Frame of reference
Short-term goal
Occupation 1
Setup
Rationale
Gradations
Occupation 2
Setup
Rationale
Gradations
FUNCTIONALLY STATED PROBLEM 2
Frame of reference
Short-term goal
Occupation 1
Setup
Rationale
Gradations
Occupation 2
Setup
Rationale
Gradations
FUNCTIONALLY STATED PROBLEM 3
Frame of reference
Short-term goal
Occupation 1
Setup
Rationale
Gradations
Occupation 2
Setup
Rationale
Gradations

Ask yourself these questions when checking your work:
1. Are all areas addressed?
2. Are the occupations suited to the client's abilities?
3. Are the goals written in functional, measurable terms?
4. Are the problems you selected part of the OT domain?
5. Are the occupations purposeful?
6. Knowing the disease process, are your goals realistic?

Performance Skill 6F

HOME ASSESSMENT

Complete a home assessment and make recommendations in a report format for the living environment where you reside. Assume that your home is the home of your client and that your client's body size and build are the same as yours. You may experience difficulty due to the inaccessibility of your environment for someone in a wheelchair, not unlike the situations in which your clients will be. Make whatever recommendations are necessary. Your client will then decide whether he or she is able to make the necessary changes for accessibility or whether he or she may need to relocate to a more amenable living situation. Type the report containing the following information, complete with a floor plan of your home:

1. Draw a floor plan of each floor of your dwelling on a separate piece of 8 × 10 inch paper.
2. Assess your dwelling by taking measurements and reflecting on your task performance in your home. Make recommendations for equipment and modifications. Use the space below to complete a draft of your work.

   a. Entrance description and measurements

   b. Recommendations for entrance equipment/modifications

   c. Kitchen description and measurements

   d. Recommendations for kitchen equipment/modifications

   e. Living room description and measurements

   f. Recommendations for living room equipment/modifications

   g. Bedroom description and measurements

   h. Recommendations for bedroom equipment/modifications

     i.   Bathroom description and measurements

     j.   Recommendations for bathroom equipment/modifications

     k.   Laundry description and measurements

     l.   Recommendations for laundry equipment/modifications

     m. Recommendations for other equipment/modifications

3.   Summarize your overall impression of the accessibility of your living situation.

HOME HEALTH

Type:
Home Health, Adult

Age:
67 years old

Sex:
Female

Culture/Religion:

Insurance Information:

Diagnosis:
Right CVA, HTN

Social History:
Emily resides with her husband in a tri-level home. She has functioned independently and owned and operated a small business. Emily has many interests, including computers, friends, music, and TV.

Medical History:
Emily has good sitting balance; oriented ×3. She has difficulty with ambulation and needs maximum assistance with dressing, bathing, and homemaking. She needs minimum assistance with eating, toileting, and ambulation. She has fair standing balance but tends to run into items on the left side. She has poor endurance. Left UE impaired to light touch, minimum flexor tone throughout arm, active elbow to 90°, slight tone in wrist, shoulder, hand.

CASE STUDY 55

SKILLED NURSING

Type:
Long-Term Care

Age:
67 years old

Sex:
Female

Culture/Religion:

Insurance Information:

Diagnosis:
ALS, diabetes

Social History:
Doris is now and will remain a resident of this long-term care facility. She has been living with her daughter and son-in-law for the past six months. It has been too difficult for them to care for her; she is a large woman.

Doris enjoys watching television, reading novels, and talking to her friends and family on the telephone.

Medical History:
Doris now requires maximum assistance of two to transfer to and from bed, toilet, and shower chair. She uses a wheelchair but is no longer able to push it. She is losing the ability to use her hands to grasp for any period of time. She is experiencing difficulty with eating, holding and dialing the phone, using the remote control, getting dressed, and bathing herself. She is becoming extremely discouraged and depressed.

OT has been ordered to see whether any increase function is possible.

CASE STUDY 56

SKILLED NURSING

Type:
Subacute

Age:
89 years old

Sex:
Female

Culture/Religion:

Insurance Information:

Diagnosis:
Blindness, debility, right hip fx., diverticulosis, osteoporosis, and anemia

Social History:
Margaret was independent with all self-care tasks and lived in independent living at a retirement community. She was a very private lady who kept to herself most of the time. She spent most of her time listening to books on tape, music, and the radio. She also listened to several soap operas on television.

Medical History:
Margaret had her hip pinned five days ago and hopes to be able to return to inde-

pendent living after rehabilitation. She is now able to ambulate from bed to bathroom with minimum assistance and verbal cues.

Margaret's UE ROM is WNL, and her strength is approximately 3+/5 throughout. On ADL evaluation she required moderate assistance, verbal cues, and setup with UEs. Her LEs required maximum assistance, verbal cues, setup, and reminder of hip precautions. Her grooming required minimum assistance, setup, and verbal cues.

Margaret is pleasant and cooperative. She is having some difficulty remembering instructions from one day to the next.

LONG-TERM CARE

Type:
Rehabilitation

Age:
78 years old

Sex:
Female

Culture/Religion:

Insurance Information:

Diagnosis:
Deconditioning, right DVT, right thigh hematoma, both THR three years ago due to DJD, NIDDM, obese, S/P cardiac cath.

Social History:
Wilma lives alone in her own home. She did all her own homemaking with the exception of yard work. She has been very social, visiting often with friends. She also has done work at the senior citizen center. She was married for forty years until her husband died. She had one son, who was killed in a car accident as a young boy.

Medical History:
Wilma is obese and walks with a walker. She was receiving OT and PT at the hospital before her admission to the rehab center. Her goals include:

1. Minimum assistance with LE dressing
2. Minimum assistance with bedside bathing
3. Minimum assistance for transfer to tub bench and adapted commode
4. CGA with toileting hygiene

ACUTE CARE

Type:
Acute Care Inpatient

Age:
66 years old

Sex:
Female

Culture/Religion:

Insurance Information:

Diagnosis:
Left knee replacement

Social History:
Sylvia lives with her husband in their own home. She works as an accountant with a large firm. Sylvia and her husband have three grown children, who all live on their own. She has four grandchildren, whom she loves to visit and often babysits. She is concerned about doing her job and staying active with her grandchildren.

Medical History:
Sylvia is one day post operative. She has a long history of osteroarthritis. She has experienced pain in her knee for several years, but lately she was experiencing difficulty with walking on stairs and just handling the constant pain. Sylvia has had no other surgeries or serious illness. She is overweight and reports that she does not exercise, even though she knows she should. She also reports trying all kinds of weight loss programs to no avail. She feels she is 40 pounds overweight.

CASE STUDY 59

ACUTE CARE

Type:
Acute Care Inpatient

Age:
67 years old

Sex:
Female

Culture/Religion:

Insurance Information:

Diagnosis:
Hypercalemic, dehydration, fell at home, r/o dementia

Social History:
Fran lives alone in a third-floor apartment, in a building that has an elevator. She reports independence in dressing but requires assistance with bathing. She has a homemaker who comes twice a week. Fran has used a walker for ambulation before admission.

Medical History:
Fran's medical history includes left CVA with right-sided weakness, rheumatoid arthritis, SOB, and what she reports as a "nervous breakdown."

On assessment she had fair endurance, was independent in eating using her left hand, is independent in UE dressing, and required moderate assistance with LE dressing. She needs assistance to stand to pull up pants and verbal and physical cues to don socks and footwear correctly.

Fran's transfers required moderate assistance of one. She was unable to maintain standing without assistance, although she attempted several times to do so.

Fran's right hand has 3/5 overall strength, and she is able to oppose all digits. During observation Fran was noticed to hold her right hand to her side and not utilize the function available.

Fran gives a sketchy history when asked how she prepares her meals and what she eats. She reports no leisure interests since her CVA except watching TV. She appears very anxious. On Allen's cognitive scale she is functioning at a 4.2 level.

SKILLED NURSING

Type:
Rehabilitation

Age:
73 years old

Sex:
Female

Culture/Religion:

Insurance Information:

Diagnosis:
Spinal sclerosis C5-6, acute facial cellulite, sepsis, hypertension, tetraplegia, profound proximal muscle weakness

Social History:
Before admission Elaine lived alone. She does have family and is uncertain whether they are willing and able to care for her. She would like to continue living alone independently.

Medical History:
Elaine's PMH includes CHF, MI, and arthritis. The CT myelogram shows complete block. She has trace biceps and trace triceps. She has no fine movement in her fingers and has bilateral hand splints.

She requires maximum assistance to feed herself using her ®UE with a universal cuff and spork. On occasion she coughs and gags when drinking liquids. She has no functional grasp and partial arm placement. She requires maximum assistance in bed mobility and moderate assistance with unsupported sitting balance. She is currently wearing a soft collar. She requires maximum assistance with sliding board transfers.

ACUTE CARE

Type:
Acute Care Inpatient

Age:
67 years old

Sex:
Male

Culture/Religion:

Insurance Information:

Diagnosis:
Left vertebral/basilar anterior aneurysm, NPO, seizure, resolving vertigo, persistent left lung collapse, pneumonia, S/P aneurysm clipping, COPD, left hemiplegia

Social History:
Jordan lives with his brother in their own home. They also have four dogs. Jordan likes to cook and garden. Jordan and his brother spend most of their time at home.

Medical History:

Jordan is alert and oriented, seems aware of his deficits, is appropriate, and interacts well with staff. On evaluation he moves his left UE in a floppy and uncoordinated pattern. He has 90° shoulder flexion and abduction; all other movements are within normal range. His sensation is normal; he does, however, display minimum left side neglect.

At this time his transfers require maximum assistance. He requires moderate assistance with grooming. He is independent in putting on a pullover shirt. He is dependent in all other care.

CASE STUDY 62

ACUTE CARE

Type:
Acute Care Inpatient

Age:
73 years old

Sex:
Male

Culture/Religion:

Insurance Information:

Diagnosis:
C6 quadriplegia

Social History:
George lives with his wife in their own home with a large yard and garden for which George is responsible. His wife is 70 years old and moderately disabled from rheumatoid arthritis. She walks with a walker and has relied on George to assist with the homemaking duties. Following his retirement, George and his wife have enjoyed traveling for the past several years.

Medical History:
George was admitted following injury to the spinal cord sustained when he was hit by a car while crossing the street. He has previously been hospitalized only once for an appendectomy. He denies smoking and drinks only on occasion.

George has not received an OT assessment at this time. He is very depressed and anxious about how he will care for himself and his wife.

CASE STUDY 63

ACUTE CARE

Type:
Acute Care Inpatient

Age:
76 years old

Sex:
Female

Culture/Religion:

Insurance Information:

Diagnosis:
Left occipital craniotomy, duroplasty, cranioplasty

Social History:
Freida lives alone, but her daughter is visiting from out of town now. She has no other children. Freida lives in her own home and has two cats. Before admission she was independent in all homemaking tasks, including yard work and flower gardening, which are her favorite hobbies.

Freida's husband died six years ago after a heart attack. She continued to be very active with their friends at church and also a group of friends with whom they played cards.

Medical History:
Freida requires moderate assistance of one to transfer and come to sitting in bed. She complains of back pain when sitting and dizziness when coming from supine to sit. She also complains of pressure on her scalp lesion.

Freida is dependent in all self-care at this time. She attempts to feed herself but appears to be having motor planning difficulties.

She also seems to be missing objects on her right side. Freida is being seen by speech therapy because of expressive communication problems, using inappropriate words. She is also being seen by PT, where she is learning to use the walker.

Freida has ROM WNL in all extremities. Her strength is WNL on the left side and fair overall on her right side. She displays fine motor problems on her right side and frequently drops items placed in her hand. Freida has intact sharp/dull; impaired localization; proprioception and stereognosis.

SKILLED FACILITY

Type:
Subacute

Age:
82 years old

Sex:
Female

Culture/Religion:

Insurance Information:

Diagnosis:
Malaise and fatigue, COPD, ovarian CA

Social History:
Miriam has moved from independent living to the nursing center because of her low tolerance for activity. She has been active in the past with volunteering for residents in the nursing center. She delivered mail and helped to fill out menus for residents. For the past two weeks Miriam has taken all her meals in her room and has refused participation in all activities.

> **Medical History:**
>
> Miriam is cognitively alert and oriented ×3. Her ROM is WFL, strength and coordination WNL. She is independent in transfers and uses a wheelchair for long distances. At this time she requires minimum assistance for bathing and grooming. She is independent in dressing and feeding.
>
> Miriam is able to tolerate ten minutes before becoming extremely tired and short of breath. She requires moderate to maximum encouragement to stay out of bed longer than two hours. Her stages of CA are advancing; she is often tearful and has secondary hair loss from chemo.

REFERENCES

American Occupational Therapy Association. latest edition. *Reference Manual of the Official Documents of the American Occupational Therapy Association.* Bethesda, MD: Author.

American Occupational Therapy Association. 1998. *Reference Manual of the Official Documents of the American Occupational Therapy Association.* Bethesda, MD: Author.

Asher, I. E. 1996. *Occupational Therapy Assessment Tools: An Annotated Index.* 2d ed. Bethesda, MD: American Occupational Therapy Association.

A/V Health Services. n.d. *Adapting the Home for the Physically Challenged.* Roanoke, VA: Author.

Bayles, K. A., and C. K. Tomoeda. 1997. *Pastimes.* San Antonio, TX: Therapy Skill Builders.

Christiansen, C. ed. 2000. *Ways of Living: Self-Care Strategies for Special Needs.* 2d ed. Rockville, MD: American Occupational Therapy Association.

Cole, M. D. 1998. *Group Dynamics in Occupational Therapy: The Theoretical Basis and Practice Application of Group Treatment.* 2d. ed. Thorofare, NJ: Slack.

Davis, C. M. 1998. *Patient Practitioner Interaction: An Experiential Manual for Developing the Art of Health Care.* 3d ed. Thorofare, NJ: Slack.

Dempsey-Lyle, S., and T. L. Hoffman. n.d. *Into Aging: Understanding Issues Affecting the Later Stages of Life.* Thorofare, NJ: Slack.

Early, M. B. 1998. *Physical Dysfunction Practice Skills for the Occupational Therapy Assistant.* St. Louis, MO: Mosby.

Emlet, C. A., J. L. Crabtree, V. A. Condon, and L. A. Treml. 1996. *In-Home Assessment of Older Adults: An Interdisciplinary Approach.* Gaithersburg, MD: Aspen Publishers.

Folstein, M. F., S. E. Folstein, and P. R. Mettugn. 1975. "Minimental State: A Practical Method for Grading the Cognitive-State of Patients for the Clinician." *Journal of Psychiatric Research,* 12: 189–198.

Holden, U., and R. T. Woods. 1995. *Positive Approaches to Dementia Care.* 3d ed. Edinburgh: Churchill Livingstone.

Hutchins, B. 1991. *Managing Dysphagia.* Tucson, AZ: Therapy Skill Builders.

Issacs, B., and A. Kinnie. 1973. The Set Test as an Aid to the Detection of Dementia in Old People. *British Journal of Psychiatry,* 123:467.

Larson, K. A., R. G. Stevens-Ratchford, L. Pedretti, and J. L. Crabtree. eds. 1996. *ROTE: The Role of Occupational Therapy with the Elderly.* Bethesda, MD: American Occupational Therapy Association.

Lewis, S. C. 1989. *Elder Care in Occupational Therapy.* Thorofare, NJ: Slack.

MacLay, E. 1977. *Green Winter: Celebration of Old Age.* New York: Reader's Digest Press.

Melvin, J. L. 1989. *Rheumatic Disease in the Adult and Child: Occupational Therapy and Rehabilitation.* 3d ed. Philadelphia: F. A. Davis.

Michelson, B. 1985. *A Slice of Life.* DeKalb, IL: Author.

Miller, M. E., C. W. Peckham, and A. B. Peckham. 1995. *Activities Keep Me Going and Going.* Vol. 2. Centerville, OH: Macro Printed Products.

Neidstadt, M. E., and E. B. Crepeau. eds. 1998. *Willard and Spackman's Occupational Therapy.* 9th ed. Philadelphia: Lippincott.

Paracheck, J. F. 1986. *Parachek Geriatric Rating Scale.* 3d ed. Glendale, AZ: Center for Neurodevelopmental Studies.

Pierson, F. M. 1999. *Principles and Techniques of Patient Care.* 2d ed. Philadelphia: W. B. Saunders.

Platt, J. V., R. Begun, and E. D. Murphy. 1992a. *Daily Activities After Your Total Hip Replacement.* Bethesda, MD: American Occupational Therapy Association.

Platt, J. V., R. Begun, and E. D. Murphy. 1992b. *Daily Activities After Your Total Knee Replacement.* Bethesda, MD: American Occupational Therapy Association.

Reed, K. L. 1991. *Quick Reference to Occupational Therapy.* Gaithersburg, MD: Aspen Publishers.

Ross, M. 1997. *Integrative Group Therapy: Mobilizing Coping Abilities with the Five-Stage Group.* Bethesda, MD: American Occupational Therapy Association.

Seaver, A. M. H. 1994. "My World Now." In *The Blair Reader.* L. G. Kriszner and S. R. Mandell. eds. Upper Saddle River, NJ: Prentice Hall.

St. Mary's Hospital Medical Center and the Board of Regents of the University of Wisconsin System. 1984. *ROM Dance.* Madison, WI: WHA Television and St. Mary's Hospital Medical Center in Madison.

Watts, J. H., C. Brollier, D. F. Bauer, and W. Schmidt. 1989. The Assessment of Occupational Therapy Functioning. 2d ed. In *Instrument Development in Occupational Therapy.* J. H. Watts and C. Brollier. eds. New York: Haworth.

Appendixes

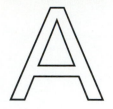 Analysis of Occupations

Occupational Analysis

Complete the following occupational analysis on a craft or occupation assigned by your instructor. Detail the materials needed, characteristics of the activity, treatment implications, steps to completion, and the identified components inherent in the craft or occupation. Fill out the outline and forms below as you go.

Occupational Analysis

Descriptors:

Activity:_____

Cost: _____

General characteristics: _____

Time: (Are different sessions needed? If so, allocate time needed for each session.)

_____

Materials needed (including tools and equipment):

Characteristics of equipment, tools, materials (resistance, control, cleanliness):

Contraindications of the occupation (precautions, danger):

Intervention implications (How could this activity best be used in each practice area?):
Pediatrics

Physical rehabilitation

Mental health

Geriatrics

Evaluation possibilities (How might this craft/occupation be used as part of the evaluation process?):

Frame of reference compatibility (With which frame(s) of reference does the activity best align?):

Steps to completion:

Fill in the following columns indicating the major steps and the necessary instructions to complete the task along with applications.

MAJOR STEPS (usually only 3 or 4 steps)	INSTRUCTIONS (details of step by step instructions)	APPLICATION (include hints, nonessential, yet helpful information)

Using the chart below as a model, create a computer-generated Performance Component and Context Chart using the terms in the latest edition of uniform terminology (AOTA). Make as many component and context boxes as needed. Determine how much the component or context is involved in the activity. Circle the amount of involvement as appropriate: minimal (min), moderate (mod), maximal (max), not applicable (N/a). In the Describe Involvement column state how that component or context is involved. In the Adapted and Graded Columns, state how the activity can be adapted and graded. Fill out the different columns as assigned by your instructor. See the following example for making a birdhouse. One component has been completed for you.

Performance Component and Context Chart

Component Title:

DESCRIBE INVOLVEMENT	ADAPTED	GRADED
Tactile		
Min / (Mod) / Max / N/a — To determine that sanding is complete, it is necessary to feel the smoothness of the wood.	Pre-sand the wood for the client.	Make a more complicated birdhouse with intricate designs.
Min / Mod / Max / N/a		
Min / Mod / Max / N/a		
Min / Mod / Max / N/a		

Context Title:

DESCRIBE INVOLVEMENT	ADAPTED	GRADED
Min / Mod / Max / N/a		
Min / Mod / Max / N/a		
Min / Mod / Max / N/a		

APPENDIX A: ANALYSIS OF OCCUPATIONS

Abbreviated Occupational Analysis Chart

Using the chart below as a model, create a computer-generated Abbreviated Occupational Analysis Chart using the latest edition of uniform terminology (AOTA). Make as many component and context boxes as needed. Determine to what degree that component or context is used in the activity marking the appropriate column. In the final column, describe how the component or context is used in the task.

ABBREVIATED OCCUPATIONAL ANALYSIS CHART					
	DEGREE TO WHICH IT IS USED				How is the Component or Context used in this task?
PERFORMANCE COMPONENTS	None	Min.	Mod.	Max.	

APPENDIX A: ANALYSIS OF OCCUPATIONS

Abbreviated Occupational Analysis/Adapted Chart

Using the chart below as a model, create a computer-generated Abbreviated Occupational Analysis/Adapted Chart using the latest edition of uniform terminology (AOTA). Make as many component and context boxes as needed. Determine to what degree that component or context is used in the activity marking the appropriate column. Indicate how the component or context is used in the task. In the final column, indicate how the task could be adapted.

ABBREVIATED OCCUPATIONAL ANALYSIS/ADAPTED CHART						
	DEGREE TO WHICH IT IS USED				How is the Component or Context used in this task?	How can this be adapted?
PERFORMANCE COMPONENTS	None	Min.	Mod.	Max.		

APPENDIX A: ANALYSIS OF OCCUPATIONS

Abbreviated Occupational Analysis/Graded Chart

Using the chart below as a model, create a computer-generated Abbreviated Occupational Analysis/Graded Chart using the latest edition of uniform terminology (AOTA). Make as many component and context boxes as needed. Determine to what degree that component or context is used in the activity marking the appropriate column. Indicate how the component or context is used in the task. In the final column, indicate how the task could be graded.

ABBREVIATED OCCUPATIONAL ANALYSIS/GRADED CHART						
	DEGREE TO WHICH IT IS USED				How is the Component or Context used in this task?	How can this be graded?
PERFORMANCE COMPONENTS	None	Min.	Mod.	Max.		

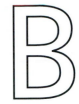

Self-Awareness

Therapeutic Use of Self-Analysis

Date: _____ I participated in: _____

In the following areas as taken from Neidstadt (1996), describe your own strengths and concerns. Include improvement strategies for each identified area of concern. Include self-reflective thoughts as well as feedback from others such as your instructor and/or peers.

AREAS	STRENGTHS	CONCERNS	IMPROVEMENT STRATEGIES
Affect, emotional tone (enthusiastic, energetic, serious, low-key)			
Attending and listening (including your ability to reflect back on and add to what the speaker has said)			
Cognitive style (detail or gestalt oriented, abstract or concrete, ability to understand diverse points of view)			
Confidence (not only what you feel, but also what you think you show to others)			
Confrontation (can you do it and with whom?)			
Empathy (for what emotions in what situation?)			
Humor (do you use it, and if so, how?)			

Leadership style (directive, facilitative, follower)			
Nonverbal communication (facial expressiveness, eye contact, voice tone and volume, gestures)			
Power sharing (need to control, comfortable with chaos)			
Probing (when are you comfortable doing it, with whom and about what?)			
Touch (do you use it automatically or unconsciously, when, where and with whom?)			
Verbal communication (vocalism, use of vernacular, ease of speaking)			

Therapeutic Use of Self Analysis areas taken from: American Journal of Occupational Therapy *50 (8), 682.*
Copyright © 1996, American Occupational Therapy Association, Inc. Reprinted with permission.

Appendix B: Self-Awareness

ANALYSIS OF SELF

Complete the following form rating yourself on each identified behavior as it relates to your performance of the assigned task. Rate yourself from 1 (lowest) to 5 (highest). Include self-generated comments about your performance as well as any feedback you received from your instructors and peers.

PROFESSIONAL BEHAVIOR
RELATED TO TASK PERFORMANCE

Name:_____ Date:_____ Task:_____

BEHAVIORS	1	2	3	4	5	COMMENTS
Managing time						
Solving problems						
Using resources						
Tolerating frustration						
Planning						
Taking risks						
Controlling impulses						
Complying with safety						
Managing the environment						
Sharing supplies						
Expending effort						
Attending to detail						
Assisting others						
Responding to feedback						

Total points: _____

Describe how the above behaviors affect clinical practice:

Describe what you will do to improve your professional behavior:

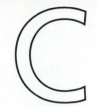

C

Professional Practice Records

Supervision Log for OTA/OT Collaboration

Supervision by an occupational therapist (OT) is required for all occupational therapy assistants (OTAs), regardless of the OTA's experience. It may be necessary to provide evidence of this supervision. In the clinic, note writing can provide the evidence. Another way to document evidence of supervision is to keep a log. The following supervision log for OTA/OT collaboration provides space to document the dates, clients, current status, and occupational therapy process recommendations. Upon completion of each entry to the log, obtain your supervisor's signature. Make photocopies of this document as needed so that it can be used over time. Modify and adapt this form to suit your specific needs.

SUPERVISION LOG FOR OTA/OT COLLABORATION

YOUR NAME: _____

DATES	CLIENTS	CURRENT STATUS/COMMENTS	RECOMMENDATIONS	SUPERVISOR'S SIGNATURE

Appendix C: Professional Practice Records
Service Competency

Service competency needs to be established when a new supervisor/supervisee relationship is formed. It is to your benefit that documentation of this process is maintained.

This is essential for occupational therapy assistants as well as beginning occupational therapists. Service competency also needs to be established when an experienced therapist or assistant changes practice areas.

The following records allow you to document the service competency process. The Service Competency in Progress Record documents a skill that is in the process of being learned. The Assessment Service Competency Record documents the assessments for which service competency has been achieved. The Intervention Service Competency Record documents the interaction techniques for which service competency has been achieved. The Physical Agent Modality (PAM) Service Competency Record documents the PAMs for which service competency has been achieved

Begin to record your service competency growth and development as you go on your Fieldwork Level II experience. Continue this record as you accept your first position as an occupational therapy practitioner. Add this to your portfolio, which will continually document your competency as a lifelong learner.

Service Competency in Progress Record

Skill _____

Document your progress toward service competency by completing the following chart. Identify the competency skill, the specific step you have completed to establish competency (use the suggested guidelines below), the date of completion of that step, and comments about your progress toward service competency. A sample has been provided for you.

RECOMMENDED STEPS TO ESTABLISH SERVICE COMPETENCY:

1. Obtain and read available literature on the identified skill.
2. Attend an inservice or workshop on the identified skill.
3. Observe other practitioner performing the identified skill.
4. Practice the identified skill on a peer or supervisor.
5. Perform the identified skill on a client with the supervisor observing.
6. Perform the identified skill on a client and collaborate with the supervisor on a frequent basis (initially).

SKILL	STEP COMPLETED	DATE	COMMENTS ON PROGRESS
Ultrasound	a. Read book on ultrasound	1-5-00	Took the self-test at the back of the chapter; obtained a 96%

Assessment Service Competency Record

List the assessments for which service competency has been achieved. Document the date and obtain your supervisor's signature on completion.

ASSESSMENT	DATE	SUPERVISOR SIGNATURE

Intervention Service Competency Record

List the intervention techniques for which service competency has been achieved. Document the date and obtain your supervisor's signature on completion.

INTERVENTION TECHNIQUE	DATE	SUPERVISOR SIGNATURE

Physical Agent Modality (PAM)
Service Competency Record

List the PAM for which service competency has been achieved. Document the date and obtain your supervisor's signature on completion.

MODALITY	DATE	SUPERVISOR SIGNATURE

Index

Page numbers in *italics* denote figures.